Iatrogenic Vascular Injury:
A Discourse on Surgical Technique

Edited by

T.J. Bunt M.D., F.A.C.S.

Clinical Associate Professor of Surgery
University of Arizona
Chief of Vascular Surgery
Maricopa Medical Center
Consulting Vascular Surgeon
Carl Hayden Veterans Administration Medical Center
Phoenix, Arizona

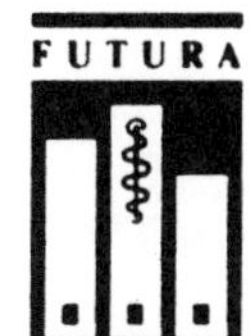

**Futura Publishing
Company, Inc.**
Mount Kisco, NY
1990

Library of Congress Cataloging-in-Publication Data

Iatrogenic vascular injury : a discourse on surgical technique /
    edited by T.J. Bunt.
        p.   cm.
    Includes index.
    ISBN (invalid) 0-87793-358-5
    1. Blood-vessels—Surgery—Complications and sequelae.
2. Surgical errors—Prevention.   I. Bunt, T.J.
    [DNLM: 1. Blood Vessels—injuries.   2. Iatrogenic Disease—
etiology.   3. Iatrogenic Disease—prevention & disease.
    4. Vascular Surgery—adverse effects.   5. Vascular Surgery—
methods.
    WG 170 I11[
    RD598.5.I22   1989
    617.4'1301—dc20
    DNLM/DLC
    for Library of Congress   89-11877
                                                                    CIP

Published by

Futura Publishing Company, Inc.
2 Bedford Ridge Road
Mount Kisco, New York 10549

L.C. No.: 89-1187
ISBN No.: 0-87793-358-5

Contributors

Bunt, T.J., M.D., F.A.C.S.   Clinical Associate Professor of Surgery, University of Arizona; Chief of Vascular Surgery, Maricopa Medical Center; Consulting Vascular Surgeon, Carl Hayden Veterans Administration Medical Center, Phoenix, Arizona

Dobrin, Philip B., M.D., Ph.D., F.A.C.S.   Associate Professor of Surgery, Department of Surgery, Loyola University Medical Center, Maywood, Illinois and Hines Veterans Administration Medical Center, Hines, Illinois

Friedman, Harold I., M.D., Ph.D., F.A.C.S.   Associate Professor of Surgery and Chief, Division of Plastic Surgery, University of South Carolina, Columbia, South Carolina

Haines, Peter C., M.D.   Assistant Professor of Surgery, University of South Carolina, Columbia, South Carolina

Littooy, Frederick N., M.D., F.A.C.S.   Associate Professor of Surgery, Loyola University, Maywood, Illinois; Chief, Peripheral Vascular Surgery, Hines Veterans Administration Medical Center, Hines Illinois

Mohammad, S. Fazal, Ph.D.   Director of Hematology, Artificial Heart Research Laboratory, Division of Artificial Organs, University of Utah, Salt Lake City, Utah

Moore, William M., M.D.   Fellow in Vascular Surgery, Ochsner Clinic, New Orleans, Louisiana

Sottiurai, Vikrom S., M.D., Ph.D., F.A.C.S.   Clinical Associate Professor of Surgery, Louisiana State University, New Orleans, Louisiana

Foreword

When meditating over a disease, I never think of
finding a remedy for it, but instead, a means of
preventing it.

Louis Pasteur[1]

Writing the wisdom of the French peasant-artisan that he was, Pasteur's words come down to us after a century admonishing us to step back from our operating table and look at what we are doing. Implied, but not stated, is that we, as vascular surgeons, must realize that we are producing injury.

In the foreword to the only monograph now in print, treating exclusively with iatrogenic vascular injury,[2] Rutherford states cogently, "...the scope and magnitude of the subject have reaching almost epidemic proportions." He was referring, of course, to diagnostic arterial and venous catheterization injury, PTLA injury, and the vascular trauma induced by orthopedic, neurosurgical, and gynecologic interventions. He was not speaking of clamp trauma, needle injury, nor the myointimal response that is common to prosthetic grafting, laser and atherectomy trauma, or carotid endarterectomy. How much more frequent are these events and the vessels wall's inevitable response to them. These are the subject of this volume.

It is the stated purpose of this book "...to delineate how and what sort of injury occurs and to advocate preventive/protective measures." As it does so, the eight contributors under the author/editor's guidance have summarized their scientific work in the perspective of other scientific contributions worldwide. This provides the reader with a literature review commentary that serves to define the present problems of vascular surgical iatrogenic injury. Paradoxically, we recognize that this injury is done in good-faith attempts to correct pathological problems. One expects that the clear definition of the problems, the display of observations collected regarding their genesis collected within these covers could provide a foundation upon which to construct solutions to the problems of a vessel wall's reaction to injury.

After 1950, the first generation of vascular surgeons developed techniques of revascularization for occlusive disease and exclusion of aneurysms to extend life and preserve limbs. The next generation applied scientific observations derived from noninvasive measurements, actuarial science, and statistical methods to standardize the variety of techniques that was their heritage. As the third generation began its explorations to minimize invasion of therapeutic interventions, a clear impediment to further progress was seen in the midst of their thoroughfare. Within this third generation of vascular surgeons are those who have mastered the skills of electron microscopy, arcane organic chemistry, fluid dynamics, and cellular biology. Their observations are in the chapters that follow. The future of vascular surgery is in their hands and in those of other scientists. It is to them that the torch is being flung to be carried forward, successfully we hope.

If vascular surgery is to progress as a specialty distinct from other surgery, the purpose of this volume must be accomplished. As the editor has said, this is to recognize "...the inadvertent production of an endothelial or medial injury by the vascular surgeon as the result of his vascular technique." Further, the specialty must find and employ methods of minimizing or preventing the injury response. I believe the information summarized in this book provides evidence that theoretical understanding and experimental skills have advanced to the point that this is possible. History will decide whether this is the observation of a realist or an unredeemed positivist. After all, it was Pasteur who believed that "there are no such things as applied sciences, only applications of science." (Il n'existe pas de sciences appliquees, mais seulement des applications de la science).

John Bergan, M.D.

References

1. Pasteur, L: Address 11 Sep 1892. Comptes Rendus des Travaux du Congres Viticole de Lyon, 9–14 Septembre 1982, page 49.
2. Bergentz, SE, Bergqvist, D: *Iatrogenic Vascular Injuries*. Berlin, Springer-Verlag, 1989.

Preface

A preface is generally conceived as an explanation for why a book was written and includes expressions of thanks to the special people in the author's life, some of whom may actually have had something to do with the writing of the book. This preface shall follow those guidelines, but even more so, shall be a small touch of insight into the "why": why indeed would anybody spend the better part of their years trying to engineer a very small book devoted to a topic that just about everybody already knows everything there is to know about the topic (just ask your favorite vascular surgeon about vascular technique!).

It should be noted that this book was never supposed to have been written at all; in fact, I wasn't supposed to have been a physician; and later on, I was very forcibly impressed upon *not* to be a surgeon; it took even longer to become a vascular surgeon. But I did anyhow, and this book, as a palpable result of what was *not* supposed to be, is dedicated to the people who allowed it all to happen. It is dedicated to the people and events of my checkered path through academia, a path I always took more or less on the outside—questioning, analyzing, and critical. As a result, I suspect I was not the most enjoyable resident to have around. There were some who could deal with my attitude—fewer still who took the time to answer the underlying questions. Ten years later, I still have strong feelings about my "education" and "training"; perhaps a little mellowed with age and experience (I think they call that maturation), particularly since I am now on the other side of that issue as a teacher and evaluator of resident attitude problems.

This book is therefore a collection of analytical thought, in this case about the most basic things that vascular surgeons do. It is written by someone who loves the field, and is in general awe of those who originated it, developed it, and now are its senior mentors. Yet, it in many ways challenges the precepts of the field. The challenge is not malevolent, but simply a reflection of the approach I have always taken in my own (self-) education and the philosophy that I try to impart to my own students—that education implies a *synthesis* of what has been taught/read/seen into one's own eclectic management style and thought process; that the student should never blindly accept anything, but should root his/her beliefs firmly in a soil of validation and not be overly reliant upon nor awed by experience or tradition.

There is a rightful place for dogma and tradition: There *must* be standards by which the craft of vascular surgery is taught and its select cadre of practitioners are measured. However, there must also be continual analysis of the dogma, modification to new ideas, and new synthesis of old thoughts. What we are all striving for is the best care that we can provide; or, for the purpose of this book, the best techniques by which we can provide it.

So, in a curious way, I dedicate this small effort in critical thought to some rather diverse people—

- to my wife, Libby; who knew from the very beginning what I was and could do, who took my dream and chose to help me fly.
- to that short-sighted portion of the attending surgeons at Florida 10 years ago, who saw in me only antiauthoritarian rebellion; but in so doing, gave me the direction and initiative to become the academician and teacher that I did not see in them.
- to my son, Christopher, who through his profound limitations with Cornelia de Lange syndrome has caused me to realize what is really important in life and worth striving for.
- to the major names in vascular surgery who were and are my "mentors-in-absentio," who have guided me in their writings and have allowed me to join the lesser ranks of vascular surgery, despite my own misgivings as to qualifications.
- and most of all, this is dedicated to my residents, the students of vascular surgery; who are as entranced by the field as I, as dedicated to learning its complexities, and who provide me the daily motivation to improve and learn more, so that I can in turn teach them.

I hope that you enjoy this book, that it makes you think and maybe even causes you to change some of what you do. Better yet, I hope that it motivates you to do a study to rethink what is opined here so that we both can learn.

Introduction

Peripheral vascular surgery is to its devotees a discipline of finely honed technical skills, one in which the difference between excellent and average operative results may be measured in small percentage point integers. Integral to this concept of vascular surgery as a highly refined technique is the important concept of *atraumatic* technique; that gentle tissue handling, careful efficient dissection, and minimal intimal injury that contribute to the most optimal technical result.

The opposing concept to atraumatic vascular technique is *iatrogenic vascular injury*. Minimization of the former is highly dependent upon a detailed knowledge of the latter. The purpose of this book is to detail the extent of the injury that may occur with inappropriate or careless technique and to thereby provide a solid, well-researched basis for recommendations as to exactly what constitutes optimal vascular technique. Iatrogenic vascular injury as we define it becomes the inadvertent production of an endothelial or medial injury by the vascular surgeon as the result of his/her vascular technique. This may stem from instrument or suture selection; dissection, suturing, or anastomotic techniques; or choice and handling/preparation of the conduits. It follows as a direct corollary that peripheral vascular surgeons must be as fully cognizant of the advantages/limitations of their instruments as they are of the physics and engineering of their conduits or how the conduits are anastomosed to vessels as the surgeon is of the anatomy/physiology and clinical pathology of the disease process for which vascular surgical operations are undertaken.

This book is directed at two audiences and thus is written with a dual purpose. It first seeks to offer students of vascular surgery a logical basis on which to select their *own* techniques, since we adhere to the teaching principle that students should not rigorously follow traditional methods (even our own teaching), but rather should form their own eclectic technique based on factual and experimental evidence. Second, it seeks to offer any practicing surgeon a complete research review of the effects of vascular technique on ultimate results. The flow of the book is thus from a thorough discussion of normal histology, ultrastructure, and physiology; through the effects of injury, age, and atherosclerosis and how the normal responses to injury may be altered in precisely those patients in whom vascular operations are usually indicated; to a discussion of specific conduit handling, dissection technique, instrument selection, etc.

A surgeon's approach to the dissection of vessels is probably as characteristic of that individual surgeon as is choice of home or car. There are the "hamhands" who dissect with blunt fingers indicative of blunter minds, as there are those who sharply and gently incise the tissues with careful precision and efficiency indicative of their concise and proper approach to life; and there are those surgeons who almost caress the vessels, standing back on occasion to marvel at the complexities and beauty of the revealed anatomy.

But metaphors (or parodies) aside and stereotypical analysis abandoned, is there any evidence that vascular dissection need be ruled out in finely delineated measures—but simply, does fine technique *matter*? It is the thesis of this book that it does matter if one is to obtain the best short-term and long-term results and avoid complications.

Gross handling of tissue is self-evidently injurious; yet there is no direct literature supporting that supposition; if for no other reason than the inferred conclusion that those who practice gross surgery obtain equally gross results and seldom find themselves in print extolling the virtues of their ways. It would seem self-evident that crude tissue dissection would lend itself to complication—venous lacerations, inadvertent enterotomies, excessive blood loss, etc.; similarly poor attention to the details of wound closure would lead to wound hematomas, seromas, lymphoceles, and ultimately to graft infections. Poorly conceived anastomoses also may lead to long-term problems as surely as poorly conceived operations, particularly as regards the formation of fibrointimal hyperplasia and pseudoaneurysms with late thromboses. Inappropriate use of embolectomy catheters, occlusive clamps, or production of excessive local ischemia may all be presumed etiologic factors in long-term stenosis formation; each of these is examined in detail.

The legal implications of such a book cannot be ignored. It should be understood by any practicing surgeon (even if such fine points of gentlemanly behavior are sometimes lost upon our legal colleagues) that there are usually three or four "right" ways to do things. Even in the most august of situations (an emeritus academic professor enumerating his years of experience [plus or minus a few prejudices]), the most clearly delineated stance does not *res ipsa loguitor* establish the *only* standard of care.

Thus, although we may firmly opine as to optimal techniques based on literature review and research analysis in the course of this writing, that does not in and of itself make these recommendations the *only* way that it should be done; and a complication occurring in the absence of observation of these techniques does not itself imply practice outside peer review norms or even outside good surgical practice. These are opinions—well researched and firmly delivered, but opinions all the same.

T.J. Bunt, M.D., F.A.C.S.

Contents

Chapter 1

Physiology of the Vessel Blood Interface

S. Fazal Mohammad and Willem Jan W. Bos

The human body is provided with vascular channels to serve the distribution of needed metabolites and to remove undesirable catabolites from the tissues. Although this is the primary function of the vascular system, blood vessels also perform a host of other functions, which are of critical importance to maintain the integrity of the multicellular organism. It is indeed true that blood vessels are more than a simple conduit.

The entire vascular system could be divided into arterial and venous sides that are separated by a network of capillaries with the heart providing the driving force to circulate the blood and thus complete the circuit. There are distinct differences in the anatomical structures of arteries and veins. This is based in part on the fact that blood circulates through the arteries at a significantly higher pressure than blood circulating through the veins. However, in addition to anatomical differences, the arteries and veins may differ in their physiological response to the circulating blood and the presence of various stimuli.

Therefore, in order to best understand the consequences of injury to the blood vessels, it is appropriate to examine the structures of arteries and veins separately, even though there are several common features between the two systems. It should become obvious from the following discussion that the arterial and the venous systems would

From *Iatrogenic Vascular Injury: A Discourse on Surgical Technique,* edited by T.J. Bunt, M.D. © 1990, Futura Publishing Inc., Mount Kisco, NY.

respond differently to a given force and that the two systems may also differ in their response to injury.

Vascular Morphology

Based on their architecture, arteries can be divided into two categories—elastic and muscular. Elastic arteries are those with large diameters where the media is composed of both smooth muscle cells and many elastic laminae (aorta, carotids), whereas smaller arteries in which the media is less elastic (fewer elastic laminae) and contains predominantly smooth muscle cells are called muscular arteries.[1] Small arteries where the media consists of only one or two layers of smooth muscle cells are called arterioles. As illustrated in Figure 1, the blood from arterioles passes through the microcirculatory bed, which

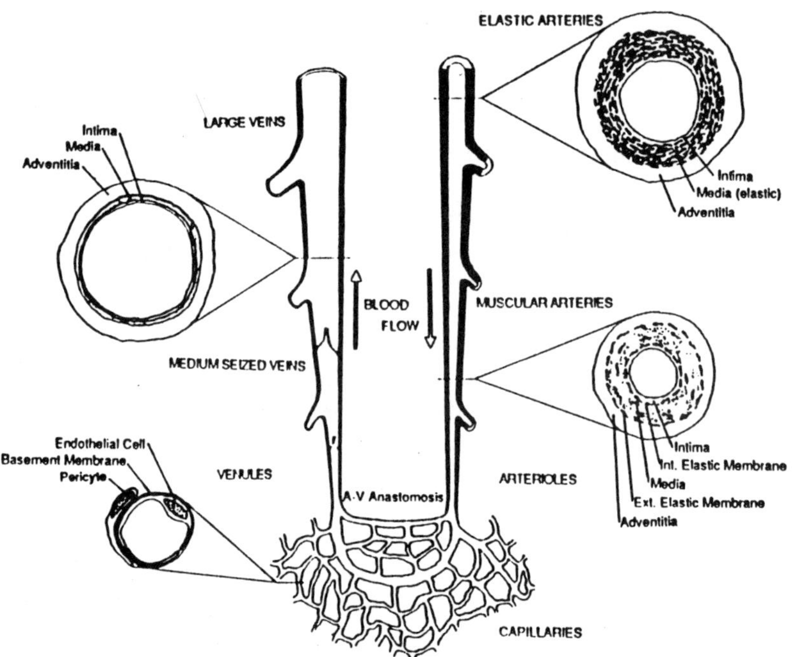

Figure 1. *Schematic illustration of arterial and venous systems. Note the relative size and thickness of the corresponding arteries and veins.*

is composed of arterioles, capillaries, postcapillary venules, and muscular venules.

The veins can be subdivided into medium sized and large veins. When compared with the arteries, the thickness of the wall is considerably smaller, and the overall diameter of the veins is relatively larger than the corresponding artery (Fig. 1).

Components of the Vascular Wall

With the exception of the capillaries in the microcirculatory bed, the wall of blood vessels consists of three distinctive layers: (1) tunica intima, (2) tunica media, and (3) tunica adventitia.[1-3] Capillaries are composed primarily of tunica intima. The tunica intima in large elastic arteries is composed of endothelium, a thin (approximately 80 μm thick) basal lamina, and a subendothelial region composed of collagenous bundles, elastic fibrils, smooth muscle cells, and in some cases, fibroblasts. In other blood vessels, the intima is composed of the endothelial cells alone or endothelium and the basal lamina.[1]

The venous wall (Fig. 2) is also composed of three layers: the tunica intima, the tunica media, and the tunica adventitia. Their boundaries are not as distinct as those seen in arteries. Moreover, there is considerable difference in venous architecture depending upon the location and size of the vein and age of the individual being studied. Medium-sized veins have a weak media with few, circularly arranged, platelike bundles of smooth muscle cells and some longitudinally arranged smooth muscle cells in the innermost part of the adventitia. In addition, smooth muscle cells and the bundles of collagen fibers may be arranged in a spiral form originating from the intima and ending in the adventitia.[4,5]

The tunica adventitia is the outermost layer of the vessel wall. Its thickness also varies considerably with vessel type and location. However, in all arteries and most veins it consists of dense fibroelastic tissue without smooth muscle cells. Some larger veins (e.g., vena cava) are exceptions, where bundles of longitudinally arranged smooth muscle cells are present in the adventitia. The adventitia also harbors vasa vasorum, the small vessels of the vascular wall that provide oxygen and nutrients to the cellular components of the vessel wall. Beside providing strength and stability, the adventitia also helps to embed the blood vessel into the surrounding tissue.[1,2]

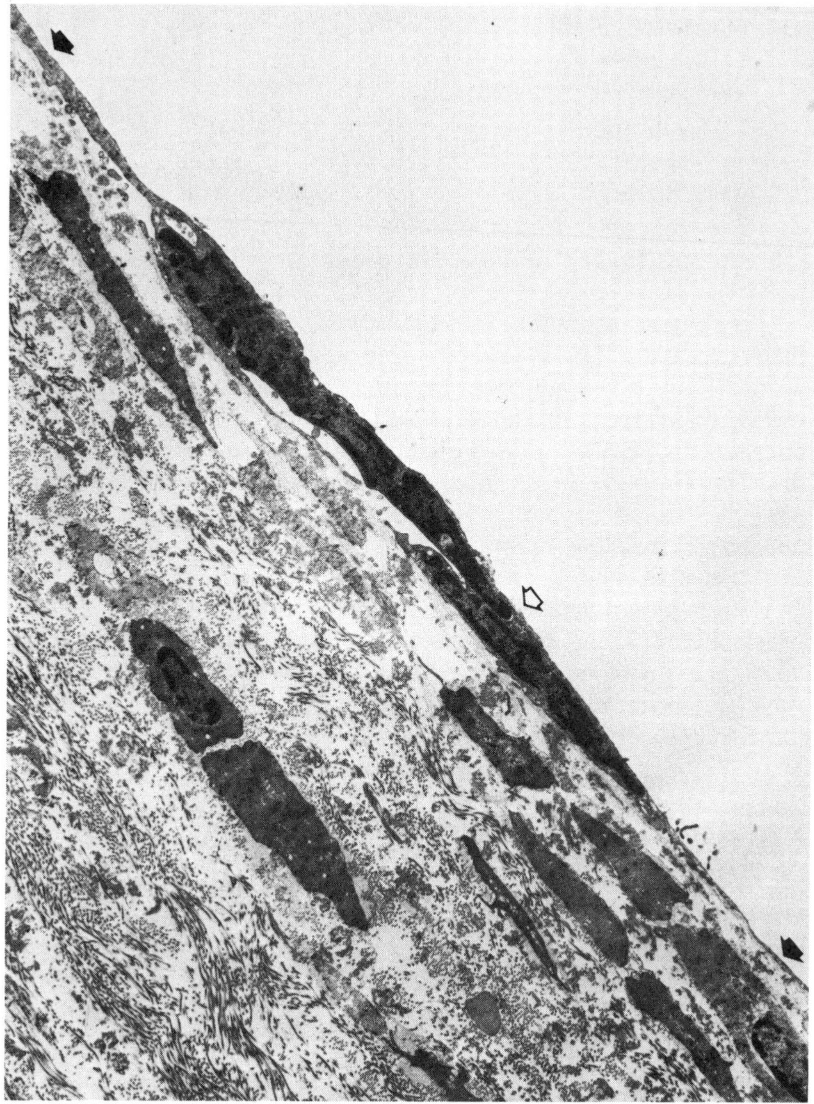

Figure 2. *Transmission electron micrograph of the intima and part of the media of a human saphenous vein. Note the junction between two endothelial cells (open arrow) and a thin layer of well-spread endothelial cell cytoplasm covering the subendothelium (solid arrows) in areas away from the nucleus (original magnification 8,167 ×).*

Differences in Large, Medium, and Small Blood Vessels

The intimal layer of elastic arteries (aorta) is composed of a simple layer of endothelial cells laid upon longitudinally arranged smooth muscle cells within the basal lamina. The media of elastic arteries could be 300 to 500 μm in thickness and composed of alternating elastic laminae and concentrically or spirally arranged smooth muscle cells. Rhodin[1] has suggested that each layer of smooth muscle cells in the media of large arteries may have a different spiral orientation. The smooth muscle cells of muscular arteries are arranged concentrically with perhaps a shorter pitch. The large veins are composed of a thin intima, only a few layers of smooth muscle cells, and a fairly thick adventitia. A medium-sized vein, however, has a slightly more distinct intima with well-defined, longitudinally arranged smooth muscle cells not seen in the large veins. The tunica media is also relatively more distinct in medium-sized veins. Veins are generally more securely embedded into the surrounding tissue compared to arteries.

One of the characteristics of veins is the presence of valves (Fig. 1), which are generally folds of intima and are composed of collagen and elastic fibers.[6] They are generally devoid of smooth muscle cells and are covered with endothelium. Valves are not present in arteries, vena cava, or some of the smaller veins. The frequency of these valves depends on the location and age of the individual.

Endothelium

The typical element at the interface between the intravascular space and tissues is the endothelial lining, a nearly continuous monolayer sheet of flat cells, covering, in humans approximately 6000 m^2 in the capillaries alone. Endothelial cells are endowed with intricate structural and functional properties. They present to the blood the most compatible interface that is known to date,[7-9] form a barrier between blood and the subendothelial structures, allow selective passage of solutes, and absorb or release a host of bioactive substances.

Since it is well recognized that the subendothelium is highly thrombogenic,[10-13] perhaps the most important function of the endothelium is to prevent the contact of blood with the subendothelium.

Not only does the endothelium form a physical barrier between blood and the subendothelium, it is actively involved in balancing and regulating hemostasis.[14] Subendothelium can initiate and support a sequence of steps that lead to the formation of a hemostatic plug; this is achieved by adhesion of platelets to the subendothelium (Fig. 3). Adherent platelets release several highly reactive products, including the arachidonic acid metabolites (endoperoxides and thromboxane A_2) and a cationic protein, platelet-derived growth factor (PDGF) that stimulates the growth of smooth muscle cells[15-17]; together, they cause vasoconstriction, aggregation of platelets, activation of coagulation and possibly complement pathways, and later, proliferation of smooth muscle cells. The activation of coagulation factors results in the formation of fibrin. Platelets enmeshed in a fribrin network are necessary for the formation of an effective hemostatic plug. Vasoconstriction helps reduce the opening and the healing process is initiated with the proliferation of smooth muscle cells (Fig. 3).

The importance of a normal hemostatic process cannot be overemphasized. A subnormal reaction leads to the risk of bleeding, whereas greater than normal adhesion of platelets or activation of coagulation factors enhances the risk of thromboembolization[18,19]—either one of these events would have serious implications. Therefore, the effect of a seemingly innocuous endothelial injury can have far-reaching consequences. This should be given due consideration during any surgical manipulation of the vascular system.

Each endothelial cell has two sides, the *luminal* side, which is exposed to the blood, and the *abluminal* side, which is anchored to the basal lamina. The abluminal surface faces no motion, while in contrast, the luminal surface faces a constant rhythmic current of plasma and uncounted billions of formed blood elements, continuous rubbing, traction, and shearing effects, not to mention turbulence at the site of bifurcation of vessels. Iatrogenic injury to the blood vessel could significantly affect these processes. The distortion of flow in the surgically manipulated areas could subject endothelial cells to undue stress and, in this manner, may alter their properties. Thus, the endothelial cells in the vicinity of the vascular injury may not be able to perform their normal hemotological functions or may be desquamated. This should be given due consideration when any blood vessel is subjected to mechanical or surgical trauma.

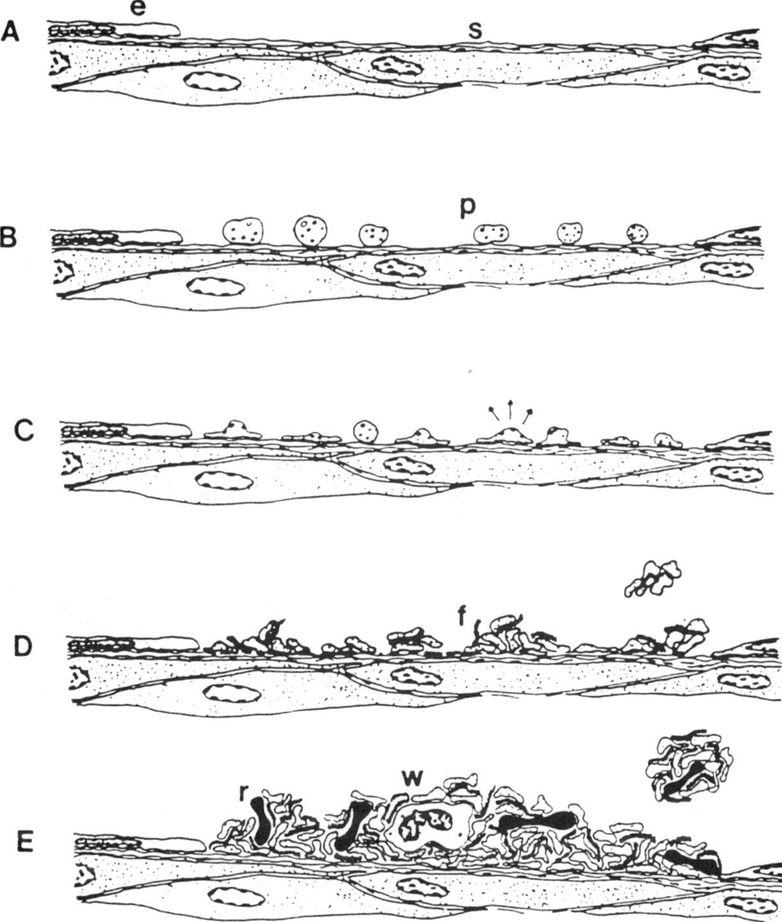

Figure 3. *Diagrammatic illustration of sequence of events following exposure of subendothelium to blood components. (A) Endothelial (e) desquamation resulting in exposed subendothelium (s); (B) platelets (p) adhere to exposed subendothelium; (C) adherent platelets are activated and their granular constituents are released (arrows); (D) substances released by adherent platelets attract more platelets and activate the coagulation pathway, resulting in the formation of fibrin (f). Adherent platelet aggregates may break loose forming microemboli; (E) Fibrin strands may enmesh adherent platelets, along with erythrocytes (r) and leukocytes (w). This mass of fibrin and blood cells can break loose and form thromboemboli.*

Morphology of Endothelium

Arterial endothelium

All arteries are lined by flattened, polygonal endothelial cells that rest on a distinct basal lamina. The luminal surface of the endothelium is not totally smooth. Instead, the center of each cell, corresponding to the nucleus, is slightly raised so that a cobblestonelike appearance results. Endothelial cells contain a prominent nucleus, occasional vesicles, mitochondria, endoplasmic reticulum, glycogen granules, and Weibel-Palade bodies (considered to be a characteristic of the endothelial cells) (Fig. 4).[20] Since this structure has not been observed in any other cell type, and therefore is unique to endothelium, these inclusions are used as a marker for endothelial cells, although it has been shown that not all endothelial cells have these cytoplasmic inclusions.[21] The Weibel-Palade bodies are generally 3 μm in length, 0.1 μm thick, and are composed of 6–20 tubules, each tubule having a diameter of approximately 150 Å

Endothelial cells appear to be aligned with their long axes parallel to the direction of the blood flow.[22–24] Certain recent studies suggest that endothelial cells assume this orientation due to radial and longitudinal contraction of the blood vessel following their removal from the body.[7,25]

Endothelial cells are connected by tight junctions, gap junctions, and intricate interfoldings of the cytoplasm of adjacent cells.[26–28] The endothelium at branch points in arteries is less uniform in its morphology and tends to be less well oriented and somewhat thicker than the endothelium remote from the branch points.[29] Endothelial cells cultured in vitro align themselves in the direction of flow when the tissue culture medium is circulated or when the cells are subjected to a controlled shear force.[30,31] The alignment of the endothelial cells at branch points and their thickening may reflect their response to the shear forces encountered at these sites. For a more detailed description of the ultra structure of arterial endothelium, the reader is referred to several excellent reviews.[22,32–34]

To form an effective barrier between the subendothelium and the blood, endothelial cells are anchored to the basal lamina underneath and interconnected with one another by tight junctions. These attachments give endothelial cells sufficient strength and tenacity to with-

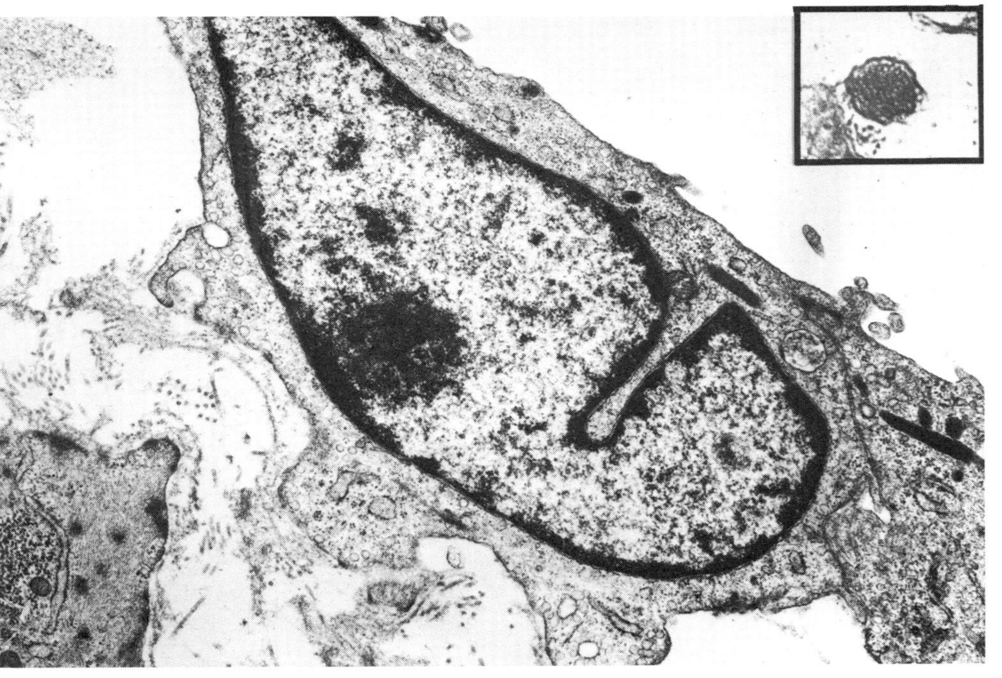

Figure 4. *Transmission electron micrograph of a human saphenous vein endothelial cell showing normal cellular structures and the unique Weibel Palade bodies (original magnification approximately 28,000 ×). Insets show a longitudinal and cross-sectional view of Weibel-Palade bodies at higher magnification.*

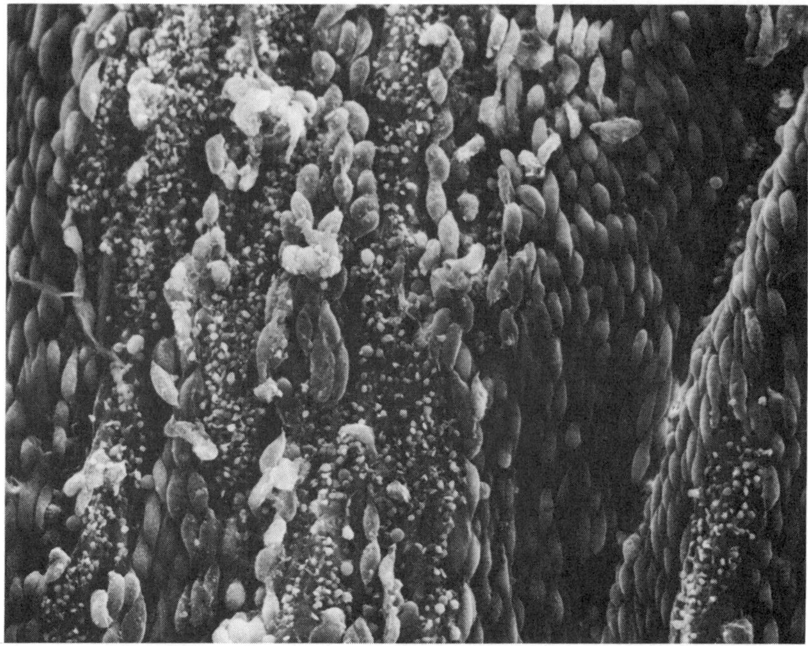

Figure 5A. *Scanning electron micrograph showing endothelial damage caused by clamping. Note endothelial desquamation and adherent platelets to exposed subendothelium. No platelets are seen adherent to areas with intact endothelium (original magnification 750 ×).*

stand the stresses normally exerted by circulating blood. Despite this tenacity, endothelial cells can be damaged by a number of chemical stimuli or physical factors. Figures 5 and 6 illustrate the fragility of the endothelial cells and demonstrate that clamping, needle punctures, and catheter tips can easily damage endothelium.

Capillary endothelium

In view of its significant role in the transport of metabolites, capillary endothelium has been studied in considerable detail. A single, curved endothelial cell forms the lining of each short segment of a capillary. A single endothelial cell may encircle the lumen and interconnect with itself as well as with adjacent endothelial cells to form a

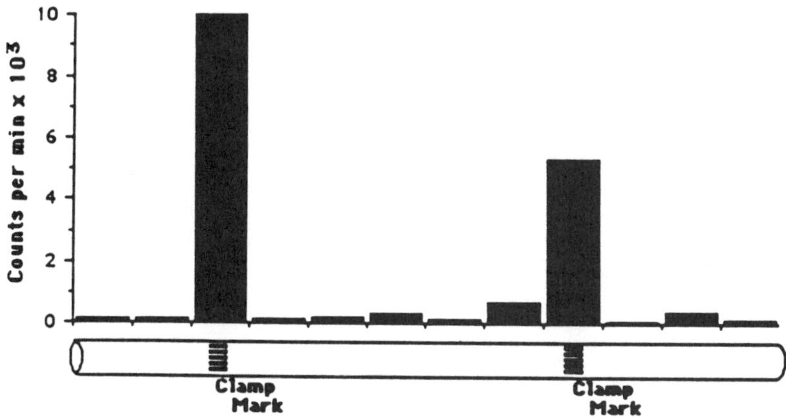

Figure 5B. *Adhesion of large number of ^{51}Cr labeled platelets to the blood vessel at the site of clamp injury. A segment of human umbilical vein was subjected to clamp injury. Subsequently fresh heparinized human blood containing ^{51}Cr labeled platelets was circulated through the vein with the help of a peristaltic pump for 30 min. at 37 °C in an atmosphere of 5% CO_2, 95% air, and 95% relative humidity. At the end of circulation, the vein was rinsed with 0.15 M NaCl until the wash was free of platelets. The vein was then divided into 1-cm segments, and the radioactivity associated with each segment was measured by gamma counting. Note the sharp increase in radioactivity in areas of clamp injury.*

capillary. The capillary endothelial cells have a more prominent nucleus than those of other segments of the vascular system and contain numerous pinocytotic vesicles.[35-37] The basement membrane of capillaries is thin and frequently appears to be interrupted. Because of their curved shape and the small diameter of the lumen, the capillary endothelial cells remain in intimate contact with the blood cells.

Venous endothelium

Postcapillary venules   The postcapillary venule is the sight of considerable activity in the vascular system. It is in these areas that leukocytes leave the vascular system by pushing their way between adjacent endothelial cells. In some part of the vascular system, the endothelium of postcapillary venules is markedly thicker with prominent nuclei. These features are particularly pronounced in lymphoid organs.[38]

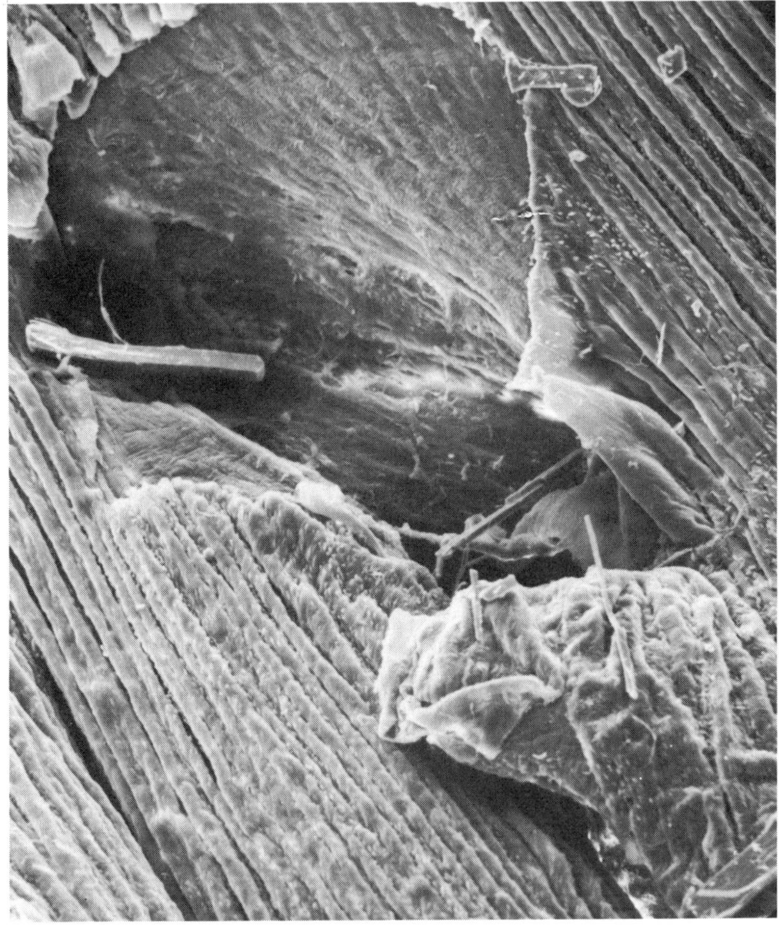

Figure 6. *Scanning electron micrograph showing the damage to the vessel wall caused by a needle puncture. The vessel was punctured in-situ with an 18-gauge needle, excised, rinsed and fixed immediately to prevent adhesion of platelets (original magnification 100 ×).*

The general morphology of venous endothelium resembles that of arterial endothelium, including a cobblestonelike appearance in which cells are arranged parallel to the direction of flow. Since segments of veins also suffer radial and longitudinal contraction when they are excised from the vascular tree and processed for electron microscopy, elongated appearance of the cells with rounded bodies may be the result of contraction suffered by the vessel segment (Fig. 7). In addition

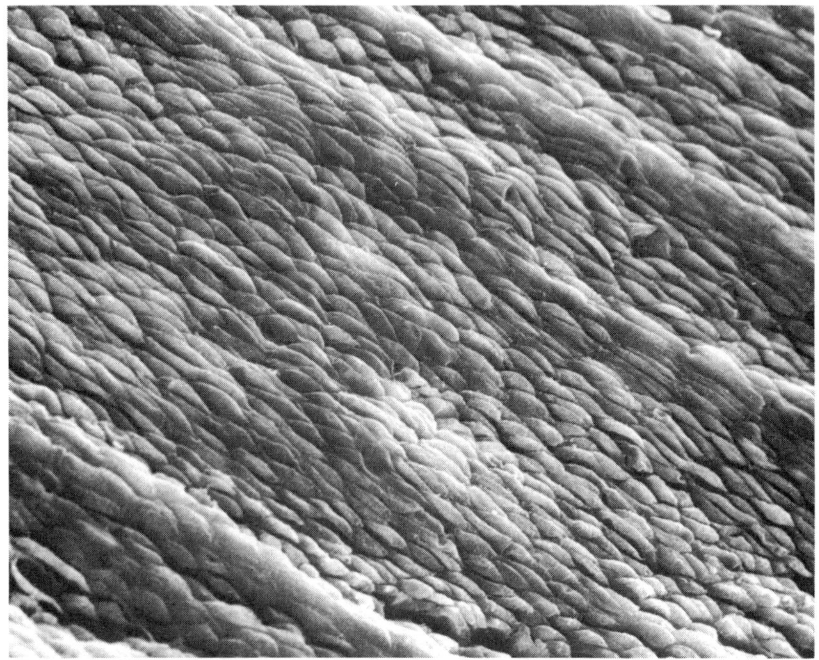

Figure 7. *Scanning electron micrograph of a dog saphenous vein. The vein suffered radial and longitudinal contraction following excision. The excised segment was rinsed with 0.15 M NaCl and fixed. Note the cobblestone appearance of the endothelial cells (original magnification 450 ×).*

to the artifacts introduced by the contraction of blood vessels, the exposure of endothelium to air or solutions with nonphysiological pH, temperature or osmolarity, and physical handling of vessel segments are likely to affect the overall morphology of the endothelium.[39,40] Complete denudation of endothelium has been noted when vessel segments are allowed to contract rapidly, particularly in cold solutions.[41] When blood vessels are fixed under conditions where minimal radial and longitudinal contraction occurs, the endothelial morphology looks quite different. In properly preserved blood vessels the endothelial cells appear flat, and the cell junctions are so uniform that it becomes difficult to identify the individual cells. Under these conditions, the scanning electron microscopic view of the endothelium shows a smooth, glasslike interface. Figures 7 and 8 show the difference between the endothelium of a well-preserved blood vessel compared to the blood vessel that suffered longitudinal and radial contraction.

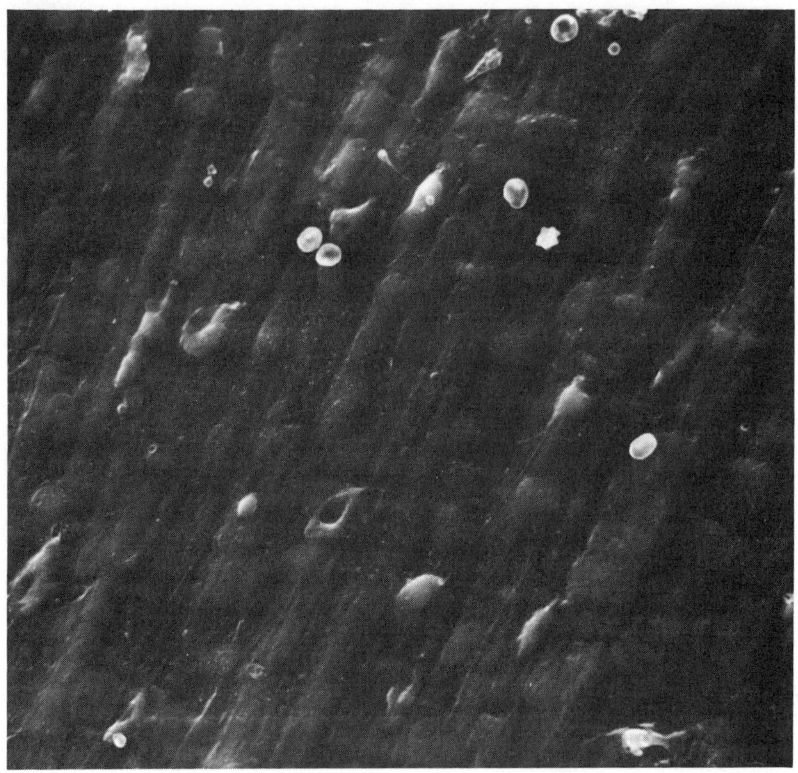

Figure 8. *Scanning electron micrograph of a dog saphenous vein, which was fixed in situ with minimal contraction. Note the smooth, glasslike appearance with no demarcation of cell borders or rounded cell bodies (A).*

Endothelial cells present to the blood a highly hemocompatible surface. This is achieved by a variety of means that include presentation of a nonreactive interface,[42] release of chemical stimuli,[7,14] and synthesis of enzymes or their precursors.[7,14,43] With the help of these features, endothelial cells collectively achieve their ultimate goal of providing an unobstructed passage for blood flow.

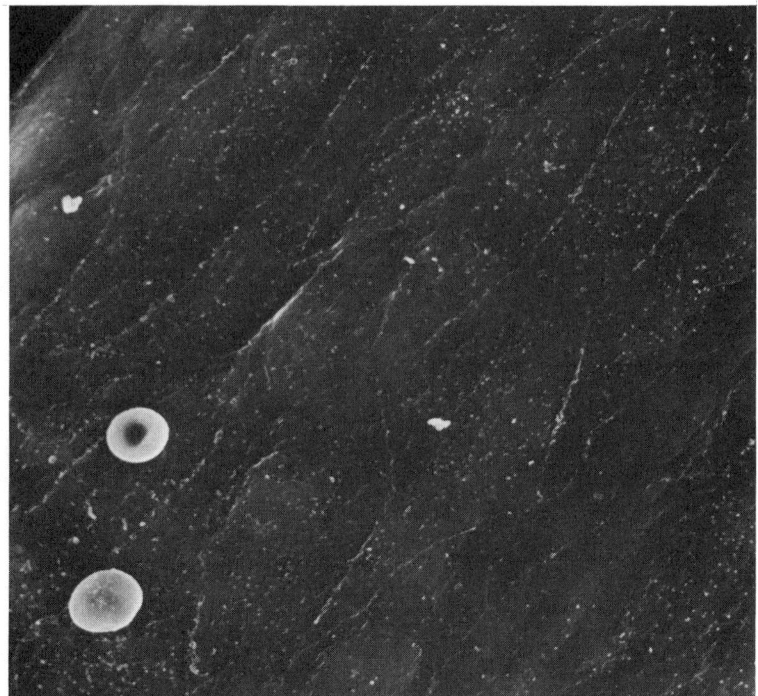

Figure 8B. *When the vein was allowed to contract slightly, demarcation of cell borders and slight rounding of cell bodies occurred (original magnifications 440 and 1,000 ×, respectively).*

Endothelial Injury

Rheologic factors

Disruption of laminar flow, increased shear stresses, and turbulent or vortical flow all contribute to injury of the endothelium.[44] Endothelial cells appear to have a shorter life span and increased vascular permeability in areas of abnormal blood flow. This condition is reflected by subendothelial edema in the area of injury and by the reactivity of injured endothelial cells with blood platelets and leukocytes.[45] Endothelium located at the branch points in the arterial system as well as areas of abnormal arterial narrowing or dilatation is altered by abnormal flow patterns of blood at these points. These cells exhibit altered polarity, swelling of cells, cytoplasmic projections, and even desquamation. Endothelial cells in this region are also more permeable, and staining with ruthenium red indicates detectable loss in the intracellular matrix. Since the rheologic factors may present one of the most common types of injury to the endothelium, the effect of such factors on endothelial cell functions has received considerable attention in recent years. Experiments with endothelial cells grown in tissue culture show that they grow as flat and polygonal cells on artificial substrates[21]; when grown in an environment where the cells experience flow, the cells become elongated and align themselves longitudinally in the direction of flow.[30,31] It is obvious that changes in the nature of blood flow would have a profound effect on the endothelium. Increased shear stresses would cause thickening of the cells, and excessively high shear stresses may potentially dislodge the endothelial cells altogether.

Anoxia and injurious gases

Endothelial cells are highly dependent on a continuous supply of oxygen.[29] Consequently, all situations that lead to anoxia (even momentarily) cause endothelial injury. Prolonged cessation of blood flow by vessel ligation, clamping, or thrombus would lead to anoxia. Ultrastructural studies following exposure of endothelial cells to anoxic conditions show that one of the early responses of endothelial cells to anoxia is the formation of cytoplasmic protrusions (Fig. 9).[29,46–49] Sustained anoxia results in the formation of blebs that may burst later, resulting in the ejection of the nucleus and the formation of a large craterlike structure on the luminal surface of the cells (Fig. 10). This is followed by a subendothelial edema if a number of endothelial cells are damaged in a particular location.

Endothelial cells can also be injured by excessively high concentrations of oxygen, nonphysiological concentrations of CO_2 and even low concentrations of carbon monoxide.[50,51]

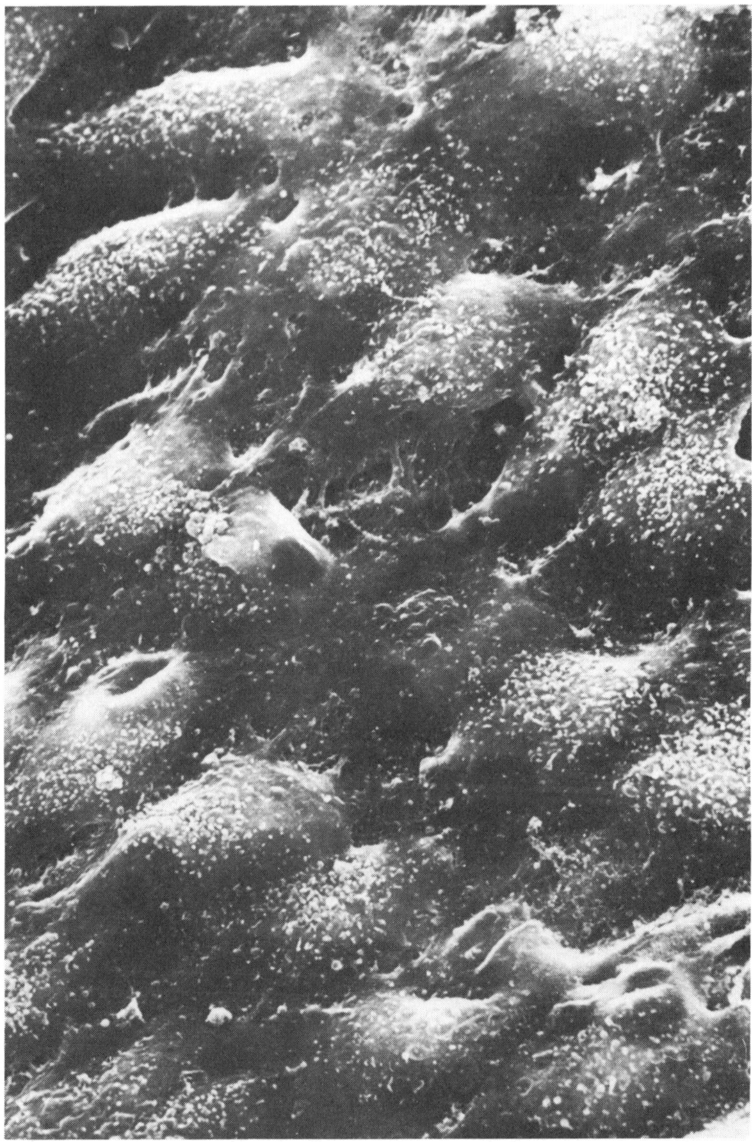

Figure 9. *Scanning electron micrograph showing protrusions on endothelial cells after anoxic injury (original magnification approximately 4,500 ×).*

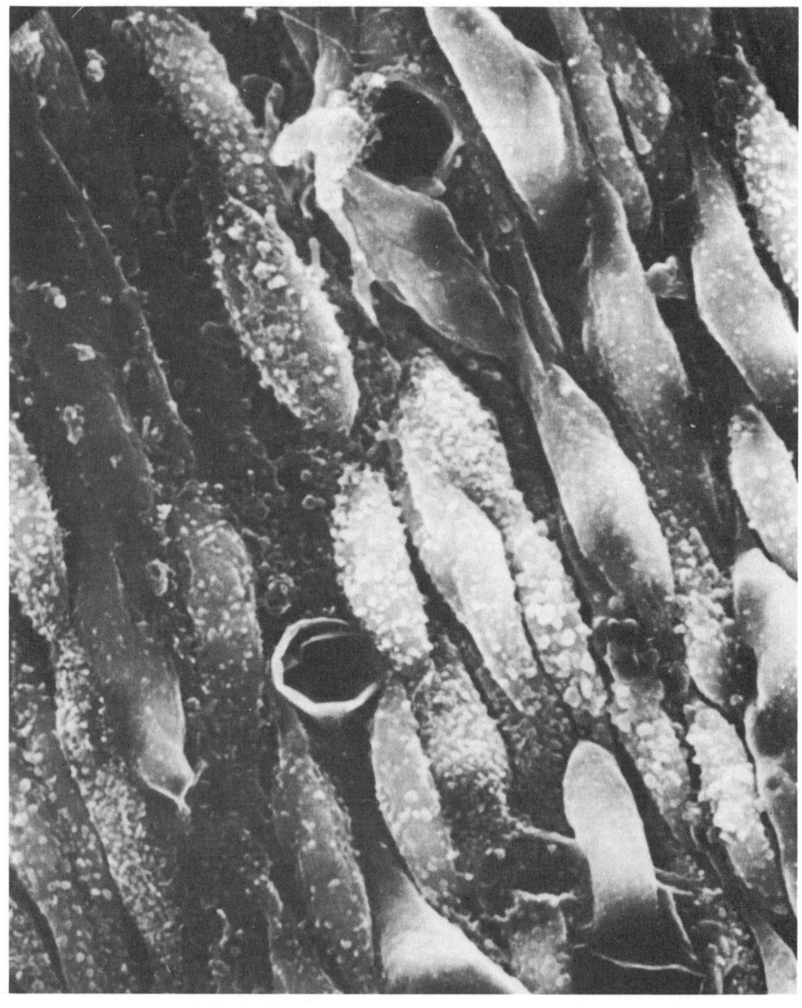

Figure 10. *Scanning electron micrograph showing protrusions as well as craterlike structures after anoxic injury (original magnification 2,200 ×).*

Mechanical injury

Although endothelial cells appear to be tenaciously adherent to the subendothelium on the abluminal side and to one another through tight junctions, these cells are extremely sensitive to mechanical injury. Endothelial cells can be damaged easily by physical manipulation of the blood vessel. Clamping of the vessel (Fig. 5), introduction of catheters, needle punctures (Fig. 6), sutures (Fig. 11), moving tips of indwelling catheters, and air bubbles cause considerable mechanical injury. In many instances the same forces that lead to endothelial injury may also damage subendothelium and the adventitia.[52–55]

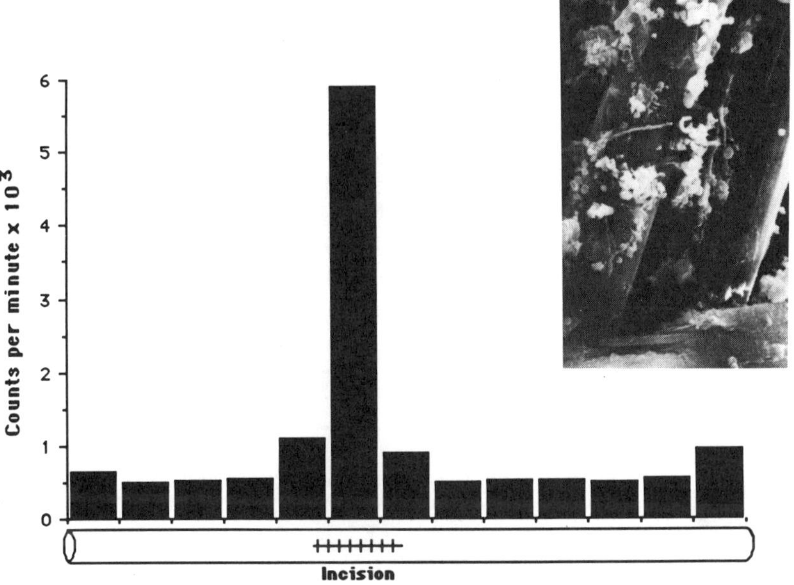

Figure 11. *Adhesion of a large number of ^{51}Cr-labeled platelets to the blood vessel at the site of a 2-cm incision in the wall of the umbilical vein, which was closed using neoprene suture material and blood-containing ^{51}Cr-labeled platelets, was circulated as described in the legend of Figure 5. Inset shows a scanning electron micrograph of platelets adherent to the suture material (original magnification 3,460 ×).*

Injury caused by other agents

Endothelial cells possess antigenic domains on their luminal surface that elicit antibody response. Several alloantigens of human endothelial cells have been characterized and are considered important in organ transplantation.[56] Reaction of these antigens with antibodies has been shown to damage endothelium. The endothelium can also be damaged by immune complexes, circulating bacteria, or bacterial toxins.[7] Viruses and rickettsiae can enter the endothelial cell cytoplasm and multiply, causing cell injury or death.[57] A number of chemical or biochemical agents also cause endothelial injury. In addition, injection of hyper- or hypotonic solutions, venoms, and certain enzymes (trypsin, chymotrypsin, and thrombin) can cause endothelial injury.[58-61] Prolonged exposure to hyperglycemia (in diabetics) and elevated levels of vasoactive substances (angiotensin, kinins, epinephrine, and certain products of prostaglandin pathway) also cause endothelial injury.[7] Hypertension, radiation, and certain drugs can also damage the endothelium.[7,46,62] One of the most important drugs from a surgical point of view is angiographic contrast media. In one experiment, exposure of cultured endothelial cells during 24 hours to different contrast media resulted in lysis of 40%–90% of the cells.[63] This effect is at least partially attributable to the hyperosmolarity of these media. Rapid dilution by continued blood flow and secondary irrigation with isotonic solutions presumably minimizes the effects seen in these in vitro experiments.[63]

Reaction of Endothelium to Injury

The response of endothelial cells to injury depends on the nature, strength, and duration of exposure to the injurious agent. Sublethal injury is manifested by edematous endothelial cells, the formation of cytoplasmic vesicles, and the development of protuberances of the plasma membrane yielding surface pits and craters. Nonlethal injury may also produce increased vascular permeability to noncellular plasma constituents.[9,64] Endothelial cells may recover from mild injury and may later exhibit normal functions. Severe injury, however, generally leads to cell death. Loss of the endothelial cell lining exposes the basal lamina to blood with several consequences. Initially, platelets adhere to the exposed basal lamina.[12] The basal lamina of capillaries in the microcirculation appears to permit platelet adhesion but does not stimulate platelet release reaction with subsequent platelet aggregation. However, exposure of the basal lamina of larger blood vessels produces platelet adhesion, release reaction, and aggregation, resulting in the development of a platelet plug and activation of blood coagulation factors that may lead to the formation of a mural thrombus (Fig. 3).[62] In addition, the loss of the endothelial lining destroys the control of vascular permeability normally exercised by this monolayer of cells. Soluble components of blood gain access to the vascular wall and adjacent tissues, thus supporting the development of edema in the area of endothelial injury.

Under normal conditions, endothelial cells appear to have a low turnover rate.[9] However, following endothelial injury, neighboring noninjured endothelial cells replicate rapidly to replace the injured cells and thus help the repair process. Following a focal endothelial injury, peripheral endothelial cells replicate from the edge and migrate inward.[65] Upon reconstitution of an intact monolayer, the reparative process ceases, and endothelial cell turnover returns to a normal slow rate.[66] This proliferative potential of endothelial cells may be influenced by a number of factors, including their ability to synthesize and secrete collagen to help anchor the cells and thus provide appropriate conditions conducive for the growth of cells. It has been suggested that endothelial cells may have a limited number of doublings, and the ability of endothelial cells to regenerate at the site of continuing injury may be restrained.[67] This has evident implications for normal/abnormal endothelial function in areas of chronic injury.

Functions of Endothelium

Endothelium plays many important roles in maintaining the vascular integrity. Beside forming a barrier between the circulating blood and the subendothelial region and presentation of a hemocompatible interface, endothelial cells regulate vascular permeability and contractility. Endothelial cells are metabolically active both in preserving their own structure and for regulation of the blood components passing the luminal surface. Endothelium actively participates in hemostatic processes by producing important biochemicals, including potent antiplatelet agents and agents that help dissolve the clot. Furthermore, the cells themselves specialize within different organs to meet specific needs.

Vascular permeability

Endothelial cells form a selective barrier between blood and the subendothelium, and in this manner, control the egress of the soluble and cellular components of blood from the vascular lumen into the surrounding tissues.[68,69] This control is exerted in several ways. Under normal circumstances, the tight junctions between endothelial cells prevent leakage of solutes or cells. These junctions are loosened, however, in response to poorly understood stimuli, permitting macromolecules and blood cells, particularly the leukocytes, to leave the vascular system.[70] It is interesting to note that endothelium regulates the transport of solutes. This is achieved by several complex mechanisms, the transport through the vesicular system being perhaps one of the most important mechanisms.[36] There are at least two different vesicular systems. In one system the cytoplasmic vesicles appear to coalesce to form tortuous channels through the endothelial cell cytoplasm that connect the luminal and abluminal surfaces of the cell, thereby forming a tunnel for the passage of macromolecules. In the second system, vesicles form on the luminal surface of the endothelial cells by invagination of the plasma membrane. These invaginations then pinch off and are transported to the abluminal surface where they attach and appear to fuse with the abluminal membrane to form openings that permit vesicular contents to enter the subendothelial space.[36] A number of factors affect permeability including blood pressure and the presence of vasoactive substances.[71–74]

Vascular integrity

Endothelial cells synthesize and secrete various components of the basal lamina, and in this manner may contribute to the integrity of the vascular wall.[75] The structural components of endothelial basal lamina differ in various parts of the vascular system. In the smaller arterioles, capillaries, and venules, the basement membrane is thin and in some areas discontinuous.[76] In these areas the basement membrane contains little elastin, but is composed predominantly of collagen, fibronectin, and a variety of glycosaminoglycans. The types of collagen synthesized by endothelial cells also vary with location. It is believed that endothelial cells synthesize and secrete subendothelial components primarily from their abluminal surface only. This is of critical concern because the presence of collagen or other subendothelial components on the *luminal* side of the endothelial cells would seriously compromise vascular integrity. The exact mechanism by which the luminal and abluminal sides of the cellular functions are differentiated is not known, but the ability of the endothelial cells to differentiate the two sides may have important implications in vascular injury and repair.

Hemocompatible interface

Endothelium appears to be the most hemocompatible surface known. Under normal conditions, endothelium neither attracts platelets nor appears to activate coagulation factors.[42] These properties are manifested by the luminal side of the endothelial cells. Although there are indications that the plasma membrane on the luminal side may be distinct from that on the abluminal side of the same cell, it is not known whether the two sides of cells are different in terms of reactivity with blood. It is also not known whether the net negative charge on the abluminal side of the endothelial cell is different from that of the luminal side of the cell. It is generally believed, however, that only the luminal surface of the endothelium is thromboresistant.

There are a number of factors that contribute to this thromboresistance. Alpha$_2$ macroglobulin on the luminal surface of the endothelium has been implicated in rendering endothelium nonthrombogenic. Other factors such as the ability to synthesize prostaglandin I_2 and plasminogen activator might play equally important roles.[9,14,75] Of particular interest is the ability of endothelial cells to secrete (1) a plasminogen activator that initiates the fibrinolytic pathway[77] and (2) an inhibitor of this activator[78] to regulate fibrinolysis. The presence of plasminogen activator on one hand and an inhibitor of this plasminogen activator on the other hand suggests that a delicate balance exists through which endothelium regulates the hemostatic processes. While endothelial cells initiate the sequence of steps that help in the dissolution of clots, this process is kept within limits with the help of inhibitors that prevent uncontrolled lysis by plasmin.[7] With these two seemingly opposed activities, endothelial cells are able to help maintain a delicate balance between hemostasis and thrombosis. Vascular or endothelial injury may result in loss of these activities and in this manner may shift the balance in favor of thrombosis in areas where endothelium is damaged.

The ability of endothelial cells to synthesize and release prostaglandin I_2 may be extremely important since it has significant antiplatelet and vasodilatory effects. Some investigators have suggested that endothelial cells continuously release small amounts of prostaglandin I_2 into the blood. These observations have led to the suggestion that prostaglandin I_2 may function as a circulating hormone.[79] However, Haslam and McClenaghan[80] concluded after careful monitoring of circulating levels of PGI_2 that the levels were too low to affect platelet aggregation and thus disagreed with the suggestion of confering hormonal status to PGI_2. In addition to Haslam and McClenaghan, other authors also questioned the physiological role of PGI_2.[81,82]

The synthesis of PGI_2 by endothelial cells can be abolished by agents (certain nonsteroidal anti-inflammatory agents, particularly aspirin) that inhibit the enzyme cyclooxygenase.[83,84] However, inhibition of prostaglandin pathway in endothelial cells has not been shown to be associated with a higher incidence of thromboembolism. This may be due in part to the fact that the administration of pharmacological agents that inhibit prostaglandin I_2 pathway would also inhibit the formation of thromboxane A_2 by the platelets. Thromboxane A_2 is one of the most potent stimulators of platelet aggregation beside being an effective vasoconstricting agent. Since thomboxane A_2 and prostaglandin I_2 have opposing effects on thrombotic processes, administration of inhibitors of prostaglandin pathway in circulating blood would result not only in the inhibition of prostaglandin I_2 synthesis but inhibition of thromboxane A_2 synthesis as well.[85] Therefore, the balance that may exist between thromboxane A_2 and prostaglandin I_2 would remain unaltered. However, the ultimate effect of pharmacological agents such as aspirin may be quite different, since aspirin inhibits prostagladin synthesis in platelets and endothelial cells. Being fragments of megakaryocyte cytoplasm, platelets are anucleated cells and are considered to be *incapable* of protein biosynthesis. Since platelets are not capable of replenishing their enzymes, their ability to produce arachidonate metabolites would be adversely affected for the remainder of their lifespan following irreversible inhibition of cyclooxygenase.[86] However, unlike platelets, endothelial cells are capable of replenishing their lost enzymes as soon as the circulating level of inhibitory drugs drop below a threshold. A careful evaluation of the effect of aspirin on endothelial cell cyclooxygenase has revealed that endothelial cells resynthesize their cyclooxygenase immediately after aspirin has been removed from the surrounding medium, and the concentration of cyclooxygenase is restored to near normal levels within hours. This is the rationale for low dose aspirin therapy. In addition to aspirin, a number of other drugs affect PGI_2 synthesis by endothelial cells. Among the commonly used drugs, indomethacine, isoproterenol, nicotine, and steroids inhibit PGI_2 synthesis whereas dipyridamole, furosemide, lidocaine, nitroglycerin, and pentoxyphylline stimulate PGI_2 synthesis.[85,87]

Mechanical Functions of the Vessel Wall

The peripheral and pulmonary circulation regulates the amount of blood delivered to the different organs. This is achieved by the following mechanisms[88]:

(1) *Changes in circulating blood volume.* This is achieved either by exchanging water and solutes with perivascular spaces or by excreting water and solutes in the kidney.

(2) *Changes in blood distribution within the vasculature.* The venous part of the splanchnic circulation has a large capacity. By adjusting the flow through this part, the amount of blood available for the rest of the circulation is regulated.[88] Blood flow through organs can be controlled individually by increasing or decreasing the tension of the smooth muscle cells in the resistance vessels (muscular arteries and arterioles).

(3) *Changes in cardiac output.* This also helps regulate the amount of blood circulating through various organs. This control is of major importance in vascular dynamics.

The vasculature itself has three main mechanical functions:

(a) it conducts the blood under different pressures,

(b) regulates the distribution of blood by increasing or decreasing the vascular resistance, or

(c) alters the compliance.[89]

Conductance

The main function of the aorta and larger arteries is to accommodate the blood ejected by the left ventricle during systole and deliver it uniformly to the arteries (Windkessel function). At the same time, these vessels expand during systole to prevent excessive blood pressures. The relative abundance of elastin in these vessels has been suggested to provide the mechanical resilience necessary for this function.[90]

Vascular Resistance

Blood flow through a particular organ is controlled almost entirely by the amount of resistance applied by small arteries and arterioles; this is dependent on the relatively large amount of smooth muscle cells in these vessels.[90,91] Upon contraction, the diameter of these vessels may decrease by as much as 20%–50%, resulting in a significant increase in resistance.[90]

Control mechanisms

Resistance to blood flow is tightly regulated to meet the needs of the areas being served by a specific blood vessel. Local as well as systemic control mechanisms are used to regulate the vascular resistance.[92]

1. *Local factors*   A number of specific stimuli may trigger localized vasoconstriction or vasodilation, depending on the needs of regional circulation. Their effect generally is confined to a limited area.

(a) *Metabolic factors.*   A number of metabolites produced by tissues have vasodilatory effects. Decreased pO_2, increase pCO_2, increased concentrations of H^+, K^+, phosphate, adenosine, adenosine nucleotides, and several prostaglandins have been shown to have vasodilatory effects.[93,94] How these factors exert their effects is not completely understood, but indications exist that they cause the release of endothelium-derived relaxing factor (EDRF).[95,96] EDRF, most likely a prostanoid,[96] is released under normal conditions by the endothelial cells after their stimulation by acetylcholine, thrombin, adenosine diphosphate (ADP), serotonin, antidiuretic hormone (ADH), and possibly other stimuli.[95] PGE_1 and thromboxane (TBX) A_2, which have antagonistic effects in the regulation of hemostatic processes, also have an antagonistic effect on the local circulation; whereas PGE_1 augments vasodilation, TBX A_2 is a strong vasoconstrictor.[93] Beside PGE_1 and thromboxane A_2, other agents released during activation of the coagulation pathways and platelets also take part in the regulation of vasoconstriction and vasodilatation. Thrombin, serotonin, ADP, and platelet-activating factor cause an increased release of EDRF, but have a contracting effect on the smooth muscle cells,[93] showing that the control of local resistance is a balanced but complicated process.

(b) *Physical factors.*   Decreased temperatures generally lower the muscular tone and decrease the vascular response to vasoconstrictors. Blood vessels in the skin represent an exception to this rule; as part of their function to control body temperature, cutaneous vessels exhibit greater vasoconstriction in response to colder temperatures.[93,97] Compression by surrounding muscular tissue also triggers a strong vasodilatory response. This response is of special importance in the heart where the subendocardial region is subjected to the highest surrounding pressures and also has the highest metabolic rate.[93]

(c) *Myogenic factors.*   A direct relationship may exist between the rate of muscle stretching and the resulting contraction of the smooth muscle cells.[93] Recently it has been proposed that endothelium-derived contracting factor (EDCF), which most likely is a prostanoid as well,[96] plays a role in this contractile response.[95,98]

2. *Systemic control.*   Unlike the effect of local factors, contraction of the blood vessels may also be regulated by systemic control. An appropriate example of systemic control is the effect of neuroregulators that produce a generalized response.

(a) *Central neural control.*   The sympathetic system provides the main pathway for neural control. The neurotransmitter in the sympathetic system is mainly norepinephrine, which binds to the alpha-receptors present on the smooth muscle cells of the blood vessels, thus initiating the vasoconstriction. The alpha-receptors are unevenly distributed in the vasculature; they are abundant in skin, skeletal muscles, splanchnic organs, and kidneys.[94] For a detailed description of the neural pathways that control the cardiovascular system, the reader is referred to references 99–101. The effect of sympathetic innervation in the heart, where it has important chronotropic and inotropic effects, is beyond the scope of this chapter.

(b) *Humoral control.*   Epinephrine,[94] norepinephrine,[94] angiotensin II,[94,102] antidiuretic hormone,[94,102] autocoids,[94,95] and thrombin[95,96,103] may participate in the humoral control of vascular resistance. Although humoral control mechanisms are included in systemic control, it is recognized that a number of stimuli listed in humoral control may also be released locally and might have a more pronounced localized effect.

Changes in resistance due to vascular pathology

The above regulatory mechanisms tightly control vascular resistance to meet the demands of the body. This control is necessary for optimal blood flow, which is critical for optimal performance of each organ and for optimal coordination among various organs. Pathological changes in the vessel wall would adversely affect its ability to respond to the above factors that control vascular resistance. Moreover, pathological changes in the vessel wall components (atherosclerosis and hypertension) may lead to inadequate release of regulatory molecules or may produce rheological changes beyond the ranges normally encountered, thus seriously affecting the vascular resistance.

(1) *Hypertension.*   Hypertension profoundly affects the vessel wall. In general, three main changes influencing the mechanical functions of the vessel wall have been observed in hypertensive subjects[90]:

(a) *Wall thickening.*   An increase in the number of smooth muscle cells and connective tissue deposits in the media in response to increased blood pressure may occur,[90,104,105] even at the early stages of the disease.[105] Increased thickness affects the elasticity of blood vessels and renders them relatively less responsive towards regulatory molecules.

(b) *Passive stiffness.*   Beside wall thickening, the vessel may become stiff and thus less able to contract and relax.[90,106]

(c) *Contractility.*   Finally, smooth muscle contractility might be increased in hypertensive subjects, which may occur due to the pathophysiological response of smooth muscle cells to increased pressure. It has been suggested that increased sympathetic activity may contribute to this phenomenon.[90,105,107] Another explanation might be that agents like serotonin, ADP, and acetylcholine, which have a vasodilating effect in normotensives, cause vasoconstriction in hypertensives. In normotensive subjects, these agents stimulate the production of EDRF by endothelium, whereas in hypertensive subjects production of EDRF is depressed.[108] The production of endothelium-derived contracting factor (EDCF) can also be stimulated by the same stimuli that normally cause the release of EDRF.[95] Therefore, given their opposing effects, EDRF and EDCF may have a significant effect on vessel wall behavior. The precise role of EDRF and EDCF in vascular pathophysiology is not well understood, and it is not clear at this time whether changes in the production of EDRF and EDCF play any role in the etiology of hypertension.

(2) *Atherosclerosis*   Although pathological changes suffered by the vessel wall in atherosclerosis are complex, intimal and medial thickening is one of the consequences of the disease, which will affect the resistance properties of the vessel in the same manner as noted in hypertensive subjects. Formation of atherosclerotic plaques results in the loss of vessel elasticity. The enhanced proliferation of smooth muscle cells in combination with plaques makes the vessel rigid and less responsive to regulatory processes as described previously.

Compliance

The main function of the venous system is to return the blood from the capillary circulation to the heart. Beside this conductive function, veins also have a capacitance function[109,110]; veins normally contain 70%–75% of the total blood volume of the body at any given time. The venous return can be influenced by adjustment in this volume of blood contained within the veins. The venous return itself is related to the right cardiac output.[111] The regulation of the amount of blood circulating through the veins is greatly influenced by the splanchnic bed, which holds a larger volume of blood than any other part of the venous system at any given time.[109,110,112]

Control of capacity

Compliance is an important component that affects the circulation of blood. There are two modes by which compliance of blood vessels can be influenced:

(1) *Passive control of compliance*   If the flow through an organ is decreased by increasing the arteriolar resistance, the pressure in the venules and veins will drop. This in turn will result in a decreased volume in the veins, thereby mobilizing the blood reserve in the areas where the inflow resistance increases.[109,110] This effect will be profound in the splanchnic bed, which has a relatively high compliance.

(2) *Active control of compliance*   The smooth muscle cells of the venous wall contract after sympathetic stimulation. Since the sensitivity to sympathetic stimulation of the vessels that hold blood reserve is higher than that of the resistance vessel, it will result in increased venous return even before the resistance in the arterioles increases.[110] Additionally, the veins van be stimulated by agents that cause vasoconstriction. Epinephrine, angiotensin, serotonin, and ADH cause the veins to contract,[112] whereas certain anesthetics, histamines, morphine, nitroprusside, acetylcholine, thrombin, and ionophore A have been shown to dilate veins.[103]

Pathological changes in compliance

Like vascular resistance, pathological changes in components of the vessel wall or changes due to flow also affect the compliance of the blood vessel. Hypertension,[109] hypotension,[112] atherosclerosis, and increased or decreased production of various regulatory molecules have significant impact on compliance.

Rheology

As a non-Newtonian fluid,[113-115] blood flow doesn't follow simple mathematical equations. This non-Newtonian character of blood is mainly due to the presence of erythrocytes. Two features of the erythrocytes are primarily responsible for this behavior: (a) their ability to form rouleaux when subjected to low shear stresses and (b) their deformability as they traverse through the vascular channels.

Because of these characteristics a nonlinear relation exists between blood viscosity and shear stress. At a low level of shear, the viscosity of blood is high because erythrocytes align themselves to form rouleaux, whereas at higher shear rates, blood behaves as a less viscous fluid because erythrocytes deform in response to shear stresses. This deformability of the erythrocytes helps in their movement away from the vascular wall during circulation; a layer of plasma separates the wall from the formed elements of blood. This effectively decreases the resistance. In addition, the plasma layer serves as a cushion to protect the endothelium from the constant rubbing action of circulating cells. The disruption of the protective effect of the laminar flow on blood vessels at branch points has been discussed in previous sections.

Mass Transportation

One of the primary functions of blood is the transportation of solutes and cells from one region of the body to another. Beside flow, two additional physical factors help blood achieve this goal: diffusion and convection. Since diffusion is relatively slow compared to the velocity of blood, its role is generally limited to areas close to the wall.[113,114] In an ideal laminar flow situation, transportation of particles to the vessel wall is minimal, until the blood vessels are small enough to enable diffusion. However, due to the presence of continuously colliding blood cells, a "Brownian motion-like" effect may cause lateral displacement.[113] Lateral movement of solutes also occurs where blood vessels curve. Finally, if a vortex occurs, the time during which a particle can contact the vessel wall increases significantly compared to the particles traveling in the midstream under laminar flow conditions.[113,114]

Intimal Injury

Under laminar flow conditions, the intima is protected from the rubbing action of blood cells. Under nonlaminar flow conditions, vessel walls experience distorted flow and excessive shear stresses. The lack of laminar flow, increased shear stresses, and areas of turbulent or vortical flow may contribute to injury of the vessel wall.[116] Of concern may be the rheologic injury at arterial branching points since these areas are particularly prone to the development of atherosclerosis.[117] As indicated in the preceding sections, endothelial cells near the arterial branching exhibit altered polarity, swelling of cells, cytoplasmic projections, and even desquamation of cells. Alteration or loss of endothelial cells in conjunction with increased probability of interaction with platelets, leukocytes, lipoproteins, and other soluble components of blood may have a causal relationship with the occurrence of atherosclerosis at these sites.[16]

Blood Cell Damage

Rheologic factors may have a profound effect on blood cells. Abnormally high shear stresses have been shown to cause the lysis of blood cells.[118–120] The threshold above which lysis occurs depends on the applied shear stress. Products leaking from one cell type may have a profound effect on other cells. To illustrate this point, ADP released from red blood cells or platelets would cause stimulation of other platelets, resulting in the formation of platelet aggregates.[113,121] Aggregates of platelets, depending on their size, would affect the circulation of blood through larger vessels and have the potential of blocking smaller blood vessels. These problems are of particular concern when blood vessels suffer iatrogenic injury or prosthetic devices (i.e., artificial heart valves, blood pumps, hemodialyzers) come in contact with blood in vivo or ex vivo.

Vascular Pathology

Any account of pathophysiology of blood vessels would be incomplete without a discussion of the diseases of the vessel wall. A blood vessel is endowed with a remarkable ability to adapt to changing environments. It can withstand a range of shear stresses, needle punctures, surgical manipulations, and changes in viscosity generally without serious pathological consequences. However, under certain conditions, the vessel wall succumbs to abnormal alteration from which it cannot recover. A host of factors, including diet, personal habits, and environmental and genetic factors may initiate or help sustain pathogenesis of the blood vessels. The following discussion is limited to atherosclerosis, which often leads to serious consequences requiring surgical intervention.

Atherosclerosis

The fundamental lesion of atherosclerosis is the atheromatous plaque. This plaque presents as a superficial fibrous cap, consisting of flat smooth muscle cells embedded in basement membrane material, collagen fibers, and proteoglycans; below this cap, smooth muscle cells and macrophages. Both cell types are often lipid laden and are surrounded by connective tissue.[122] There may be necrotic debris, cholesterol crystals, and areas of calcification[16]; organized thrombus is often associated with this lesion.[122]

Another atherosclerotic lesion is the fatty streak, which is generally found in children. At least in coronary arteries, the fatty streak seems to be a direct precursor of later fibrous plaques. In the aorta, however, evidence for this relation is less clear. Differences in anatomical location, sex, and race also have been reported.[123] The fatty streaks consist of fatty acid containing smooth muscle cells and macrophages within the intima. Extracellular lipids, proteoglycans, collagen, and elastic fibers are present in variable amounts.[124–126]

The most widely accepted theory regarding the pathogenesis of atherosclerosis is the "response to injury" theory as originally proposed by Ross and his colleagues.[16,127,128] Injury to endothelium and platelet adhesion play a central role in this hypothesis. Once endothelium is damaged, different pathways may lead to the stimulation of smooth muscle cells, thereby initiating the proliferative response in which platelet-derived growth factor (PDGF) may play an important role.[16] This growth factor, or related substances, can be secreted by platelets, monocytes/macrophages, smooth muscle cells, and endothelium.[127,129] Platelets might play an important role in releasing mitogenically active substances following their adhesion to subendothelial structures that became exposed when endothelial cells are damaged or dislodged. Under appropriate circumstances, in collaboration with other factors (e.g., low density lipoproteins), these early events cause pathological sequelae that are beyond the scope of this discussion. Readers are referred to several excellent review articles on this subject.[16,127,130]

Concluding Remarks

From the above discussion it becomes apparent that blood vessels have a complex organization. In order to perform their primary function as a blood conduit, blood vessels must adapt to changes in pressure and flow; as a supply line for nutrients, they must reach almost every cell; as a life line they must assure that blood keeps flowing with minimal risk of obstruction. At the same time, blood vessels must also assure that in the event of injury, minimal blood loss occurs and the damage is repaired efficiently to obviate future risk of bleeding at the site of injury. The blood, with all its 'defensive' and 'offensive' components is contained within the vascular system, ready to unleash on invading organisms or other emergencies facing the body. Following injury, blood will clot but only to the extent that bleeding is arrested; powerful enzymes are released to dissolve the clot and then vanish; mitogenic factors are released to help in the reparative processes and then disappear when this goal is accomplished. During all this time, blood generally flows unobstructed and the need of each organ of the body is met.

The remarkable ease with which blood vessels perform their assigned tasks is an example of biological efficiency. By understanding their composition and a number of factors they use to provide uninterrupted blood flow, a necessary prerequisite for homeostasis, a great deal has been learned about cardiovascular diseases. This has paved the way for significant advances in vascular surgery, and has helped evolve appropriate strategies to prevent/arrest debilitating diseases. Recognizing that this may only be the beginning, equipped with the tools of biochemistry and molecular biology, the future promises considerable breakthroughs that would affect not only our understanding of vascular pathophysiology, but also how this knowledge is applied to treat or prevent vascular diseases.

References

1. Rhodin, JAG: Architecture of the vessel wall. In DF Bohr, AA Somlyo, HV Sparks (eds): *Handbook of Physiology, Section 2: The Cardiovascular System, Vol II: Vascular Smooth Muscle*. Bethesda, 1983, American Physiological Society, pp 1–31.
2. Bader, H: The anatomy and physiology of the vascular wall. In WF Hamilton (ed): *Handbook of Physiology, Section 2: Circulation Vol II*. Washington D.C., American Physiological Society, 1963, pp 865–889.
3. Rhodin, JAG: The fine structure of the vascular wall in mammals, with special reference to smooth muscle components. *Physiol Rev* 42(suppl 5):48–87, 1962.
4. Kuegelgen, A: Von, Weitere Mitteilungen ueber den Wandbau der grossen Venen des Menschen unter besonderer Bereucksichtigung ihrer Kollagenstrukturen. *Z Zellforsch Mikroskop Anat* 44:121–174, 1956.
5. Goerttler, K: Ueber den Einbau der grossen Venen des menslichen Unterschenkels. *Z Anat Entwicklungsgeschichte* 116:591–609, 1953.
6. Bloom, W, Fawcett, DW: A textbook of histology, chapter 13: Blood and lymph vascular systems. Philadelphia, W.B. Saunders Co, 1975, pp 386–426.
7. Mohammad, SF, Mason RG, Eichwald, EJ, et al: Healthy and impaired vascular endothelium. In A Lasslo (ed): *Blood Platelet Function and Medicinal Chemistry*. Amsterdam, Elsevier Biomedical, 1984, pp 129–173.
8. Salzman, EW, Merrill, EW: Interaction of blood with artificial surfaces. In RW Colman, J Hirsh, VJ Marder, et al (eds): *Hemostasis and Thrombosis: Basic Principles and Clinical Practice*. Philadelphia, JB Lippincott Co, 1987, pp 1335–1347.
9. Mason, RG, Mohammad, SF, Saba, HI, et al: Functions of endothelium. *Pathobiol Ann* 9:1–48, 1979.
10. Stemerman, MB: Vascular intimal components: precursors of thrombogenesis. *Prog Hemost Thromb* 2:1–55, 1974.
11. Sakariassen, AK, Bolhuis, PA, Sixma, JJ: Human blood platelet adhesion to artery subendothelium is mediated by factor VIII-von Willebrand factor bound to the subendothelium. *Nature* 279:636–638, 1979.
12. Huang, TW, Benditt, EP: Mechanism of platelet adhesion to basal lamina. *Am J Pathol* 92:99–110, 1979.
13. Cazenave, JP, Dejana, E, Kinlough-Rathbone, R, et al: Platelet interaction with the endothelium and subendothelium: The role of thrombin and prostacyclin. *Haemostases* 8:183–192, 1979.
14. Bull, HA, Machin, SJ: The hemostatic function of the vascular endothelial cell. *Blut* 55:71–80, 1987.

15. Dilley, RJ, McGeachie, JK, Prendergast, FJ: A review of proliferative behaviour, morphology and phenotypes of vascular smooth muscle. *Atherosclerosis* 63:99–107, 1987.
16. Ross R: The pathogenesis of atherosclerosis—an update. *N Engl J Med* 314:488–500, 1986.
17. Heldin, CH, Westermark, B, Wasteson, A: Platelet-derived growth factor: Purification and partial characterization. *Proc Natl Acad Sci USA* 76:3722–3726, 1979.
18. Feinstein, DI: Acquired inhibitors against factor VIII and other clotting proteins. In RW Colman, J Hirsh, VJ Marder, et al (eds): *Hemostasis and Thrombosis: Basic Principles and Clinical Practice.* Philadelphia, JB Lippincott Co, 1987, pp 825–840.
19. Hirsh, J, Genton, E: Thrombogenesis. In: *Physiological Pharmacology.* New York, Academic Press, 1974, pp 99–133.
20. Weibel, ER, Palade GE: New cytoplasmatic components of arterial endothelia. *J Cell Biol* 23:101–112, 1964.
21. Haudenschild, CC: Morphology of vascular endothelial cells in culture. In EA Jaffe (ed): *Biology of Endothelial Cells.* Dordrecht, Martinus Nijhoff Publishers, 1984, pp 129–154.
22. Majno G: Ultrastructure of the vascular membrane. In W F Hamilton, P Dowe (eds): *Handbook of Physiology, Vol. 3, Sec. 2, Circulation.* Baltimore, Williams and Wilkins, 1965, pp 2293–2375.
23. Peine, CI, Low, FN: Scanning electron microscopy of cardiac endothelium of the dog. *Am J Anat* 142:137–158, 1974.
24. Mason, RG, Mohammad, SF: A human model for study of blood vascular wall interactions. *Arch Surg* 115:952–958, 1980.
25. Clark, JM, Glagov S: Luminal surface of distended arteries by scanning electron microscopy: Eliminating configuration and technical artifacts. *Br J Exp Pathol* 57:129–135, 1976.
26. Rhodin, JAG: Ultrastructure of mammalian venous capillaries, venous capillaries, venules and small collecting veins. *J Ultrastruc Res* 25:452–500, 1968.
27. Smith, U, Ryan, JW: Electron microscopy of endothelial and epithelial components of the lungs: Correlations of structure and function. *Fed Proc* 32:1957–1966, 1973.
28. Simionescu, M, Simionescu, N, Palade, GE: Segmented differentiation of cell junctions in the vascular endothelium: The microvasculature. *J Cell Biol* 67:863–885, 1975.
29. Mason, RG, Balis, JU: Pathology of the endothelium. In BF Trump, AU Arstilla (eds): *Pathobiology of Cell Membranes, Vol II.* New York, Academic Press, 1980, pp 425–471.
30. Eskin, SG, Navarro, LT, O'Bannon, W, et al: Behavior of endothelial cells cultured on silastic and dacron velour under flow conditions in-vitro: Implications for prelining vascular grafts with cells. *Artif Org* 7:31–37, 1983.
31. Eskin, SG, Ives, CL, McIntire, LV, et al: Response of cultured endothelial cells to steady flow. *Microvasc Res* 28:87–94, 1984.
32. Joris, I, Majno, G: Atherosclerosis and inflammation. *Adv Exp Med Biol* 104:227–243, 1978.

33. Palade, GE: Blood capillaries of the heart and other organs. *Circulation* 24:368, 1961.
34. Ryan, JW, Ryan, US: Pulmonary endothelial cells. *Fed Proc* 36:2683–2691, 1977.
35. Rhodin, JAG: The ultrastructure of mammalian arterioles and precapillary sphincters. *J Ultrastruc Res* 18:181–223, 1967.
36. Wagner, RC, Casley-Smith, JR: Endothelial vesicles. *Microvasc Res* 21:267–298, 1981.
37. Simionescu, M, Simionescu, N, Palade, GE: Morphometric data on the endothelium of blood capillaries. *J Cell Biol* 60:128–152, 1974.
38. Butcher, EC, Kraal, G, Stevens, SK, et al: A recognition of endothelial cells: Directing lymphocyte traffic. In HL Nessel, HJ Vogel (eds): *Pathobiology of the Endothelial Cell*. New York, Academic Press, 1982, pp 409–424.
39. Davies, PF, Bowyer, DE: Scanning electron microscopy: Arterial endothelial integrity after fixation at physiological pressure. *Atherosclerosis* 21:463–469, 1975.
40. Gertz, SD, Rennels, ML, Forbes, MS, et al: Preparation of vascular endothelium for scanning electron microscopy: A comparison of the effects of perfusion and immersion fixation. *J Microsc* 105:309–313, 1975.
41. Lo Gerf, FW, Quist, WC, Crawshow, HM, et al: An important technique for preservation of endothelial morphology in vein grafts. *Surgery* 90:1015–1024, 1981.
42. Rodgers, GM, Greenberg, CS, Shuman, MA: Characterization of the effects of cultured vascular cells on the activation of blood coagulation. *Blood* 61:1155–1162, 1983.
43. Nossel, HL, Vogel HJ: Pathobiology of the Endothelial Cell. New York, Academic Press, 1982.
44. Flaherty, JT, Pierce, JE, Ferrans, VJ, et al: Endothelial nuclear patterns in the canine arterial tree with particular reference to hemodynamic events. *Circ Res* 30:23–33, 1972.
45. Hertzer, NR, Beven, EG, Benjamin, SP: Ultramicroscopic ulcerations and thrombii on the carotid bifurcaton. *Arch Surg* 112:1394–1402, 1977.
46. Johnston, WH, Latta, H: Glomerular mesangial and endothelial cell swelling following temporary renal ischemia and its role in the no-reflow phenomenon. *Am J Pathol* 89:153–166, 1977.
47. Fonkalsrud, EW, Sanchez, M, Zerubavel R, et al: Serial changes in arterial endothelium following ischemia and perfusion. *Surgery* 81:527–533, 1977.
48. Bhawan, J, Joris, I, DeGirolami, et al: Effect of occlusion of large vessels I. A study of the rat carotid artery. *Am J Pathol* 88:355–380, 1977.
49. Kjeldsen, K, Thomsen, HK: The effect of hypoxia on the fine structure of the aortic intima in rabbits. *Lab Invest* 33:533–543, 1975.
50. Teplitz, C: The core pathobiology and integrated medical science of adult acute respiratory insufficiency. *Surg Clin North Am* 56:1091–1133, 1976.
51. Kjeldsen, K, Astrup, P, Wanstrup, J: Ultrastructural intimal changes in the rabbit aorta after a moderate carbon monoxide exposure. *Atherosclerosis* 16:67–82, 1972.

52. Gertz, SD, Rennels, SM, Forbes, MS, et al: Endothelial cell damage by temporary arterial occlusion with surgical clips. Study of the clip side by scanning and transmission electron microscopy. *J Neurosurg* 45:514–519, 1976.
53. Hirsch, EZ, Robertson, AL: Selective acute arterial injury and repair: I. Methodology and surface characteristics. *Atherosclerosis* 28:271–287, 1977.
54. Bjorkerud S: Injury and repair in arterial tissue. Experimental models: Types and relevance to human vascular disease—A survey. *Angiology* 25:636–648, 1974.
55. Warren, BA, Philip, RB, Inwood, MJ: The ultrastructural morphology of air embolism: Platelet adhesion to the interface of endothelial damage. *Br J Exp Pathol* 54:163–172, 1973.
56. Vetto, RM, Burger, DR: The identification and comparison of transplantation antigens on canine vascular endothelium and lymphocytes. *Transplantation* 11:374–377, 1971.
57. DeBrito, T, Hoshino-shimizu, S, Pereira, MO, et al: The pathogenesis of the vascular lesions in experimental rickettsial disease of the guinea pig (Rocky Mountain spotted fever group). *Virchows Arch (Pathol Anat)* 358:205–210, 1973.
58. Constantinides, P, Robinson, M: Ultrastructural injury of arterial endothelium: I Effect of pH, osmolarity, anoxia, and temperature. *Arch Pathol* 88:99–105, 1969.
59. Suzuki, AO, Ohashi, M: The spurting of erythrocytes through junctions of the vascular endothelium treated with snake venom. *Microvasc Res* 10:208–215, 1975.
60. Constantinides, P, Robinson, M: Ultrastructural injury of arterial endothelium: I Effects of enzymes and surfactants. *Arch Pathol* 88:113–117, 1969.
61. Mohammad, SF, Mason, RG: A human model for a study of blood vascular wall interactions: Effect of enzymatic treatment of intima. *Arch Pathol Lab Med* 105:62–65, 1981.
62. Mustard, FJ, Kinlough-Rathbone, RL, Packham, A: The vessel wall in thrombosis. In RW Colman, J Hirsh, WJ Marder, et al (eds): *Hemostasis and Thrombosis: Basic Principles and Clinical Practice.* Philadelphia, J. B. Lippincott Co, 1987, pp 1073–1088.
63. Laerum, F: Cytotoxic effects of six angiographic contrastr media on human endothelium in culture. *Acta Radiol* 28:99–105, 1987.
64. Zweifach, BJ: Integrity of vascular endothelium. In BM Altura (ed): *Advances in Microcirculation, Vol. 9: Vascular Endothelium and Basement Membranes.* S. Karger, Basel, 1980, pp 206–225.
65. Sholley, MM, Gimbrone, MA Jr, Cotran, RS: Cellular migration and replication in endothelial regeneration: A study using irradiated endothelial cultures. *Lab Invest* 36:18–25, 1977.
66. Haudenschild, C, Schwartz, SM: Endothelial regeneration II. Restitution of endothelial continuity. *Lab Invest* 41:407–418, 1979.
67. Ross R: Atherosclerosis: A problem of cell biology of arterial wall cells and their interactions with blood components. *Arteriosclerosis* 1:293–311, 1981.

68. Klynstra, FB, Bottcher, CJ: Permeability patterns in pig aorta. *Atherosclerosis* 11:451–462, 1971.
69. Landis, EM, Pappenheimer, JR: Exchange of substances through the capillary walls. In WF Hamilton, P Dow (eds): *Handbook of Physiology, Vol. 2, Sec. 2, Circulation*. Baltimore, Williams and Wilkins, 1965, pp 961–1034.
70. Gosselin, RE, Stibitz, GR: The diffusive conductance of slits between endothelial cells in muscle capillaries. *Microvasc Res* 14:363–382, 1977.
71. Luft, JH: Capillary permeability. 1. Structural considerations. In BW Zweifach, L Grant, RT McGlusckey (eds): *The Inflammatory Process, Vol 2*. New York, Academic Press, 1973, pp 47–93.
72. Bundgaard M, Frokjaar-Jensen J, Crone C: Endothelial plasmalemmal vesicles as elements in a system of branching invaginations from the cell surface. *Proc Natl Acad Sci USA* 76:6439–6442, 1979.
73. Thorgeirsson, G, Robertson AL: The vascular endothelium—Pathobiologic significance. *Am J Pathol* 93:803–848, 1978.
74. Robertson, AL, Khairallah, PA: Arterial endothelial permeability and vascular disease. The "trapdoor" effect. *Exp Mol Pathol* 18:241–260, 1973.
75. Kefalides, NA: Biochemical aspects of the vessel wall. In RW Colman, J Hirsh, VJ Marder, et al (eds): *Hemostasis and Thrombosis: Basic Principles and Clinical Practice*. Philadelphia, J.B. Lippincott Co, 1987, pp 793–803.
76. Murphy, ME, Johnson, PC: Possible contribution of basement membrane to the structural rigidity of blood capillaries. *Microvasc Res* 9:242–245, 1975.
77. Bachmann, F: Plasminogen activators. In RW Colman, J Hirsh, VJ Marder, et al: *Hemostasis and Thrombosis: Basic Principles and Clinical Practice*. Philadelphia, J.B. Lippincott Co, 1987, pp 318–339.
78. Philips, M, Juul, AG Thorsen, S: Human endothelial cells produce a plasminogen activator inhibitor and a tissue type plasminogen activator inhibitor complex. *Biochim Biophys Acta* 802:99–110, 1984.
79. Moncada, S, Korbut, R, Bunting, S, et al: Prostacyclin is a circulating hormone. *Nature* 273:767–768, 1978.
80. Haslam, RJ, McClenaghan, MD: Measurement of circulating prostacyclin. *Nature* 292:364–366, 1981.
81. Steer, ML, MacIntyre, DE, Levine, L, et al: Is prostacyclin a physiologically important circulating anti platelet agent? *Nature* 283:194–195, 1980.
82. Pace-Asciak, RC, Carrara, MC, Levine L, Nicolaou KC: PGI 2 specific antibodies administered in vivo suggest against a role for endogenous PGI2 as a circulating vasodepressor hormone in the normotensive and spontaneously hypertensive rat. *Prostaglandins* 20:1053–1066, 1980.
83. Burch, JW, Stanford, N, Majerus, PW: Inhibition of platelet prostaglandin synthesis by oral aspirin. *J Clin Invest* 61:314–319, 1978.
84. Marcus, AJ: The role of prostaglandins in platelet function. *Prog Hematol* 11:147–171, 1979.
85. Lasslo, A, Quintana, RP: Interaction dynamics of blood platelets with medicinal agents and other chemical entities. In A Lasslo (ed): *Blood Platelet Function and Medicinal Chemistry*. Amsterdam, Elsevier Biomedical, 1984, pp 229–315.

86. Roth, GJ, Stanford, N, Majerus, PW: Acetylation of prostaglandin synthetase by aspirin. *Proc Natl Acad Sci USA* 72:3073, 1975.
87. Forster, W, Sarembe, B, Mentz, P (eds): Prostaglandins and Thromboxanes, Part I, Prostaglandins and Thromboxanes in the Cardiovascular System. Oxford, Pergamon Press, 1980, pp 261–352.
88. Green, JF: Determinants of systemic bloodflow. In AC Guyton, DB Young (eds): *Cardiovascular Physiology III, International Review of Physiology*. Baltimore, University Park Press, 1979, pp 33–66.
89. Green, JF: Fundamental cardiovascular and pulmonary physiology; an integrated approach for medicine. Philadelphia, Lea and Febiger, 1982, pp 101–110.
90. Dobrin, PB: Vascular mechanics. In JT Shepherd, FM Abboud (eds): *Handbook of Physiology Section 2: The Cardiovascular System, Vol III, Peripheral Circulation and Organ Blood Flow, Part 1*. Bethesda, American Physiological Society, 1983, pp 65–102.
91. Burton, AC: Relation of structure to function of the tissues of the wall of blood vessels. *Physiol Rev* 34:619–642, 1954.
92. Johnson, PC: Principles of peripheral circulatory control. In PC Johnson (ed): Peripheral Circulation. New York, John Wiley and Sons, 1978, pp 111–140.
93. Olsson, RA: Local factors regulating cardiac and skeletal muscle bloodflow. *Ann Rev Physiol* 43:385–395, 1981.
94. Rowell, LB: General principles of vascular control. In: Human Circulation During Physical Stress. New York, Oxford University Press, 1986, pp 8–43.
95. Vanhoutte, PM: Endothelium dependent contractions in arteries and veins. *Blood Vessels* 24:141–144, 1987.
96. Vanhoutte, PM, Rubanyi, GM, Miller, V, et al: Modulation of vascular smooth muscle contraction by the endothelium. *Ann Rev Physiol* 48:307–320, 1986.
97. Rowell, LB: Cardiovascular adjustment to thermal stress. In JT Shepherd, FM Abboud (eds): *Handbook of Physiology Section 2: The Cardiovascular System, Vol III, Pheripheral Circulation and Organ Blood Flow, Part 1*. Bethesda, American Physiological Society, 1983, pp 967–1023.
98. Harder, DR: Pressure-induced myogenic activation of cat cerebral arteries is dependent on intact endothelium. *Circ Res* 60:102–107, 1987.
99. Shepherd, JT, Abboud, FM (eds): *Handbook of Physiology Section 2: The Cardiovascular System, Vol III, Peripheral Circulation and Organ Blood Flow, Part 2*. Bethesda, American Physiological Society, 1983.
100. Zanchetti, A, Tarazi, RC (eds): *Handbook of Hypertension. Vol 8: Pathophysiology of Hypertension*. Amsterdam, Elsevier Science Publishers, 1986.
101. Shepherd, JT, Mancia G: Reflex control of the human cardiovascular system. *Rev Physiol Biochem Pharmacol* 105:1–99, 1986.
102. Schmid, PG, Sharaba, FM, Phillips, MI: Peptides and blood vessels. In JT Shepherd, FM Abboud (eds): *Handbook of Physiology Section 2: The Cardiovascular System, Vol III, Peripheral Circulation and Organ Blood Flow, Part 1*. Bethesda, American Physiological Society, 1983, pp 815–835.

103. Seidel, CL, La Rochelle, J: Venous and arterial endothelia: Different dilator abilities in dog vessels. *Circ Res* 60:626–630, 1987.
104. Rorive, GL, Carher, PG, Fordart, JM: The structural responses of the vascular wall in experimental hypertension. In A Zanchetti, RC Tarazi (eds): *Handbook of Hypertension. Vol 7: Pathophysiology of Hypertension.* Amsterdam, Elsevier Science Publishers, 1986, pp 427–453.
105. Kaplan, NM: *Clinical Hypertension.* Baltimore, Williams and Wilkins, 1986.
106. Cox, RH: Basis for the altered arterial wall mechanics in the spontenously hypertensive rat. *Hypertension* 3:485–495, 1981.
107. Brody, MJ, Haywood, JR, Touw, KB: Neural mechanisms in hypertension. *Ann Rev Physiol* 42:441–453, 1980.
108. Lee, TJF, Shirasaki, Y, Nichols, GA: Altered endothelial modulation of vascular tone in aging and hypertension. *Blood Vessels* 24:132–136, 1987.
109. Rothe, CF: Physiology of venous return: an unappreciated boost to the heart. *Arch Intern Med* 146:977–982, 1986.
110. Hainsworth, R: Vascular capacitance: its control and importance. *Rev Physiol Biochem Pharmacol* 105:101–173, 1986.
111. Guyton, AC: Determination of cardiac output by equating venous return curves with cardiac response curves. *Physiol Rev* 35:123, 1955.
112. Rothe, CF: Venous system: physiology of the capacitance vessels. In JT Shepherd, FM Abboud (eds): *Handbook of Physiology Section 2: The Cardiovascular System, Vol III, Peripheral Circulation and Organ Blood Flow, Part 1.* Bethesda, American Physiological Society, 1983, pp 397–452.
113. Goldsmith, HL, Turitto, VT: Rheological aspects of thrombosis and hemostasis: Basic principles and applications. *Thromb Haemost* 55:415–435, 1986.
114. Fluid dynamic and hemorheologic considerations. In: Guidelines for Blood-Material Interaction. Report of the National Heart, Lung, and Blood Institute Working Group. 1985, pp 65–83.
115. Milnor, WR: *Hemodynamics.* Baltimore, Williams and Wilkins, 1982.
116. Flaherty, JT, Pierce, JE, Ferrans, VJ, et al: Endothelial nuclear patterns in the canine arterial tree with particular reference to hemodynamic events. *Circ Res* 30:23–33, 1972.
117. Reidy, MA, Bowyer, DE: Scanning electron microscopy of arteries. The morphology of aortic endothelium in hemodynamically stressed areas associated with branches. *Atherosclerosis* 26:181–194, 1977.
118. Leverett, LB, Hellums, JD, Alfrey, CP, et al: Red blood cell damage by shear stress. *Biophys J* 12:257–273, 1972.
119. Wurzinger, LJ, Opitz, R, Blasberg, P, et al: Platelet and coagulation parameters following millisecond exposure to laminar shear stress. *Thromb Haemost* 54:381–386, 1985.
120. Dewitz, TS, McIntire, LV, Martin, RR, et al: Enzyme release and morphological changes in leukocytes induced by mechanical trauma. *Blood Cells* 5:499–512, 1979.
121. Hardwick, RA, Gritsman, HN, Stromberg, RR, et al: The biochemical mechanisms of shear-induced platelet aggregation. *Trans Am Soc Artif Int Organs* 29:448–452, 1983.

122. Ross, R, Wight, TN, Strandness E, et al: Human atherosclerosis I, Cell constitution and characteristics of advanced lesions of the superficial femoral artery. *Am J Pathol* 114:79–93, 1984.
123. McGill, H: Persistent problems in the pathogenesis of atherosclerosis. *Arteriosclerosis* 4:443–451, 1984.
124. Robbins, SL, Cotran, RS, Kumar, V: Pathologic basis of disease. Philadelphia, W.B. Saunders Co, 1984.
125. Faggioto, A, Ross, R, Harker, LA: Studies of hypercholesterolemia in the non-human primate. I Changes that lead to fatty streak formation. *Arteriosclerosis* 4:323–340, 1984.
126. Faggioto, A, Ross, R: Studies of hypercholesterolemia in the non-human primate. II Fatty streak conversion to fibrous plaque. *Arteriosclerosis* 4:341–356, 1984.
127. Scharf, RE, Harker, LA: Thrombosis and atherosclerosis: Regulatory role of interactions among blood components and endothelium. *Blut* 55:131–144, 1987.
128. Haust, MD: Pathogenesis of atherosclerosis: Current status. In G Schlierf, H Moerl (eds): *Expanding Horizons in Atherosclerosis Research*. Berlin, Springer-Verlag, 1987, pp 3–12.
129. Westermark, B, Heldin, CH: Structure and function of platelet derived growth factor. *Act Med Scand*, 715 (Suppl):19–23, 1987.
130. Oppenheimer, MJ, Oram, JF, Bierman, EL: Downregulation of high density lipoprotein receptor activity of cultured fibroblasts by platelet derived growth factor. *Arteriosclerosis* 7:325–332, 1987.

Chapter 2

Vascular Injury from Vascular Occlusive Devices

William M. Moore and T.J. Bunt

Iatrogenic vascular injury is unfortunately a common if unrecognized accompaniment of an otherwise beautifully orchestrated, carefully researched, and technically painstaking vascular operation. Injuries are encountered at both medial and endothelial levels, and are related to all aspects of the dissection and anastomosis; however, the most significant potential for injury is related to the utilization of various vascular occlusion devices. The long-term and short-term sequelae of such injuries are significant factors in the success of a particular revascularization; it therefore follows that a vascular surgeon must be as fully cognizant of the limitation of his/her instrumentation as he/she is of the anatomy/physiology of the vessels repaired or of the physics and engineering effects of the grafts utilized on those same vessels. Put succinctly, the vascular surgeon should know the advantages and disadvantages of the clamps he/she chooses to utilize and how to make the best use of them. This chapter deals with the injury patterns incurred by various vascular occlusive devices and makes general recommendations as to the optimal use of each.

Classification of Occlusive Devices

In a prior collective review, we proposed a classification scheme to include the various occlusive devices under general descriptive titles; this is further explained in Table 1 to include newly introduced de-

Table 1.
Classification Scheme for Occlusive Devices

Description	Examples
1. Crossmembered Metallic Clamps	
A. Nonserrated jaws	—
B. Noncoinciding serrated jaws	Senning, Potts, Wylie, Green
C. Interdigitating serrated jaws	DeBakey, Glover, Bailey, Satinsky
2. Spring-loaded Opposing Clamps	Deithrich, Blalock, DeBakey, and Glover Bulldogs
3. Crossmembered Metallic Clamps with Protective Surfaces	Fogarty Softjaw Fogarty Hydrogrip Brown Occluder
4. Loop Tourniquets	Vesseloops Umbilical Tapes Fogarty Occluder
5. Intraluminal Balloon Occluders	Fogarty Inahara-Pruitt Edwards Becton-Dickinson
6. Miscellaneous	
A. Berlin clamp	
B. Dunn inflatable occluder	
C. Adler	

Noninclusive representative samples of the various classes of vascular occlusive clamps. (Modified from Bunt et al: Iatrogenic vascular injury. *J Vasc Surg* 2:491–497, 1985.)

vices. Noninclusive representative examples of commonly employed clamps are also given. For purposes of this review, this classification is used to describe generic groups.[1–3]

Classification of Arterial Injury

Assessment of the degree of arterial injury incurred by clamps has been heavily weighted toward examination of the endothelium simply because three of the four studies giving classification schemata were studies focusing on the endothelial injury with scanning electron microscopy (SEM). We collated the prior and slightly differing schemata into one classification. This proved useful for comparison of SEM studies of clamp injury.

A more complete classification might include severities of arterial wall laceration and secondary manifestations such as embolus, dissection, thrombus adherence, or frank arterial disruption. Such a revised classification scheme is given in Table 2.[1-3]

Table 2.
Classification of Arterial Injury
Incurred by Vascular Instruments

0 No injury
1 Endothelial imprint without disruption
2 Separation endotheliam, intimal flap 3 mm
3 Endothelial denudation, exposed subendothelium, endothelial shredding
4 Medial laceration, medial hemorrhage, necrosis
5 Adventitial laceration or crush
6 Arterial disruption, dissection, pseudoaneurysm

A complete scheme of possible vessel injury incurred by vascular occlusive devices. (Modified from Bunt et al: Iatrogenic vascular injury. *J Vasc Surg* 2:491–497, 1985.

Definitions

Crossmembered clamp: A metallic design single-action device in which ratchet-controlled closure of the handles causes opposition to the clamp jaws; jaw surfaces may have serrations but are metallic without overlaid protective cushions.

Protective surface: A metallic design single-action device in which ratchet-controlled closure of the handles causes incomplete opposition of the clamp jaws, the remaining space being filled by opposed surfaces of protective cushions on each jaw.

Loop tourniquet: A doubly encircled tape or loop that is secured with, and occlusive pressure controlled by a hemostat applied either to a Rumel sheath or to both ends of the loop that then are applied to the drapes.

Intraluminal occluder: An inflatable balloon catheter introduced intraluminally whose inflation occludes the internal lumen.

Holding pressure: Henson and Rob first defined this as the clamp pressure just sufficient to prevent slippage. Harvey and Gough numerically described this as a pressure sufficient to prevent horizontal distraction of the applied clamp by 9.81 N or the equivalent of 1 kg plus gravity force.[4,5]

Occlusive pressure: Henson and Rob initially defined this, and most authors have utilized their convenient designation, as just sufficient applied clamp force to overcome intraluminal forward propulsive pressure. Harvey and Gough have numerically defined this as the pressure just sufficient to occlude intraluminal flow through an artery perfused at 200 mmHg pressure.[4,5]

Literature Review

Henson and Rob in 1956 studied the effects of placing a variety of standard crossmembered clamps and looped tourniquets on the right gastroepiploic artery at the time of subtotal gastrectomy, utilizing 15-minute reperfusion; the clamped segment was then harvested en bloc and analyzed with light microscopy. All type I clamps inflicted severe medial and endothelial injury on the vessels (Class 4 injuries) as did a 2-0 silk ligature doubly looped as a tourniquet. However, one centimeter cotton umbilical tapes applied as tourniquets caused negligible injury. They theorized that this differential spectrum of arterial injury might best be related to the concentration of applied force on a very small surface area of the vessel. Thus, the small silk ligature caused more injury than the wide umbilical tape. Similarly, narrow bladed type I clamps caused more injury than wider bladed clamps of otherwise similar crossmembered design. This early study did not specifically address endothelial injury, although such injury may be inferred from examination of their photomicrographs. It may also demonstrate a more marked injury pattern for each studied clamp, based on the small caliber and nonmuscular nondiseased characteristics of the gastroepiploic vessels chosen for study. It did point out, however, very early in the development of peripheral vascular surgery, that there was a distinct potential for iatrogenic vascular injury when crossmembered clamps were utilized and the potential for less injury with loop tourniquets.[5]

Hickman and Mortenson in 1981 studied a variety of vascular clamps applied to the canine thoracic aorta for 30 minutes with 2 hours of reperfusion: specimens were prepared for light microscopy evaluation after reperfusion time of 2 hours and again at 10 days. They noted that, in general, the occlusive pressure of various type I clamps was essentially equal to the holding pressure, e.g., that initial clamp application obtained maximal holding pressure. In addition, they noted that there was an increased severity of injury incurred by increasing closure of the clamp. Serrations on such clamps provided a more secure holding pressure but also were associated with an increased severity of injury.[6]

Harvey and Gough in 1981 studied a variety of clamps applied to ex vivo canine vessels occluded for 5 minutes, reperfused for 5 minutes, and then studied with light and SEM. They noted that some type I clamps had a modest range of absolute pressures afforded by increasing ratchet closure of the clamp and that holding pressure usually was obtained at minimal ratchet closure: In contrast, a type III clamp usually required maximal occlusive pressure to obtain adequate holding pressures. Thus, they suggested that the minimal ratchet closure that provided luminal occlusion for any given vessel would afford adequate holding pressure capabilities, and would tend to minimize the injury inflicted.

They confirmed the severe injury patterns associated with type I clamps but noted a marked reduction in injury severity with type III clamps. They also examined the specimens with trypan blue supravital dye staining techniques to evaluate endothelial viability as demonstrated by dye uptake. These studies revealed a much more diffuse endothelial injury than was apparent with light microscopy on SEM alone, with the devitalized endothelium corresponding to the clamp imprint. This data suggests that there is probably an endothelial injury in all occlusive device applications even if histologic or SEM disruption is not seen; the injury seen may relate to temporary endothelial ischemia secondary to direct external pressure and/or isolation from nutrient luminal flow during the period of clamp application.

Harvey and Gough also detailed the more complex nature of injuries incurred by occlusive clamps, looking at medial injury expressed as a medial penetration ratio (medial penetration/medial depth). Type I clamps were noted to have ratios of 0.4 to 0.7 whereas type II clamps showed zero ratios, and type III, 0.1. This would infer that type I clamps essentially cause a Class 4 injury on routine usage.[4]

DePalma et al. studied the effects of various type I and type II clamps applied at full ratchet force to canine aorta, carotid, or femoral arteries for 3-minute occlusion times; specimens of the clamped areas were then examined at 10 days and 13 months. In addition, they looked at the effect of an atherogenic diet on the healing and/or pathogenetic potential of the clamp-injured vessel. Specimens harvested at 10 days demonstrated evident medial injuries in that the clamped areas could be easily visualized as compressed areas on the external surface: SEM examination was noteworthy for flattened endothelium and persistent transition zones between clamped and unclamped endothelial areas. Histologic examination demonstrated endothelial injury, medial hemorrhage, and inflammatory exudates throughout. There was also disruption of the internal elastic lamellae. Specimens harvested at later intervals demonstrated a progression to fibrous scar with smooth muscle proliferation in the injury area at 13 months. An atherogenic diet caused a significant atheromatous degeneration of the clamp-injured vessels, with lipid insudation and foam cells as well as fibromuscular proliferation. The most marked changes were seen at the femoral artery location.

DePalma's study also addressed two related points: the force exerted by various clamps and the relation of that force to the size of the clamped artery. Type III clamps had fairly constant force at all jaw apertures, whereas type I clamps were noted to have rapid linear increases with increasing size of the vessel, so that the same clamp applied to an aorta might exert twice as much force as when applied to a femoral artery.[7]

Guidoin et al. performed successive studies on ex vivo nonperfused canine aortas to which clamps were applied and the specimen then resected en bloc: occlusion times ex vivo were maintained for 5, 30, or 120 minutes and the specimens then examined with SEM. A second study applied infrarenal aortic clamps while aortic grafting was performed and then examined the clamp sites at en bloc resection of the graft segment at 2, 24, and 48 hours, at 1 and 4 weeks, and at 6 months.

Their studies noted profound endothelial and medial injuries incurred by type I and significant injuries by type III clamps. They also noted visible external imprints from all clamps on the adventitial surfaces. Initial endothelial injuries were accompanied by fibrin/platelet deposition that progressively increased over 48 hours; medial necrosis, hemorrhage, and inflammatory exudates were then noted. Re-endothelialization occurred within 1 week and was complete within 1 month; however clamp imprints could still be visualized.[8,9]

Confirmatory evidence for the injury potentials of vascular clamps has come from a variety of papers. Slayback noted that there was a linear increase in the severity of endothelial injury with increasing clamp pressure when rabbit arteries subjected to various microvascular arterial clamps were visualized with SEM.[10] Richling studied neurosurgical clips in a microvascular setting utilizing SEM and noted incidentally that more injury was incurred at the site of Heifetz clamp application proximal and distal to the clip. They also noted an increasing severity of injury as occlusion time increased from 10 and 30 minutes, through 60 and 180 minutes. Similarly there was a linear correlation between the severity of injury and the force applied; varying the springload pressure from 20 and 35 g through 45 and 65 g linearly increased the injury. It is of interest that they were able to correlate the severity of injury with the length of occlusion, suggesting that the injury is not simply one of physical crushing force but also is related to ischemia of the crushed and/or isolated segment.[11] Fonkalsrud provides related evidence in this regard, noting ischemic injury to the vessel isolated between occluding clamps.[12]

Our own studies on type I, II, and III clamps are confirmatory of other authors in both a canine aortoiliac model simulating normal nonatherosclerotic vessels and then extended to a human model of diseased femoropopliteal arterial segments. We utilized 20- to 30-minute occlusion and 5- to 10-minute reperfusion interval for clamps applied serially to canine infrarenal aortic segments, studying the harvested segments with SEM. Diseased vessels were obtained at time of above-knee amputation in humans, applying the clamps to perfused in situ popliteal artery segments and resecting the specimens en bloc for SEM analysis (Fig. 1).

Type I clamps caused visible adventitial imprints (Figs. 2A–2D) and Class 3 to 4 endothelial and medial injuries. Type III clamps also caused adventitial imprints but endothelial injury was limited to Class 1. A medial crush injury was also obviously occurring, but it was not specifically looked for in these studies (Figs. 3A-D). Type II clamps caused no definable external imprint and a Class 1 injury (Figs. 4A,B).[2,3]

The salient findings in our studies were twofold. First, that clamp injuries observed by other authors in normal laboratory animal vessels were equally, if not more, severe in human atherosclerotic vessels; and second, silastic loop tourniquets when appropriately applied caused no visible or SEM apparent injury. "Appropriate" use is critical, however, since we were able to demonstrate Class 1 injuries if the loop was inappropriately cinched up and the vessels elevated out of the operative plane (Fig. 3D). It is evident that there are limitations to the

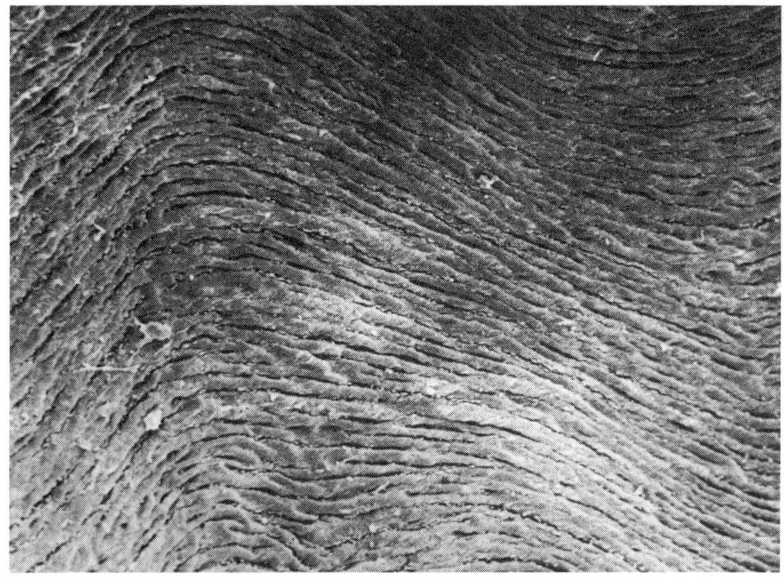

Figure 1A. *Demonstrates scanning electron micrograph of control endothelial surfaces of a canine artery at 100 ×.*

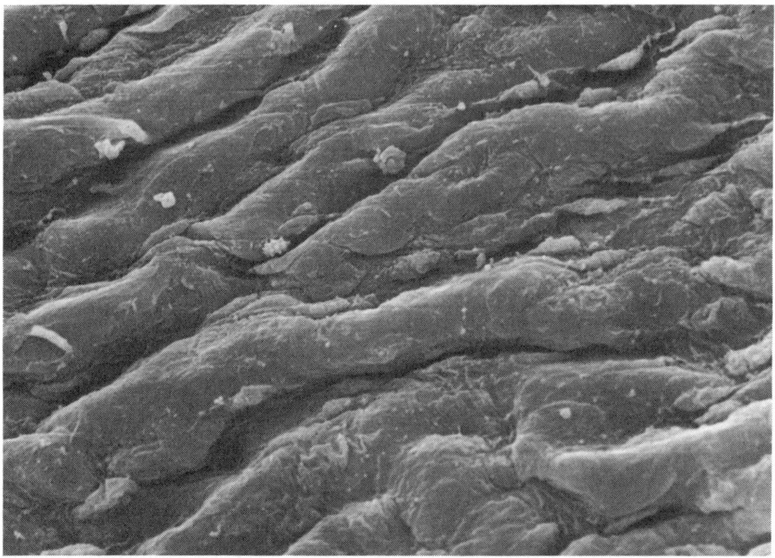

Figure 1B. *Demonstrates scanning electron micrograph of control endothelial surfaces of a canine artery at 800 ×.*

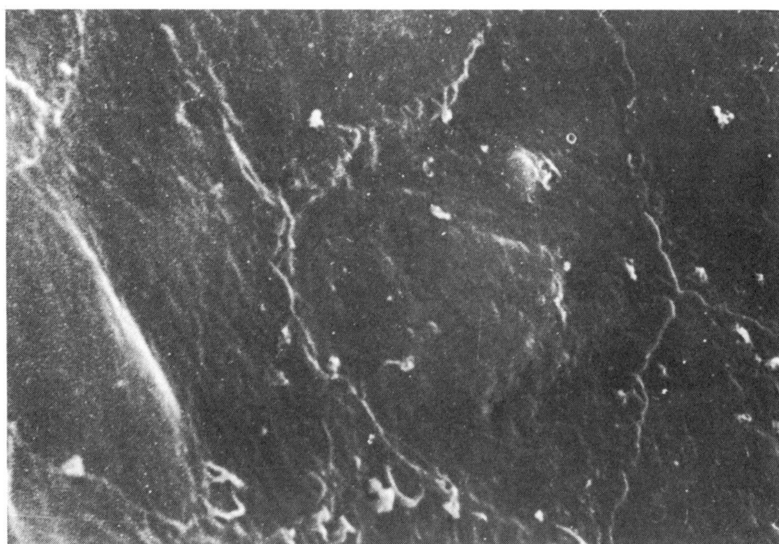

Figure 1C. *Demonstrates scanning electron micrograph of human popliteal artery at 2000 ×. (Figs. 1A-C, with permission from either Moore, WM, Manship, LR, Bunt, TJ: Differential endothelial injury caused by vascular clamps and vessel loops: Part I, Normal vessels. Am Surg 51:392–400, 1985, or Manship, LR, Moore, WM, Bunt, TJ: Differential endothelial injury caused by vascular clamps and vessel loops: Part II, Atherosclerotic vessels. Am Surg 51:400–403, 1985.)*

use of such loops; larger vessels and heavily diseased thick-walled or calcific vessels do not occlude well with gentler pressures, and in these situations an alternate device should be considered.

We have also described an in vivo model for assessing the relative force applied to the intima by an externally applied occlusive device.[13] The model involves an intraluminal pressure transducer that measures the change in pressure when a clamp is applied to an intact vessel under constant perfusion pressure. Table 3 outlines the absolute values of pressures, and Figure 5 gives a graphic demonstration of the increase in applied pressures as one progresses from type IV toward type I devices. These values are reproducible and generally follow the outline expected from prior studies. Concomitant SEM studies confirmed the equivalent progression of endothelial injury.[13]

Other types of occlusive devices have been presented briefly in the literature. We have studied three of these in our laboratory in the same model as our previous studies; the data is summarized in Table 4.

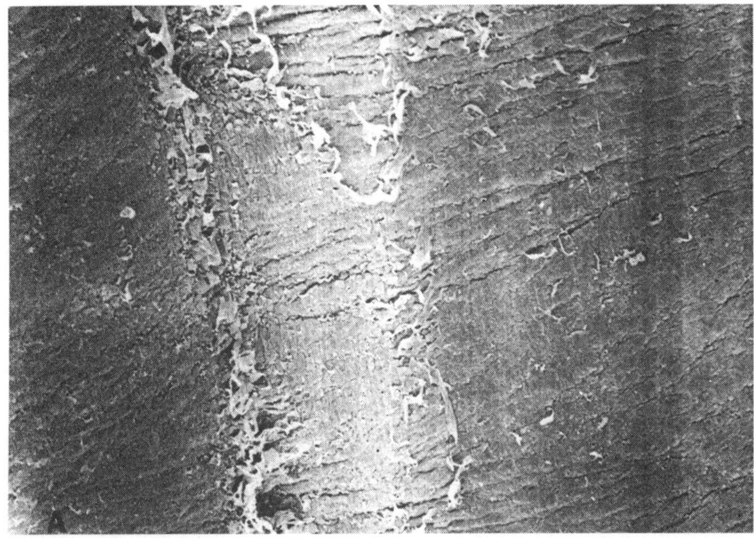

Figure 2A. *Demonstrates a scanning electron micrograph of the endothelial surface of a vessel occluded for 5 minutes with a type I device; A through D are canine artery at 72 × , canine artery at 600 × , human artery at 72 × , and human artery at 600 × , respectively. (With permission from either Moore, WM, Manship, LR, Bunt, TJ: Differential endothelial injury caused by vascular clamps and vessel loops: Part I, Normal vessels. Am Surg 51:392–400, 1985, or Manship, LR, Moore, WM, Bunt, TJ: Differential endothelial injury caused by vascular clamps and vessel loops: Part II, Atherosclerotic vessels. Am Surg 51:400–403, 1985.)*

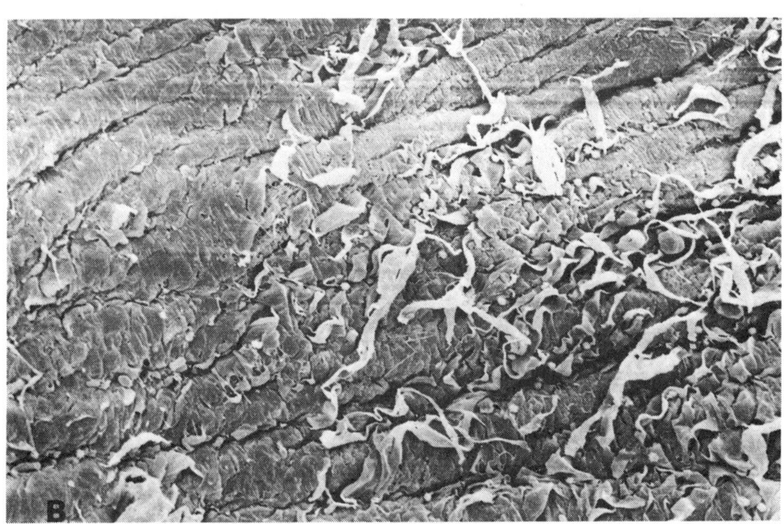

Figure 2B.

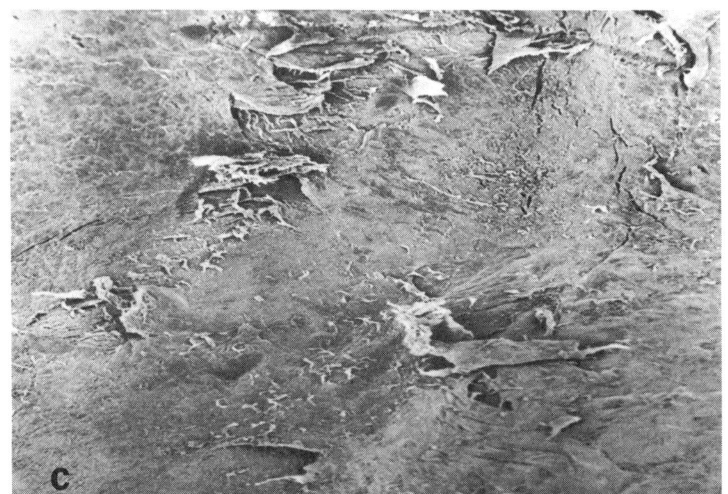

Figure 2C.

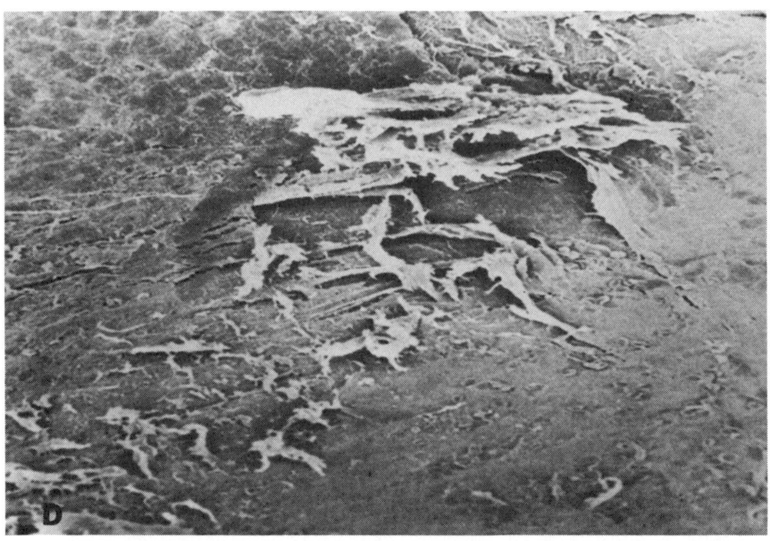

Figure 2D.

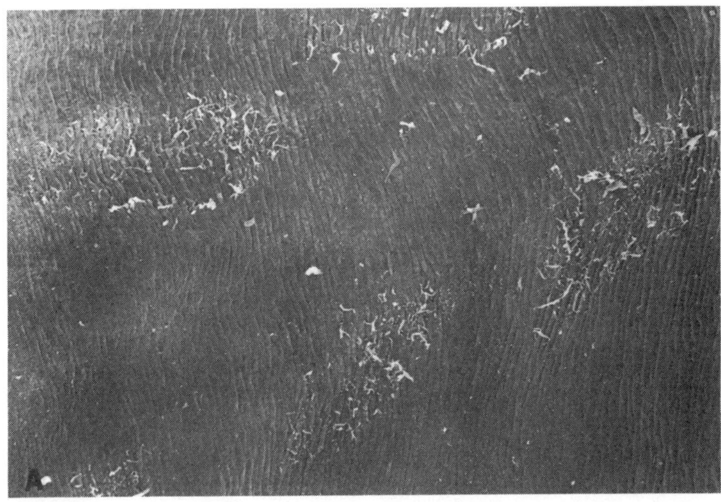

Figure 3A. *Demonstrates a scanning electron micrograph of the endothelial surface of a vessel occluded for 5 minutes with a type III device. A through D are canine artery at 60×, canine artery at 600×, human artery at 60×, and human artery at 1000×, respectively. (With permission from Moore, WM, Manship, LR, Bunt, TJ: Differential endothelial injury caused by vascular clamps and vessel loops: Part I, Normal vessels. Am Surg 51:392–400, 1985, and Manship, LR, Moore, WM, Bunt, TJ: Differential endothelial injury caused by vascular clamps and vessel loops: Part II, Atherosclerotic vessels. Am Surg 51:7:400–403, 1985.*

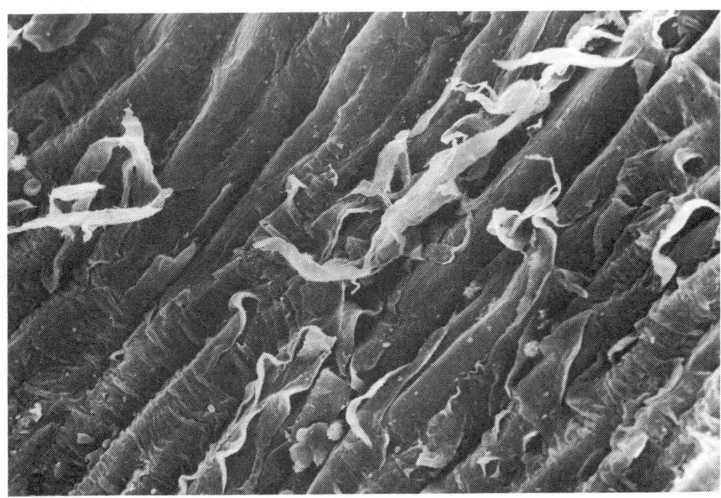

Figure 3B.

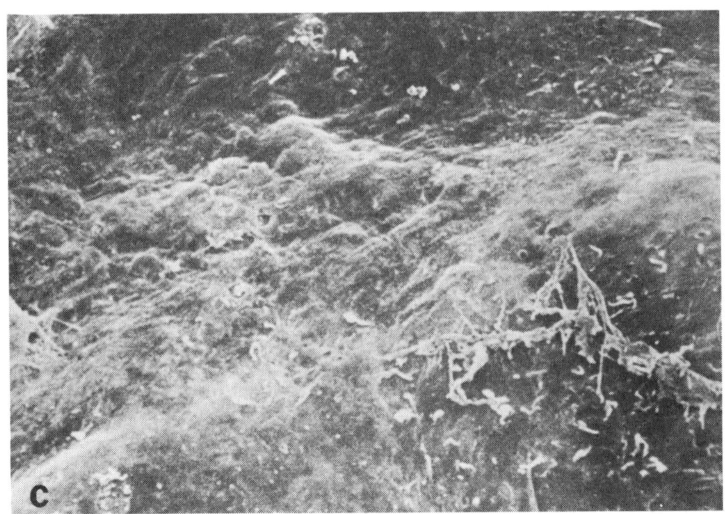

Figure 3C.

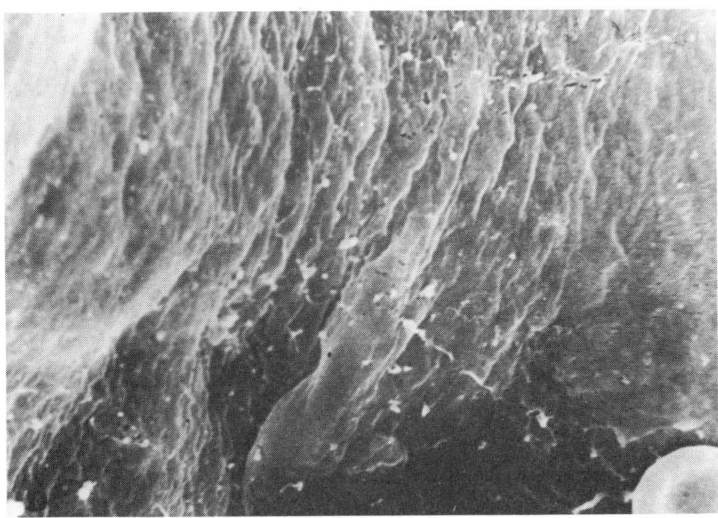

Figure 3D.

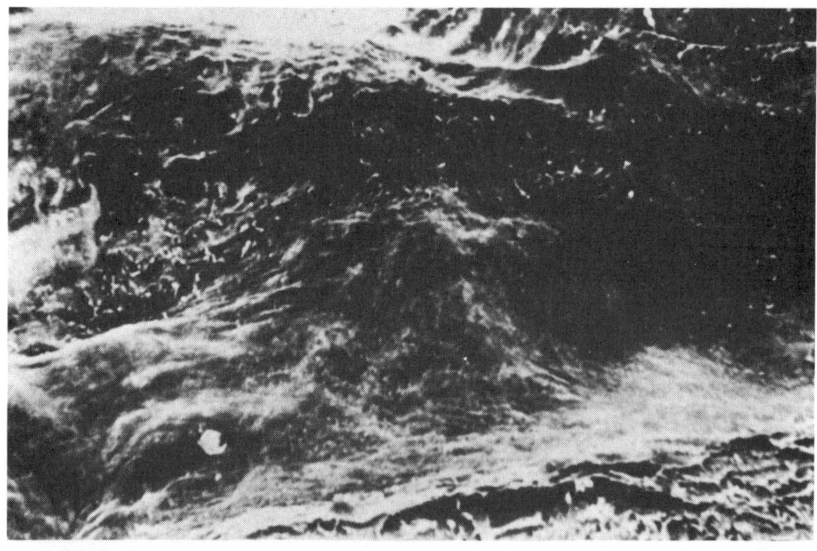

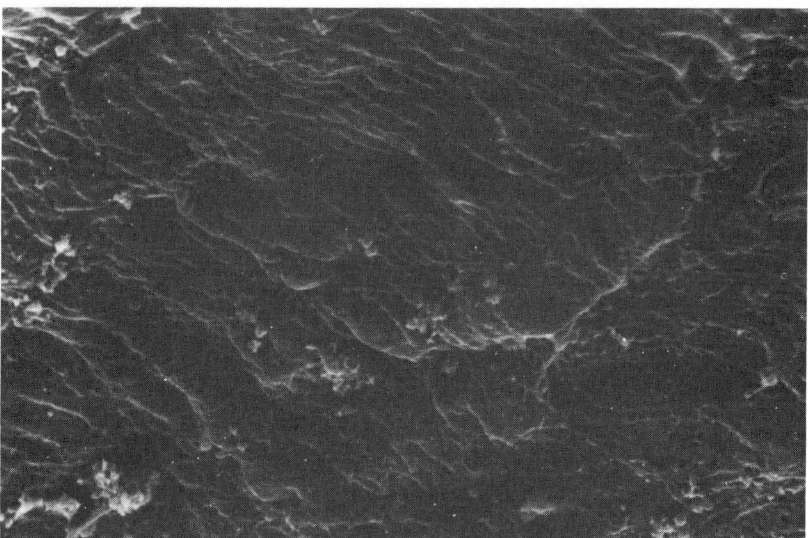

Figure 4. *Demonstrates a scanning electron micrograph of the endothelial surface of a vessel occluded for 5 minutes with a type II device; canine artery at 60 × (A, top), canine artery at 600 × (B, bottom). (With permission from either Moore, WM, Manship, LR, Bunt, TJ: Differential endothelial injury caused by vascular clamps and vessel loops: Part I, Normal vessels. Am Surg 51:7:392–400, 1985, or Manship, LR, Moore, WM, Bunt, TJ: Differential endothelial injury caused by vascular clamps and vessel loops: Part II, Atherosclerotic vessels. Am Surg 51:7:400–403, 1985.)*

Table 3. Correlation of Clamp Type, Transmural Force Index, and Intimal Injury Grade

Type	Occlusive Device Design	Transmural Pressure (mmHg)	Transmural Force Index (dynes/cm^2)	Intimal Injury Grade
I	Cooley	106	1.4×10^5	2–4
I	DeBakey	83	1.1×10^5	2–4
I	Satinsky	76	1.0×10^5	2–4
II	Fogarty Spring Bulldog	38	5.1×10^4	0–1
III	Fogarty Soft Jaw	97	1.3×10^5	1–2
IV	Silastic Vessel Loop	10	1.3×10^4	0
IV	Fogarty Occluder Pad	13	1.7×10^4	0
—	Berlin	28	3.7×10^4	0

Transmural applied forces were measured utilizing an intraluminal pressure monitor. Relative applied forces from applied vascular clamps were then correlated with vascular injury patterns. (From Moore, WM, Bunt, TJ, Herman, D, et al: Assessment of transmural force during application of vascular occlusive devices. *J Vasc Surg* 8:422–427, 1988, with permission.)

Table 4. Injury Potential of Various Vascular Occlusive Devices

Type	Injury Grade	Reference
Type I: Crossmembered Metallic Opposing		
DeBakey	2-3 ?4	
Cooley	2-3 ?4	17
Potts	3	8
Satinsky	2-3	7
Type II: Spring-loaded Opposing		
Blalock	0-1	8
Pilling	1-2	12
Heifetz	1-2	12
Diethrich	1	5
Glover Bulldog	1	7, 5
DeBakey Bulldog	1	7, 5
Type III: Crossmembered Metallic Protective Surface		
Fogarty	1	12, 17
Berlin	0-1	
Type IV: Loop Tourniquets		
Umbilical Tapes	0	
Silastic Vessel Loops	0	5, 7
Silk Ligature	3	6, 18
Fogarty Occluder	0-1	

The potential for vascular injury is given for representative devices from each classification, based on a literature review: injury grades are from Table 2. (Modified from Bunt et al: Iatrogenic vascular injury. *J Vasc Surg* 2:491–497, 1985.)

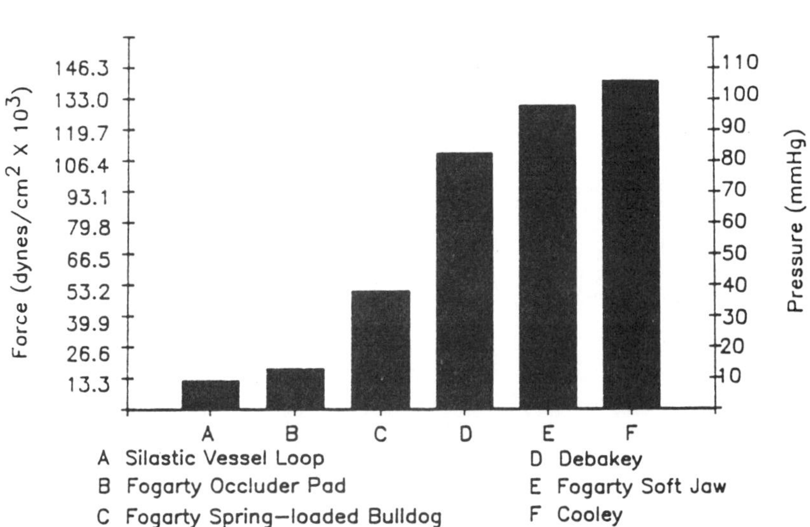

Figure 5. *Depicts graphically the applied transmural force expressed as pressure registered by the transducer (right side) or as calculated force (left side). (With permission from Moore, WM, Bunt, TJ, Herman D: Assessment of transmural force during application of vascular occlusive devices,* J Vasc Surg *8:422–427, 1988.)*

Internal balloon occluders: The data on these may best be extrapolated from that presented in Chapter 4 by Dobrin. Injury may occur during catheter insertion from the catheter tip, during balloon inflation, and during either inadvertent slippage or withdrawal of the inflated balloon without adequate balloon deflation. The most important variable is that of intraluminal pressure, with injury occurring at 100 mmHg lateral pressure, which is essentially the maximum pressure required for secure occlusion. Prevention of injury is a function of the technique outlined in Chapter 4.

Fogarty occluder: This device was introduced by Fogarty in 1985 as a loop tourniquet device with built-in holding power and decreased potential for injury due to use of a wider tubing. Its basic design tenet is that of a type IV device. The injury potential is minimal, with Class 0 to 1 injuries being noted on our studies (Figs. 6A, B, C).

Berlin clamp: Berlin introduced this device in 1978 as a potentially noninjurious device, although his original article did not specify any laboratory confirmation of same. He conceived its action to be analogous to the forefinger/thumb pinch grasp of the surgeon, with ability to limit occlusive power to only that sufficient to cause cessation of flow. In addition, the opposing surfaces of the device are protected with silastic cushions.[14] Berlin has laboratory evidence, and we have confirmed the noninjurious potential of the device in our own lab.

Since 1984 the Adler Company has marketed a variable pressure, metallic jaw clamp that is malleable for positioning and has variable spring-loaded compressive pressures. There are no serrations on the jaws therefore holding power is not optimal; but studies in our laboratory demonstrate that it is noninjurious when applied with appropriate low pressures (Figs. 7A, B).

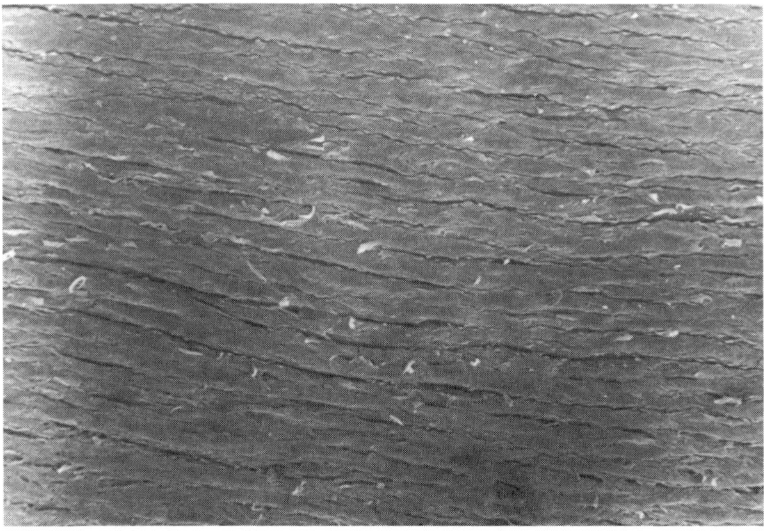

Figure 6. *Demonstrates a scanning electron micrograph of the endothelial surface of a canine vessel occluded for 5 minutes with a Fogarty occluder pad®. A, B indicate magnification at 200× and 1000×, respectively, and C, a human atherosclerotic vessel at 780×.*

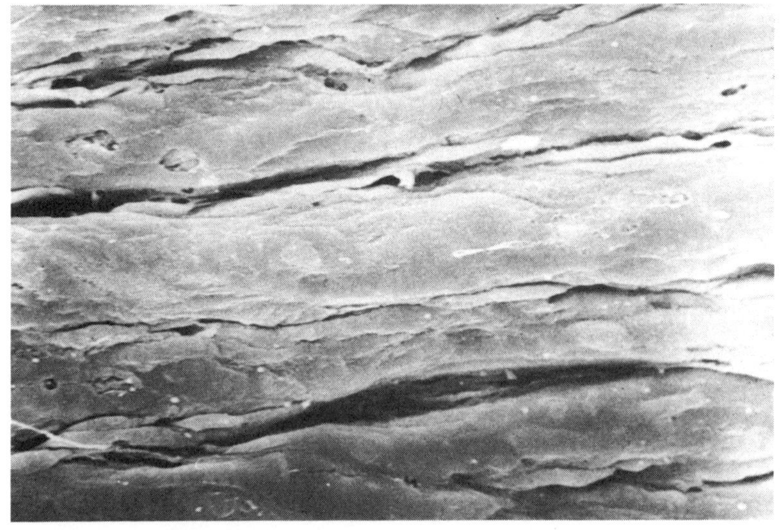

Figure 6B.

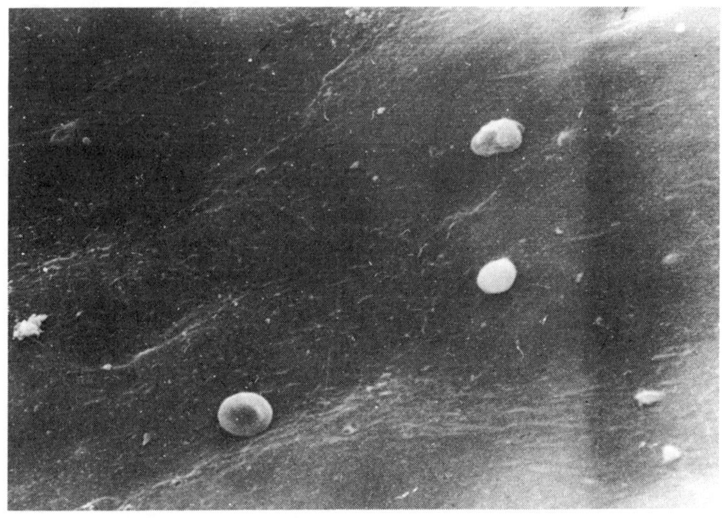

Figure 6C.

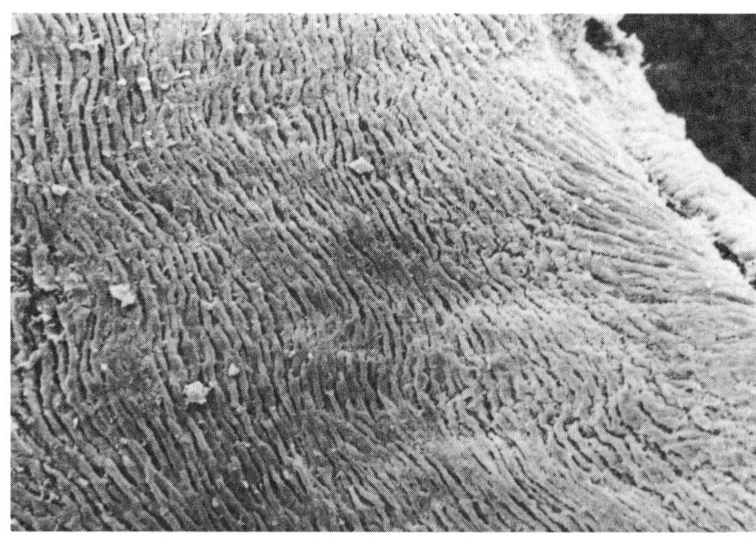

Figure 7A. *Demonstrates a scanning electron micrograph of the endothelial surface of a vessel occluded for 5 minutes with an Adler clamp®. A, B indicate magnification at 78× and 2000×, respectively.*

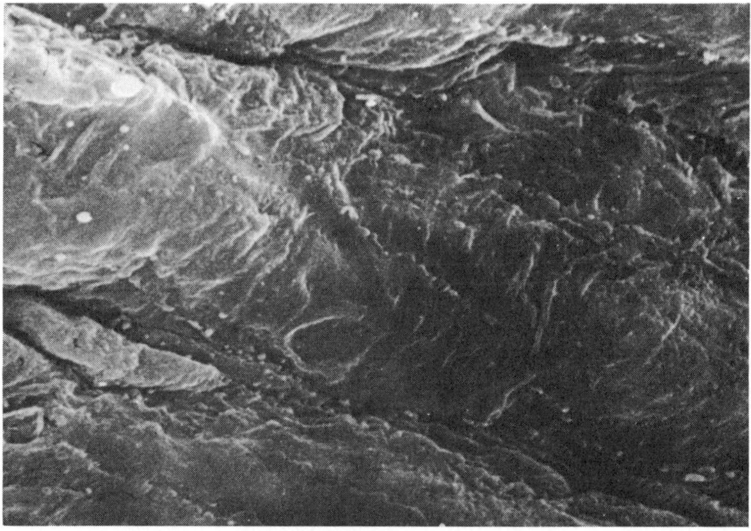

Figure 7B.

Vascular Injury Patterns

A review of the inputs from various authors and extensive experience in our combined laboratories has allowed a fairly complete compilation of the detrimental effects of various vascular occlusive devices on vascular and/or endothelial integrity. Earliest research efforts were confined to light microscopy. Later studies utilizing SEM have demonstrated that even if the arteries appeared macroscopically undamaged, endothelial injury of ultrastructurally extensive proportions was occurring. Furthermore, even when there is no ultrastructural injury, supravital dye staining has revealed that there is virtually always an endothelial injury at sites of clamp application. Furthermore, from the photographs of external vascular injury from our laboratory and review of the data from intraoperative angiography studies that demonstrate acute clamp injuries, it appears that medial and/or adventitial crush injury often occurs even when the endothelium appears to be intact at SEM.

Discussion

Normal vascular endothelium presents as thrombo-resistant flow surface to intraluminal blood. Mechanical disruption of that surface by such iatrogenic measures as vascular clamp application must inevitably lead to platelet aggregation and/or thrombus formation. Direct evidence of this process is apparent in those studies that looked at specimens after a sufficient elapsed time period (2–24 hours) for platelet deposition to have occurred. Platelet deposition may in itself be a source of distal embolization, may provide the subsurface for local thrombosis (particularly in small vessels), or may initiate the local endothelial injury leading to late atheroma formation.

Platelet adherence may furthermore be the initiating event to more long-term complications in which mitogenic factors released by adhered platelets initiate local neointimal hyperplasia and also may potentiate the formation of new atherosclerotic plaques at the injured segment. The evident long-term consequence is a local stenosis with possible late thrombosis.

Full thickness crushing injuries with type I clamps can be shown to fracture the elastic lamella. The reformation of that elastin is not of the same physical strength nor orientation—possibly leading or predisposing to local aneurysm and/or pseudoaneurysm formation. Evidence for this process is given by the relatively long-term canine studies of Krippanaehe, DePalma, and Guidoin[1,7,9] who have been able to identify the site of prior type I clamp application and crush injury by the persistence of underlying fibrous plaque at periods from 3 to 24 months following injury.

The scenario of iatrogenic vascular clamp injury is as follows: application of the clamp results in adventitial crushing, medial crushing, and hemorrhage leading to medial necrosis and variable degrees of endothelial shredding, laceration, or crush. Even if the endothelium remains intact by SEM or histology, there is an ischemic injury as demonstrated by supravital staining. The extent of the injury appears directly related to factors whose amelioration is at least potentially within the surgeon's control; the type of clamp utilized, the forcefulness of ratchet closure, the repetitiveness of clamping, the time interval that the artery is clamped, and possibly pharmacological manipulation of the platelet-derived secondary thrombotic and mitogenic responses.

The endothelial injury appears to heal by re-endothelialization from the surrounding edges, with the process complete at 1 to 4 weeks. However, by SEM and late histology the endothelium appears flattened—whether it is functionally intact is unknown and open to question. Medial necrosis of the vessel heals by inflammatory infiltration, fibrous scarring, and proliferation of smooth muscle with the end result being a fibrous plaque. Such a plaque will reliably show the location of prior clamp application.

Early postoperative thrombosis and embolization are interrelated processes dependent on fibrin and platelet deposition on the exposed subendothelium and/or sites of ischemia/injured endothelium. Thrombosis seems to be a major problem only in small caliber vessels. Embolus may be common but subclinical. In certain clinical situations (femorotibial, carotid revascularization), however, this might be a source of major postoperative problems. Medial laceration may precipitate acute dissection, particularly at aortic levels. Pseudoaneurysm formation may in part relate to the fracture of the elastin, and the fracture may allow vessel dilatation with an increase stress due to both diameter and compliance mismatching between graft and artery. Finally, early arterial infection may be related to the endothelial denudation, as intact endothelium appears to provide protection against bacteremic seeding.

The depth and extent of medial injury relates to physical characteristics of the clamps used, particularly the absolute force generated, and whether or not serrations concentrate the administered force on discrete portions of the vessel. Elastin injury is commonplace, with fracture of the internal elastic lamellae. Healing of the injury appears to proceed in an orderly sequence. The end result is not optimal for vessel function or patency in that there is production of a fibrous scar or fibroproliferative plaque. Furthermore, in the presence of an atherogenic serum, progressive atherosclerotic degeneration may also be presumed. The observed healing process gives hints as to primary etiologies for a number of possible short-term and long-term complications, namely, postoperative thrombosis, embolism, recurrent stenosis, pseudoaneurysm formation, and later arterial infection.

Recommendations

The general purpose of this book is twofold: to delineate how and what sort of injury occurs and to advocate preventitive/protective measures. It is apropos to this to state that standard commercially available vascular occlusive devices are marketed and generally considered to be relatively atraumatic, when the experimental evidence is predominantly to the contrary. However, careful use and consideration of their limitations may at least minimize the injury.

Type I Crossmembered Metal Vascular Clamps

Crossmembered metal vascular clamps as a group exert excessive forces at the jaws with steadily increasing forces as the size of the clamped vessel increases. Serrations on the jaws that are necessary for accurate holding also focus the applied force and are therefore associated with deeper medial penetrations and medial injuries. Holding pressure usually is adequate at the lowest ratchet closure, which should be utilized. Clamp utilization should be restricted to situations in which holding power is mandatory (transected vessels with limited control) or large vessels (aortoiliac) where other methods may not provide control. They should be applied once (not repeatedly) and to the lowest ratchet closure that provides occlusion. Similarly, the time interval of occlusion should be minimized. An injury will be reliably produced, but one can at least try to minimize it.

In certain situations where production of a clamp injury could be catastrophic to the technical result of the revascularization, we feel type I clamps are contraindicated, especially since other occlusive methods with markedly less injurious potential are available. Thus, we see no indication for use of a type I clamp on the internal carotid where embolization, the creation of intimal flaps, or the potential for thrombosis is undesirable. Thus, we feel that type I clamps should not be used in carotid endarterectomy or femoral tibial bypass grafting; for control of the saphenous vein when used as a conduit for any reason; and on pediatric vessels, which are undiseased and essentially normal; or on relatively undiseased muscular visceral vessels. In all these situations there are good reasons to perferentially advise type II, III, or IV devices as dictated by size of vessel or necessity for holding power. Our first choice would be a type IV, but the new Fogarty, Adler, and Berlin occluders would certainly seem appropriate also.

Type II Clamps

Type II clamps as a class are relatively noninjurious, with the severity of injury being linearly related to the force of maximal spring-loaded closure—from minimal endothelial injury with 30 to 50 g Heifetz, Pilling, Yasergel, etc., through a grade 1 to 2 injury with Glover and DeBakey bulldogs. It is useful to be familiar with the particular clamp used. Specific clamps within this category exact a much higher applied force and as such they are associated with an increased potential for injury. One should use the clamp with the least applied force that will give reliable occlusion. Obviously, the larger the vessel, the larger the clamp that will be necessary and therefore the greater occluding force to be transmitted.

Theoretically, the only difference between the type I and type II clamps is the amount of delivered force, since the jaw and serration designs are otherwise quite similar. The control a surgeon exerts is in selecting the lower pressure clamps for smaller undiseased vessels or for venous occlusion and reserving the higher pressure clamps for larger or more diseased vessels.

There is an outside limit to the utility of type II clamps. The elastic resilience or the fibrous resistance of larger or more diseased vessels may prevent adequate occlusion. As a result, practically speaking, type II clamps are restricted to small muscular arteries (profunda femoris, external carotid, renal, visceral, etc.).

Type III Clamps

Type III clamps as a generic class use the design tenets of a type I clamp but protect the vessel from concentrated applied force at the jaws by not allowing jaw-to-jaw apposition, but instead interposing various protective surfaces in that space for a more gentle and widely dispersed force. Thus, two design trends are responsible for the decreased injury potential—decreased applied force at the jaws and a wider area of dispersed force without specific concentration at discrete sites. The disadvantages of this design are that there is reduced holding power and a necessity to apply full ratchet force (occluding force) to obtain maximal holding power—thus insuring the maximal injury potential for each clamp. The Fogarty clamp somewhat ameliorates the first design facet by including a serrated bar on one side and a protective elastomere on the other.

Therefore, type III clamps are useful in a multitude of situations involving small- to medium-sized arteries/veins in which there is adequate exposed length for their application. The reduced holding power makes utilization on the aorta or on transected vessels at least worrisome if not frankly hazardous.

Type IV Occluders

Type IV occluders include a variety of commercially marketed and "makeshift" tourniquets used as doubly looped tourniquets. In general, these provide adequate occlusion of small to medium vessels with little injury potential if they are utilized correctly; that is, they are placed without excessive force, the loop is sufficiently wide to disperse the applied force, they are not cinched up excessively in a vain effort to obtain occlusion, and they are not cinched up repeatedly but are placed accurately and only once (Fig. 8). The bottom line to their appropriate usage is simple—if control cannot be obtained gently, it is better to use another occlusive device.

The generic disadvantages of these devices are: they may be difficult to apply and maintain in position without obstructing the fields, they cannot be used in a position where vessel control in the deeper planes is not perpendicular to the skin incision plane (e.g., distal internal or proximal common femoral); and control on thick-walled diseased vessels is difficult.

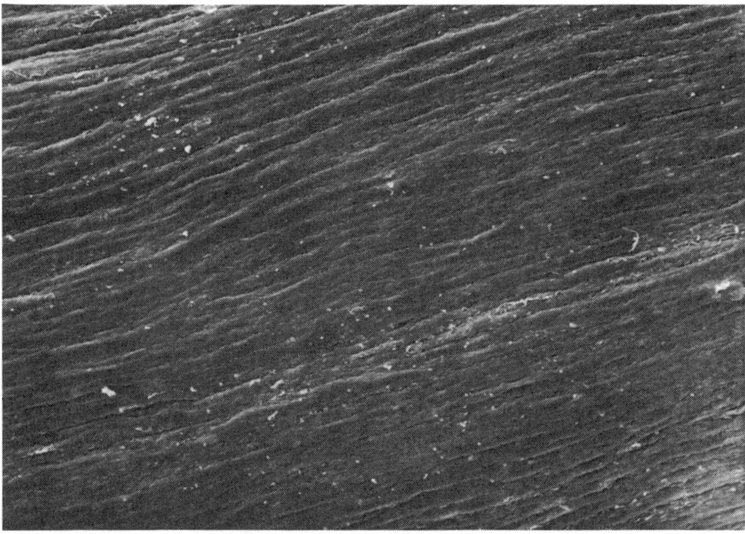

Figure 8A. *Demonstrates a scanning electron micrograph of the endothelial surface of a vessel occluded for 5 minutes with a type IV device. A through D are canine artery at 60×, canine artery at 780×, human artery at 2000×, and human artery at 2000× with an overzealously cinched application, respectively.*

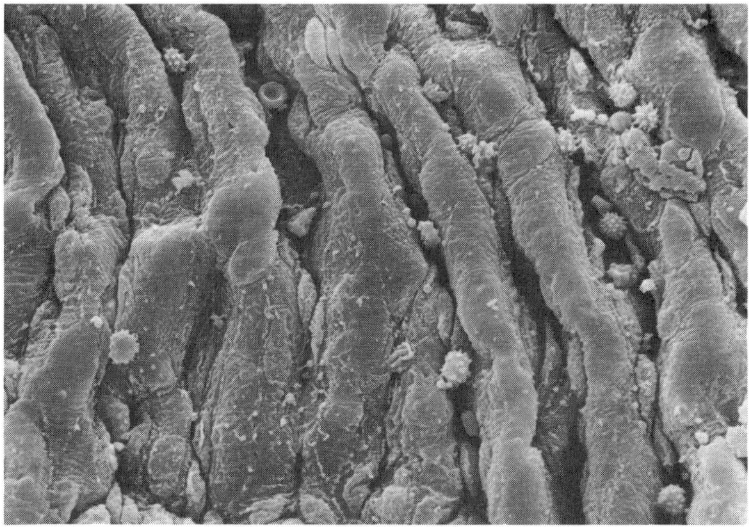

Figure 8B.

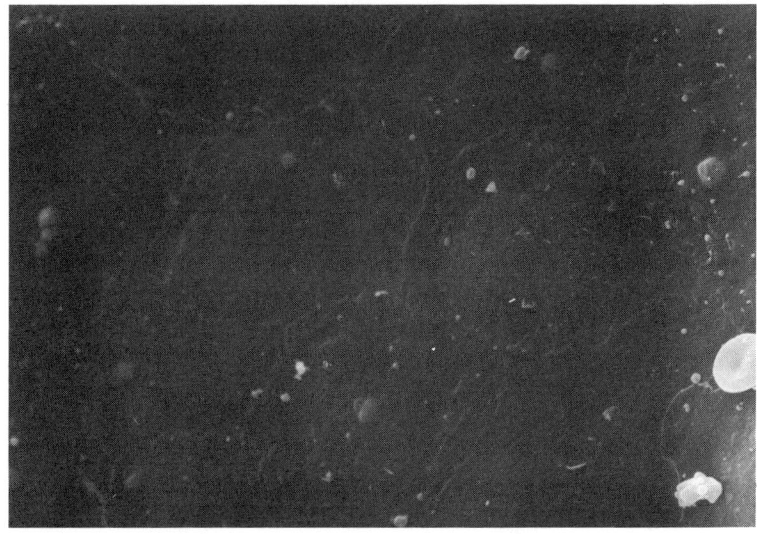

Figure 8C.

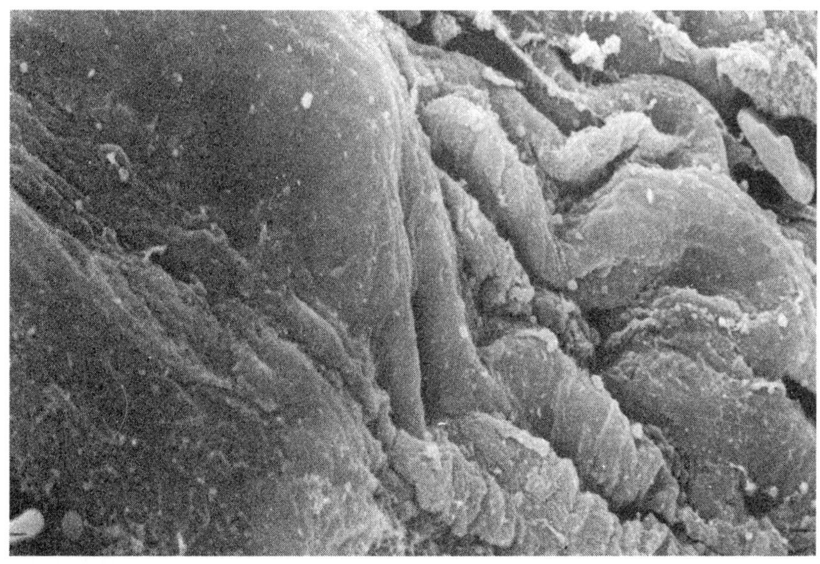

Figure 8D.

The size of the tape would seem to be very important. The force applied by the tape is both compressive and potentially a shear force as it is tightened, and both forces would presumably be concentrated on a smaller area by the smaller diameter tourniquets or conversely are dispersed over a greater area by wider tourniquets. This in large part explains the greater degree of injury seen with silk suture loops as opposed to commercial tapes.

The Fogarty occluder provides a number of desirable features in this regard—it is wide enough to disperse the force because it is a tubing; excessive cinch forces are dispersed in crushing the tube rather than selectively compressing the artery; it has a method of maintaining constant pressure control by the velour lock.

Type V Occluder

Intraluminal balloon occluders as commercially marketed offer reliable occlusive power at the relative expense of being somewhat cumbersome in the operative field. They are remarkable for the rapid and easy intraluminal control of aneurysms or pseudoaneurysms, obviating extensive proximal and distal dissection for standard circumferential arterial control. The major disadvantage is that the potential for arterial injury cannot be reliably controlled by the surgeons; there is no way to measure the force applied to the intima by the inflated balloon. The surgeon *can*, however, control injury potentials related to overinflation, withdrawal shear stresses, etc.

Dobrin notes six potential injuries from balloon catheters: (1) puncture of the distal artery by the catheter tip; (2) arterial disruption by overdistention of the vessel with balloon distention; (3) antegrade dissection of an atherosclerotic plaque during catheter introduction with intimal flap and thrombosis/dissection; (4) intimal flap raised during retrograde introduction of the catheter; (5) balloon rupture with distal embolization of balloon fragments; and (6) detachment and embolization of the balloon. All of these are equally possible iatrogenic misadvantages with intraluminal balloon occluders.

Care in introduction of the catheter, particularly in terms of visualization of the intima/lumen, and nonforceful advancement are critical measures. Dobrin's outlined measures (Table 1, Chapter 4) are also pertinent. The catheter should be inflated during retrograde withdrawal to where one "feels" lateral wall engagement and then slightly deflated from that maximal pressure. It should be fully deflated prior to withdrawal to minimize shear stresses at the arteriotomy. Inflation with liquid is preferable to air insufflation, and eccentric balloons should not be used.

Ideally the pressure for intraluminal occlusion should be monitored to assure pressures less than 200 mmHg. However, this is neither commercially available nor particularly convenient to perform.

Detrimental Effects

Demonstration of the injurious potential of vascular occlusive devices has been primarily a function of the research laboratory, with heavy reliance on the use of scanning electron microsurgery of normal canine vessels. Table 3 collates the research literature on various clamps and their injury potential, utilizing the injury classification scheme presented earlier.

There is surprisingly little documentation of clinical injuries, which may be a function of nonrecognition as well as a misinterpretation of angiographic findings. For example, early embolus or thrombosis may not be recognized as being secondary to clamp injury, but ascribed to technical problems such as intimal flap or platelet embolus of indeterminate source. Furthermore, it has been well documented that intraoperative angiography frequently underestimates the extent or severity of intimal injury. In this regard, Coelho has studied a variety of type I and II clamps on ex vivo diseased human iliac arteries in a perfusion apparatus administering pulsatile flow of saline and subjected to a 5-minute occlusion time. He then studied the vessels with real-time ultrasound and angiography in a situation, which, by its very nature, should have provided optimal resolution for either modality (no movement, no intervening tissue, constant focal lengths, etc.). Ninety-five percent of normal nonatherosclerotic vessels showed no macroscopic injury. However, 14% of arteriosclerotic arteries showed intimal tears and 26% showed intimal crush injuries, for a total 40% incidence of microscopic injury in diseased vessels. The study thus underscores the major potential for microscopic injury and its understatement by routine angiography.[15]

Review of clinical follow-up studies, particularly those involving repeat angiography, do reveal a fairly constant incidence (4% to 8%) of pathological features that are consistent with prior clamp injuries.[16,17]

Review of the literature and collation of the photomicrographs of several researchers have been used to underscore the frequency and potential severity of often unrecognized vascular injury incurred by vascular clamps. It should be recognized that iatrogenic vascular injury is a commonplace, if seldom fully realized, technical complication of peripheral vascular surgery. More importantly, the severity of the injury is in part surgeon controlled in that it is dependent on the clamp utilized and the manner in which it is used or abused. Macroscopic crush injuries are fairly readily visually apparent, endothelial and medial injuries are also occurring: Such injuries may be expected to contribute to both short-term and long-term complications such as embolism, thrombosis, pseudoaneurysm formation, and local stenoses. Intraoperative or postoperative angiography is less likely to demonstrate the injury than ultrasonography. The bottom line is prevention and that is the role and responsibility of the operating surgeon.

References

1. Bunt, TJ, Manship, LR, Moore, WM: Iatrogenic vascular injury. *J Vasc Surg* 2:491–497, 1985.
2. Manship, LR, Moore, WM, Bynoe, R P, Bunt, TJ: Differential endothelial injury caused by vascular clamps and vessel loops. Part II: Atherosclerotic vessels. *Am Surg* 51:400–406, 1985.
3. Moore, WM, Manship, LL, Bunt, TJ: Differential endothelial injury caused by vascular clamps and vessel loops: Part I: Normal vessels. *Am Surg* 51:392–400, 1985.
4. Harvey, JG, Gough, MH: A comparison of the traumatic effects of vascular clamps. *Br J Surg* 68:267–272, 1981.
5. Henson, GF, Rob, CQ: A comparative study of the effects of different arterial clamps on the vessel wall. *Br J Surg* 43:561–564, 1956.
6. Hickman, GA, Mortenson, JD: A comparative evaluation of vascular clamps. *J Thorac Cardiovasc Surg* 44:561–569, 1962.
7. DePalma, RG, Chidi, CC, Sternfeld, WL, et al: Pathogenesis and prevention of trauma—provoked atheromas. *Surgery* 82:429–437, 1977.
8. Guidoin, R, Martin, L, Levaillant, P, et al: Endothelial lesions associated with vascular clamping—surface micropathology by scanning electron microscopy. *Biomater Med Devices Artif Organs* 6:179–197, 1978.
9. Guidoin, R, Doyon, B, Blais, P, et al: Effects of traumatic manipulations on grafts, sutures, and host arteries during vascular surgery procedures. *Res Exper Med* 179:1–21, 1981.
10. Slayback, JB, Bowen, WW, Hinshaw, DB: Intimal injury from arterial clamps. *Am J Surg* 132:183–188, 1978.
11. Richling, B, Griesmayr, G, Lamet, S, et al: Endothelial lesions after temporary clipping. A comparative study. *J Neurosurg* 51:654–661, 1979.
12. Fonkalsrud, EW, Sanchez, M, Lassaletta, L, et al: Arterial endothelial changes after ischemia and perfusion. *Surg Gynecol Obstet* 142:715–721, 1976.

13. Moore, WM, Bunt, TJ, Hermon, D, et al: Assessment of transmural force during application of vascular occlusive devices. *J Vasc Surg* 8:422–427, 1988.
14. Berlin, RB: Vascular clamping: A new concept with manometric studies comparing available instruments with a novel design. *Vasc Surg* 12:108–112, 1978.
15. Coelho, JCV, Sigel, B, Flanigon, DP, et al: Arteriographic and ultrasonic evaluation of vascular clamp injuries using an in vitro human experimental model. *Surg Gynecol Obstet* 155:506–512, 1982.
16. Stanley, JC, Ernst, CB, Fry, WJ: Fate of 100 aortorenal vein grafts; characteristics of late graft expansion, aneurysmal dilatations, and stenosis. *Surgery* 74:931–944, 1973.
17. Szylagyi, DE, Elliott, JP, Hageman, JH, et al: Biologic fate of antogmous vein implants as arterial substitutes: Clinical, arteriographic, and histopathologic observations in femoropopliteal operations for atherosclerosis. *Ann Surg* 178:232–240, 1973.
18. Dunn, DC: The use of the arterial sling tourniquet in surgical practice. *Br J Surg* 60:594–596, 1973.
19. Brown, L: A vascular clamp utilizing sponge rubber. *Arch Surg* 83:177–178, 1961.

Chapter 3

Saphenous Vein Preparation

Vikrom S. Sottiurai

Despite salient morphological and physical differences between veins and arteries, saphenous vein remains the preferred substitute for lower extremity revascularization, secondary only to autogenous artery. This can be attributed to factors of morphological adaptability, contractile capability, reduced compliance mismatch with the artery, minimal kinking, resistance to infection, and operative accessibility through the same incision in the lower extremity.

Several precautions should be taken to achieve optimal results from the saphenous vein graft. Worthy of attention are vein size selection, various techniques of vein harvesting and preparation, vein storage/preservation, and techniques of anastomosis.

Anatomy of Human Saphenous Vein

The great saphenous vein begins at the ankle just anterior to the medial malleolus and terminates at the saphenofemoral junction. Twenty-five percent of great saphenous veins have a bifid system at the juxtagenu area. This anatomical variance can affect the suitability of the saphenous vein as a bypass graft when the caliber of the bifid vein is less than 2 mm.

Histologically, there are three layers in the wall of the saphenous vein. The intima includes a monolayer of endothelial cells with a varying number of subintimal myoblasts. The media consists of inner

From *Iatrogenic Vascular Injury: A Discourse on Surgical Technique*, edited by T.J. Bunt, M.D. © 1990, Futura Publishing Inc., Mount Kisco, NY.

longitudinal and outer circular smooth muscle cells. The adventitia is the thickest of the three layers. Longitudinally arranged smooth muscle cells, vasa vasorum, and nerve fibers are the dominant elements encountered in this bulky fibroelastic stratum. Sottiurai has reported the coexistence of venous and arterial vasa vasorum networks in the venous adventitia. The more numerous venous vasa vasorum emerge from the side branches of the vein and surround the vein circumferentially. Arterial vasa vasorum are derived from the adjacent artery and have a rhomboid configuration of distribution along the axis of the vein.[1]

The great and small saphenous veins contain comparatively more smooth muscle cells than other superficial veins. This may be attributed to the higher pressure that exists in the veins of the lower extremity. Because of the thick longitudinal muscular layers in the intima and media of the great saphenous vein, a characteristic longitudinal folding of the intima occurs in the nondistended vein.[2-5]

Although the comparative morphology of the proximal great saphenous vein at the groin and that of the distal saphenous vein near the medial malleolus has not been fully studied, significant morphological discrepancy exists and may have functional implication. Contrary to the distal portion of the great saphenous vein, the proximal segment of the great saphenous vein in humans contains more longitudinally oriented smooth muscle cells in the intima (Figs. 1, 2). Whether

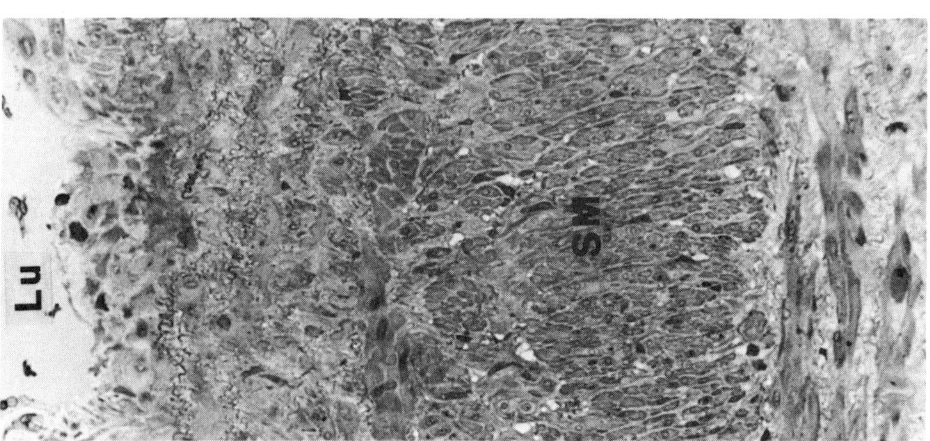

Figure 1. *Light micrograph of a 1-μm thick cross section of the proximal human saphenous vein showing the abundant longitudinal orientation of intimal smooth muscle (SM) bundles. ×275. Stained with basic fuschin and methylene blue. Lu = lumen.*

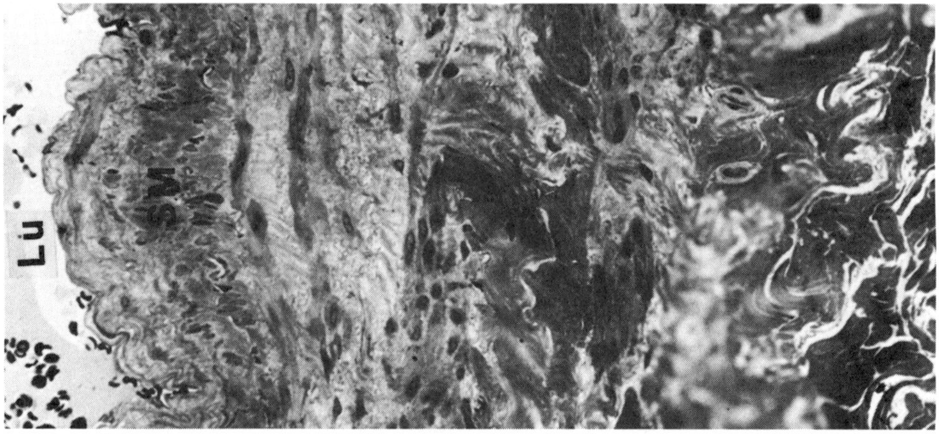

Figure 2. *Light micrograph demonstrating a paucity of intimal smooth muscle (SM) cells in a transverse section of the distal human saphenous vein from the same patient as in Figure 1. ×275. Stained with basic fuschin and methylene blue.*

the intimal smooth muscle cells in the proximal segment of the great saphenous vein affect the tensile strength of the vein graft has not been fully investigated. Based on his studies, Sottiurai indicates however that there is no demonstrable discrepancy in the bursting strength between these vein segments.[6]

Vein Preparation and Morphological Alteration

Ultrastructural revelation of vein histocytomorphology following various techniques of preparation has kindled interest in vein graft preservation. A great deal of attention is focused on proper media selection, control of pH, temperature, osmolality, osmolarity, and duration of vein storage.[7] Storage media differing from the property of the autogenous blood have the tendency to produce striking morphological changes.[7,8] However, most of these vein grafts remain patent when utilized, despite some morphological derangement. Only severe and extensive physical damage to the vein graft creates a critical thrombogenic surface to produce acute graft occlusion.

Endothelial injury occurs from ischemia or injury due to abnormal pH, abnormal temperature, abnormal osmolality, or direct physical abrasion. Intact endothelium provides a barrier between the negatively charged blood elements and the positively charged subendothelium while maintaining its own negative charge. It also prevents exposure of the subendothelial elements, particularly collagen, that are known to enhance platelet adherence and precipitation of the coagulation cascade phenomenon. Functional endothelium secrete plasminogen-activating factors, prostacyclin, and heparinoid compound. Plasmino-gen-activating factors mediate local thrombolysis; prostacyclin inhibits platelet aggregation; the heparinoid compound is the locus for anti-thrombin III or heparin cofactor binding. Loss of the venous endothe-lium has obvious direct effects on the immediate thrombogenicity and can alter graft patency.[3,9–15] Without the endothelial barrier, the under-lying myoblasts are susceptible to the influence of platelet-derived growth factors.

Medial injury appears to be largely the result of mechanical disten-tion of smooth muscle cells. During vein preparation, any derange-ment of pH or osmolality also may contribute to medial damage. Prolonged storage in the preparation media may also contribute to medial damage. Medial injury will result in smooth muscle cell de-generation or augmented extracellular matrix synthesis. The sequelae of such pathological change results in replacement of media with fibrocollagenous extracellular substances. In canine models, such mor-phological changes were demonstrable in 2-3 weeks. The precise mechanisms responsible for the pathomorphogenesis of media-intimal fibroplasia is not well defined. However, the stimulation of the smooth muscle cells from mechanical stretching and the potential influence of platelet-derived growth factor after breakdown of the endothelial barrier are factors worthy of consideration.[10,16,16a,16b]

Literature Review

Wyatt studied reversed vein grafts in humans and noted a univer-sal disruption of the endothelium and vasa vasorum at initial implanta-tion. The vasa vasorum were restored within 72 hours. However, only 30% of the endothelium remained intact at the same time interval.[17] Reichle reported that reversed saphenous vein in femoropopliteal grafts needed four to six weeks for complete re-endothelialization.[18] In canine in situ and human reversed saphenous vein grafts, Bush noted a similar time interval was required for endothelial regeneration. However, the enzymatic secretory capacity was markedly impaired when compared to autologous artery or to control vein segment.[10]

Comparing canine vein grafts harvested at various intervals,

Brody demonstrated that in coronary bypass grafts, medial myocytes and subendothelial fibrosis were the sequelae of medial ischemia.[19]

Abbot, in subjecting canine jugular veins to multiple treatments before measuring the compliance of the vein, arrived at the following conclusions. Warm immersions caused more injury than cold. Neutral pH was preferred and colloid medium had theoretical advantage in maintaining proper osmotic effect. Excessive distention (>300 mmHg) of the vein caused a decrease in compliance.[20,20a]

Ramos also noted more endothelial injury with saline than blood preparation, using silver nitrate staining, he showed that there was greater endothelial death than seen histologically.

To emphasize the long-lasting adverse sequelae produced by mechanical injury and improper media usage, Ramos studied grafts implanted up to 3 months and elegantly depicted marked endothelial denudation, elastic lamellae, and adventitial collagen fiber fragmentation as the sequalae of vein distention. Despite re-endothelialization of the denuded endothelia at one to two weeks, there was progressive and excessive subendothelial fibrosis occurring in essentially all distended grafts as early as six weeks.[4]

In quantitating the various pressure produced by different modes of vein distention, Bouchek reported that normal syringe inflations could reach 700 mmHg. It was also noted that although 500 to 600 mmHg could overcome the spasm of the vein segment, severe endothelial injury was a frequent complication. To obviate overdistention, Bouchek devised an interval balloon (Shiley Labs, Irvine, CA) to be inserted between the syringe and the catheter to control the inflation pressure at either 300 or 400 mmHg to minimize overdistention injury to the vein graft.[21]

Gundry in 1980 studied human saphenous vein in an immersion model studying four different solutions. He noted that warm saline or warm blood at 28°C caused a severe endothelial loss while cold saline or blood at 4°C fully preserved the endothelium. However, distention to 300 mmHg caused a significant endothelial injury despite utilization of the cold solutions. The injury incurred by distention was worse with saline than it was with blood.[22]

In a canine cephalic vein model, Bauman correlated the degree of endothelial injury with the amount of vein contraction caused by dissection or by irrigating and immersing solutions. In addition, he noted large cytoplasmic extrusions of subendothelial smooth muscle cells through the gap junctions of the endothelial cells. He emphasized the significance of these findings, in that they are identical to the process normally seen in the closure of a patent ductus arteriosus. It was also recognized that marked vein contraction with its resultant histologic endothelial changes was a prethrombotic process. In testing various solutions, he noted that cold blood produced more contraction and therefore more endothelial loss. The contraction was less balanced with electrolyte solutions and was totally ablated by addition of papaverine to the solution. He therefore recommended using papaverine to specifically counteract the severe contraction in vein preparation.[2]

Malone in 1981 studied a canine jugular vein model at steadily increasing levels of controlled 5-minute distention periods. He correlated the histologic and scanning electron microscopic picture with an assay of fibrinolytic activity. Malone also noted that there was a linear increase in endothelial injury at pressures greater than 300 mmHg. Scanning electron microscopy confirmed cellular changes at pressures less than 300 mmHg. Fibrinolytic activity was significantly decreased ($P < .004$) in all distended veins as opposed to control segments. When the veins were implanted into the arterial circulation, both nondistended and distended veins had a reduction in fibrinolytic activity for twelve hours prior to returning to the arterial levels, but never reached the control levels in vein.[13]

Similar evidence has been proposed by Bush, who studied the biochemical functions of harvested reversed canine veins by measuring thromboxane and prostacyclin production and correlating them with endothelial histology. Prostacyclin production was lower than prearterialization levels in both in situ and reversed vein grafts. In situ veins had higher levels than harvested veins. Normothermic blood solution could preserve function better than cold saline. Thromboxane production followed a different pattern. Only veins prepared with blood showed a significant increase in thromboxane after harvesting. However, by 1 week, all veins (regardless of preparation) showed a universal rise in thromboxane production, which persisted for 6 to 12 weeks. Despite the extensive endothelial injury encountered in veins distended to more that 200 mmHg using cold saline solution, all grafts, irrespective of preparative techniques, demonstrated a normal endothelialized surface within 6 weeks. A correlation exists in prostaglandin-6-keto-PgG-1 alpha level and the proper preparation of the intima and media. Bush theorized that protection of medial smooth muscle cells allowed continuous prostacyclin production. The latter affects adherence and subsequent thromboxane production.[9,10]

Cambria comparing in situ grafts to nondistended reversed grafts and reversed vein grafts distended to 500 mmHg with Ringer's lactate solution at room temperature in a canine model demonstrated the following observations. Endothelial injury at 2 hours following implantation was 3.9% to 6.7% of the surface area in the in situ grafts, 18.6% ± 5.9% in reversed nondistended veins, and 35.3% ± 5.4% with reversed distended veins (P <.001). At 24 hours, all grafts showed more endothelial destruction, 15.2% ± 9.5% for in situ and 25.1% ± 23.4% for reversed grafts. No differences in fibrinolytic activity could be detected at 24 hours or at 6 weeks. At 2 weeks, both groups showed less than 5% surface area endothelial injury.[11]

Vein distention is also important in terms of preservation of the vasa vasorum and side branch ligation. Gundry has noted that flush ligation of side branches caused more luminal stenosis from extrusion of a nipple of media and intima into the lumen. Gundry also reported application of forceps on the vein produced linear injury to the endothelium. Similar findings were noted with the application of vascular clamps at the end of the vein.[22]

The choice of vein size has been noted to be significant and affect graft patency. Szilagyi noted a marked decrease in patency when a less than desirable vein was used for distal infrapopliteal bypass—a 65% two-year patency in "good" grafts versus a 30% two-year patency with "bad" grafts.[22a] Sladen has more recently echoed that finding, noting that failures of reversed saphenous vein femoropopliteal bypass grafts were most frequently due to utilization of a vein with inadequate size.[23]

Sottiurai has performed extensive experiments to examine all of the various techniques of vein preparation. He has delineated the effect on the media in particular, whereas most authors have confined their observations to the immediate endothelial injury.[5,14–16,24] Sottiurai has noted that storage media with properties differing from those of autogenous blood or blood derivative have a distinct tendency to produce striking adverse morphological changes in vein graft. Despite the latter, most of the vein grafts in the experimental studies have remained patent. It would appear that perhaps only severe and extensive physical damage to the vein graft creates a sufficiently critical thrombogenic surface to produce an acute graft occlusion.

Crystalloid solution has long been the standard media used in vein preparation. However, it has been demonstrated that crystalloid solution can produce irreversible medial smooth muscle cell injury (Figs. 3–6) leading to intimal and medial fibroplasia (Figs. 7, 8). Such pathology occurs despite complete restoration of the overlying en-

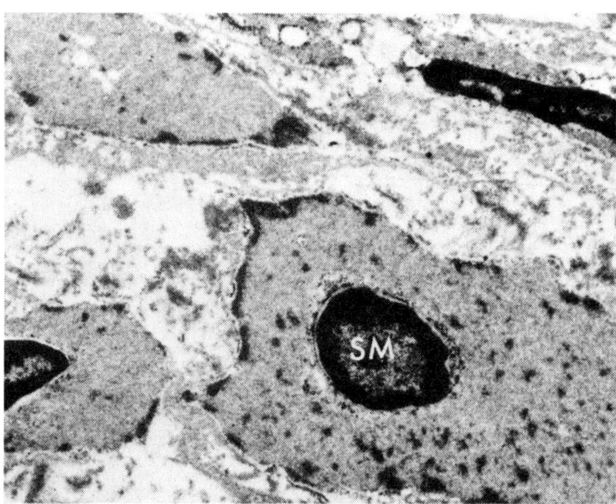

Figure 3. *Vein segment stored in lactated Ringer's solution for 30 min. There are no identifiable smooth muscle (SM) perinuclear organelles. Nucleus appears pyknotic in these cells, and myofilaments are dense and homogenous. Moderate intercellular swelling and connective tissue dissociation are present.* ×18,000

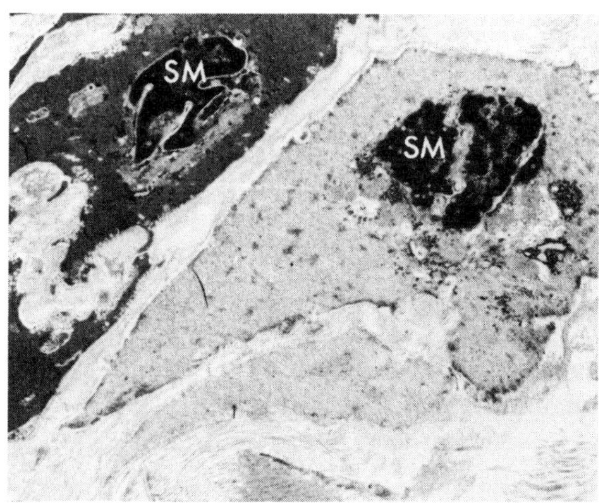

Figure 4. *Vein segment stored in lactated Ringer's solution at 4°C for 30 min. Nuclei of smooth muscle (SM) cells are homogenous and mummified. Moderate intercellular swelling and collagen fiber disruption are present.* ×18,000

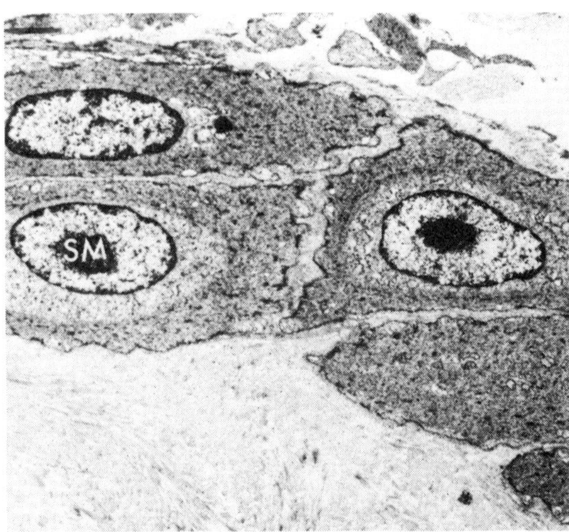

Figure 5. *Vein stored in heparinized whole blood at 4°C for 30 min. Perinuclear swelling in smooth muscle (SM) cell is present. Intercellular edema is not noted.* × *18,000*

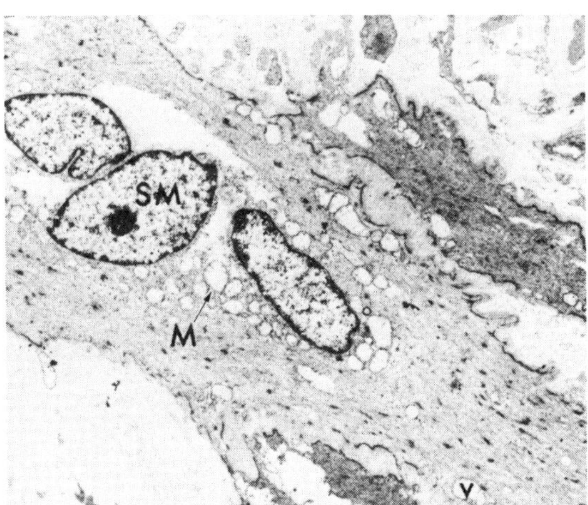

Figure 6. *Vein segment stored in heparinized whole blood at 4°C for 60 min. Perinuclear vacuoles in smooth muscle (SM) cells are apparent. Peripheral vacuoles (v) are also present. Mitochondria (M) are swollen and have lost their cristae. Myofilaments appear normal and well organized. No significant interstitial edema.* × *20,000*

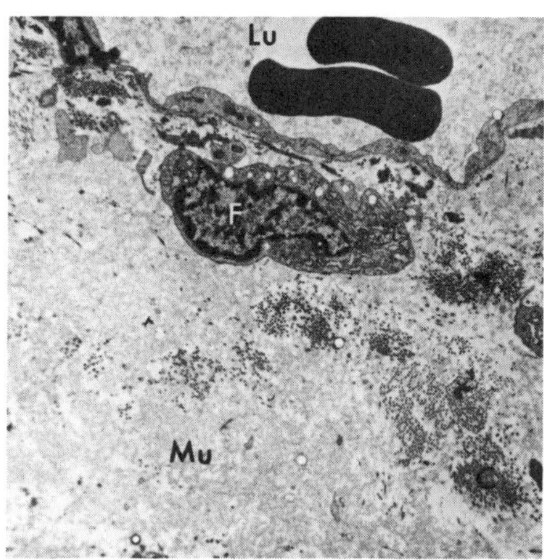

Figure 7. *Vein segment stored in lactated Ringer's solution prior to arterial grafting. Endothelial cells are normal in appearance. Myofibroblasts are evident in subintimal space. Homogenous connective tissue matrix (Mu) occupies the subendothelial regions and has replaced smooth muscle cells in this area. F = fibroblast; C = collagen bundles; Lu = lumen. ×10,000.*

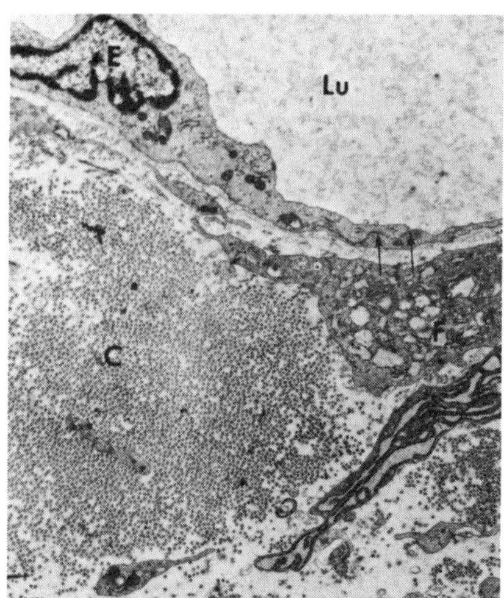

Figure 8. *Vein segment stored in lactated Ringer's solution prior to arterial grafting, harvested 6 months later with complete regeneration of endothelial cells (E). Cellular organelles and their distribution appear normal. There is an intact tight junction of two endothelial cells (arrows). Extensive subendothelial fibroplasia consisting of collagen fibers (C) is a frequent finding in vein segments stored in lactated Ringer's solution. Remnants of myofibroblasts (F) are apparent. Lu = lumen. ×10,000*

dothelium (Figs. 7, 8). This has significant implication for long-term vein graft patency. In Sottiurai's comparative studies of the various methods of vein preparation, it was noted that crystalloid solutions with deranged pH and osmolality not only induce endothelial cell disruption, disassociation, and sloughing (Fig. 9), but also caused irreversible medial smooth muscle injury (Fig. 4). This is characterized by a pyknotic nucleus, mummification of the myofilaments, cytoplasmic necrosis, and vacuolation (Figs. 3, 4). Although the endothelial injury was often restored in 10 to 14 days following vein graft insertion, injury to the media was generally irreversible and resulted in long-term intimal and medial fibroplasia (Figs. 7, 8).

Improvement of cell morphology and maintenance of vein integrity can therefore be obtained by storage of the vein in a solution with normal osmolality, normal osmolarity, appropriate temperature, appropriate pH, and for as short a duration as possible. Optimization of these parameters results in preservation of the integrity of the endothelia, smooth muscle cells, and the ground substances of the vein graft (Figs. 5, 6, 10–12).

Whole blood, blood byproducts, tissue culture media, and other colloid solutions have been demonstrated to produce better vein preservation than crystalloid solution. This can be ascribed to the neutral

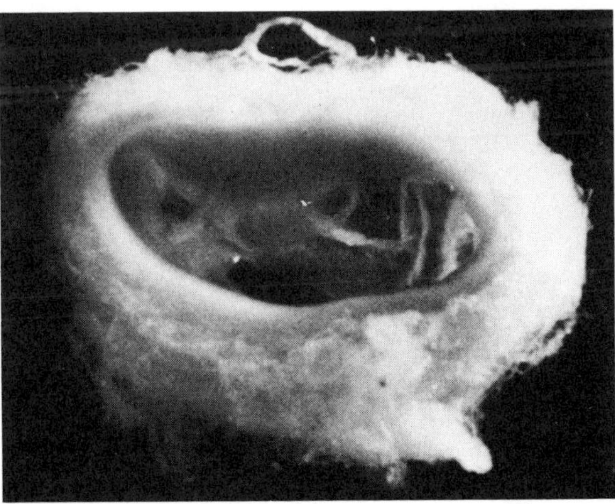

Figure 9. *Vein segment preserved in lactated Ringer's solution "slush" at approximately 4°C for 2 hr. Adventitial swelling and intimal sloughing are apparent (arrow).* × 23

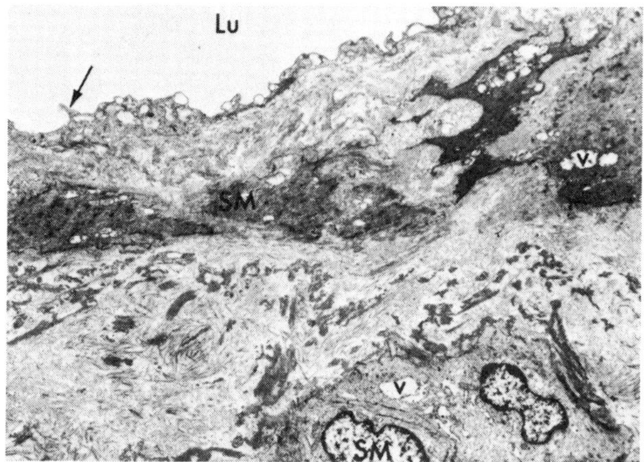

Figure 10. *Vein segment stored in heparinized whole blood for 60 min. Endothelial cells are intact, as are their microvilli (arrow). Except for small cytoplasmic vacuoles (v), subendothelial smooth muscle (sm) cells are essentially normal. Lu = lumen.* × 9,000

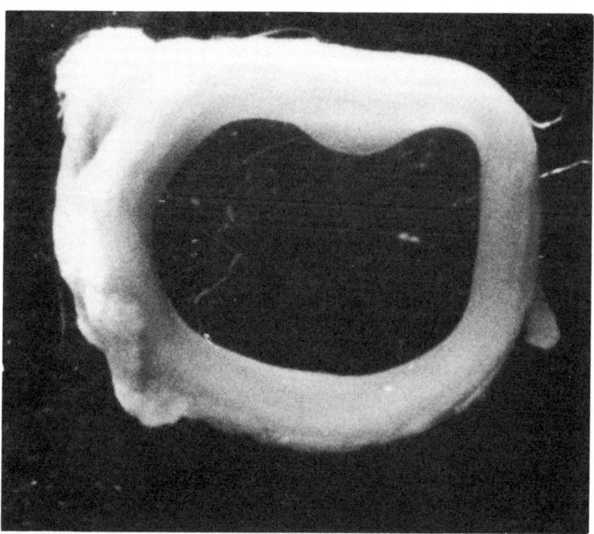

Figure 11. *Vein segment preserved in heparinized whole blood at 4 to 6°C for 2 hr. All layers of the vessel wall are intact and well preserved.* × 23

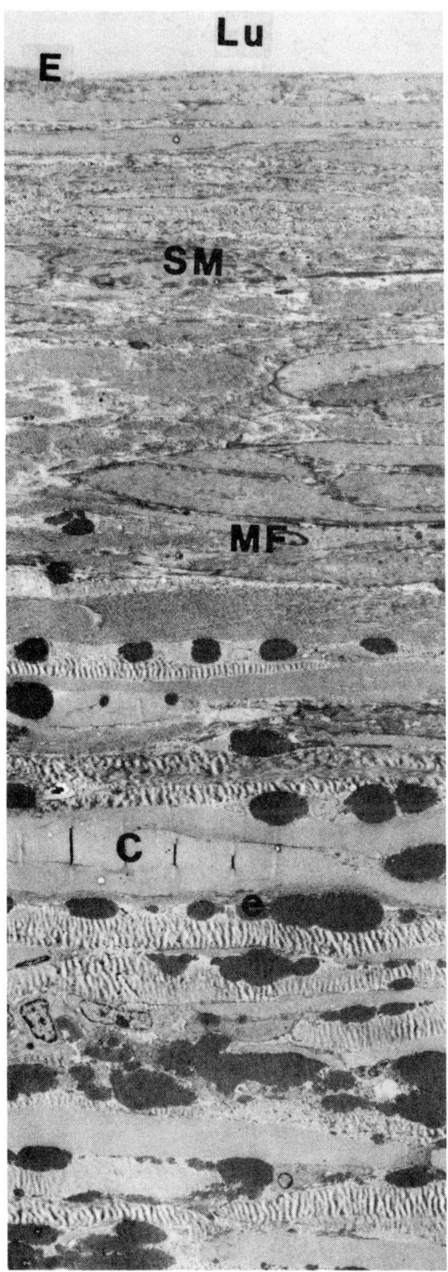

Figure 12. *Electron micrograph of vein segment distended to 150 mmHg plasmanate plus papaverine before implantation. Extensive intimal and medial cellular hyperplasia and outer media fibroplasia with abundant elastic tissue characterize arterialization of vein graft 9 months after arterial circulation. Lu = lumen; E = endothelium; SM = smooth muscle cell; MF = myofibroblast; C = collagen bundles; e = elastic tissue. × 1265*

pH, proper tonicity, osmolarity, and osmolality of the medium. With colloid solution, injury to the endothelium is limited to cell swelling, loss of microvilli, vacuole formation, and infrequent sloughing (Figs. 5, 6, 10, 11). Morphological alterations of the smooth muscle cell resulting from vein preparation are usually reversible with colloid solutions. The histomorphological derangement is characterized by paranuclear and cytoplasmic vacuole formation, cellular edema, myofilament rarification, and reduction of paranuclear orgnelles (mitochondria, Golgi complexes, and rough endoplasmic reticula) (Figs. 5, 6, 10, 11). The morphological changes are not apparent macroscopically other than mild intimal swelling and diminished compactness of the vessel wall (Figs. 11, 13, 14).

Mechanical distention of the vein segment produces gross and severe trauma to all layers of the vessel wall. Papaverine has a distinctly positive effect on cellular preservation of the vein graft. Sottiurai has shown that the relaxant effect of papaverine plays a vital role in averting both cellular injury and stimulation of myocytes during

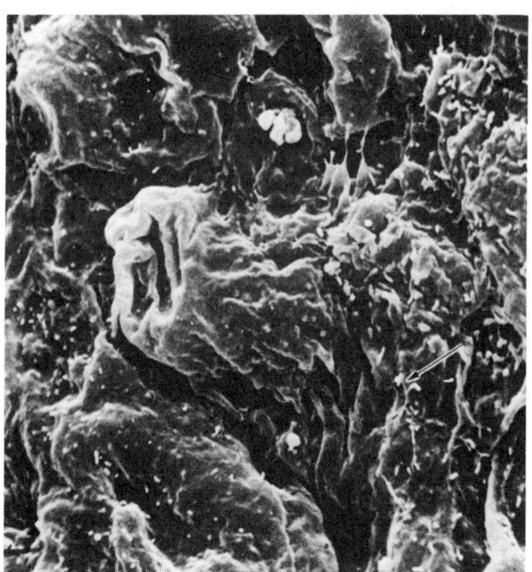

Figure 13. *Vein stored in lactated Ringer's solution for 60 min revealing swollen endothelial cells with extensive loss of microvilli (SEM).* ×6,000

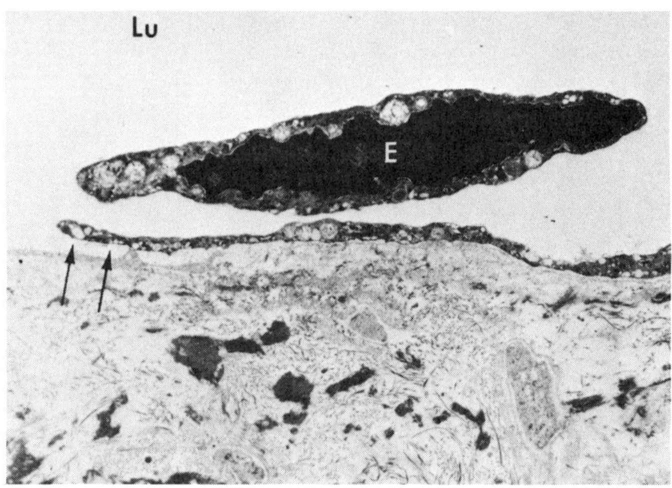

Figure 14. *Vein segment stored in lactated Ringer's solution at 4°C for 60 min. Note dissociation of endothelial cells from underlying connective tissue (arrows). Subendothelial tissue appears disorganized with diffuse intercellular edema. Lu = lumen; E = endothelial cell.* ×12,000

mechanical distention. It has been demonstrated in an in vitro study that mechanical stretching transforms myoblasts to myofibroblasts, with marked increase in cellular rough endoplasmic reticular and resultant protein synthesis. Neutralizing the mechanical distention effects with papaverine has been reported as preventing extracellular matrix formation.[1,5,6,14–16,24–26]

Arterialization of vein grafts that have been pretreated with papaverine is characterized by intimal and medial cellular *hyperplasia*, rather than intima and medial *fibroplasia* (Figs. 12, 15). Data obtained from a well-controlled vein preparation study using different treatments rendered to varying portions of a single vein segment (Fig. 16) have unequivocally demonstrated this unique vascular smooth muscle response to muscle relaxant and mechanical stimulation. Sottiurai therefore theorizes that, utilizing this mode of preparation, it would be feasible to convert a vein to a myofibrous conduit that morphologically more closely resembles an artery.[1,5,6,14–16,24–26] (See Table 1.)

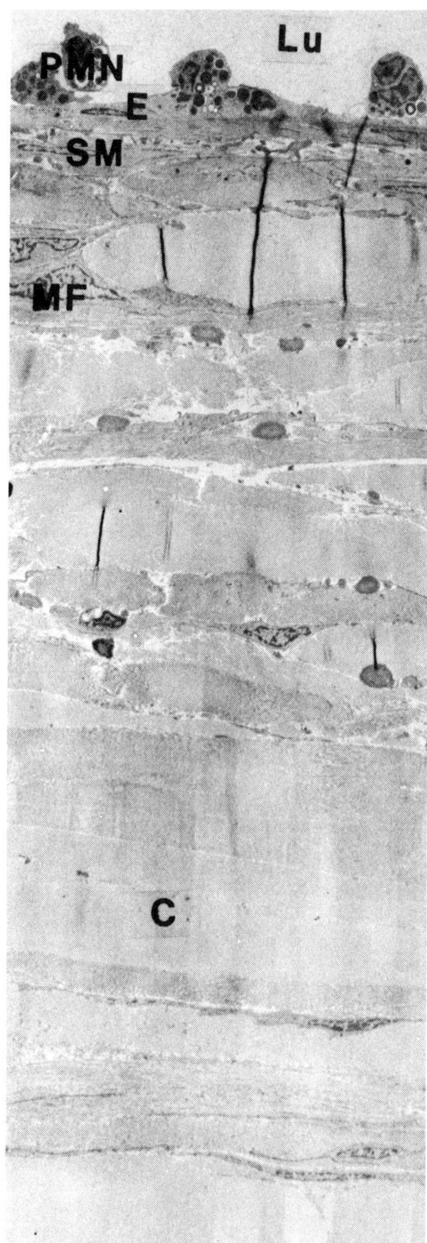

Figure 15. *Electron micrograph of vein segment distended with plasmanate to 150 mmHg before implantation. Polymorphonuclear (PMN) leukocytes adherent to endothelium (E) and marked fibroplasia to intima and media with paucity of cellular components characterize mechanically distended vein graft harvested 9 months following arterial circulation. SM = smooth muscle cells; Lu = lumen; MF = myofibroblast; C = collagen bundles. × 1,265.*

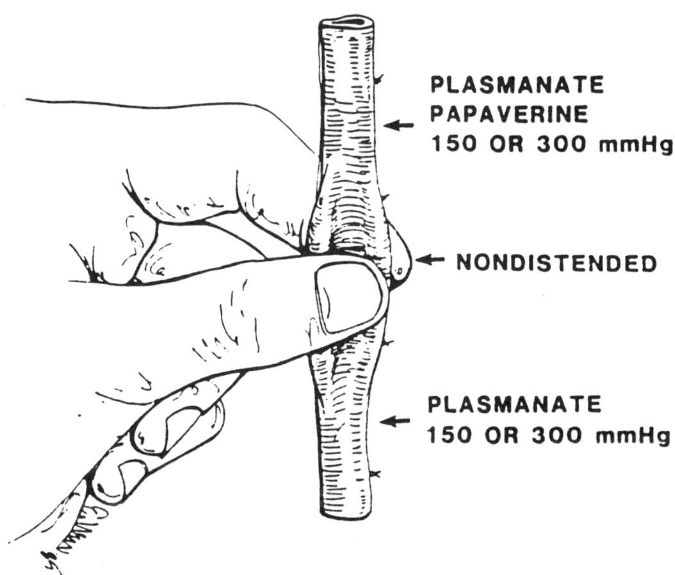

Figure 16. *Digital compression of mid-portion of vein segment to avoid mechanical distention while two end portions are mechanically distended with 300 mmHg. Prolene sutures marked arbitrary division of vein segment into three equal portions.*

Table 1.
Effect of Preparation
Technique on Venous Histology

Author	Model	Specifics	Degree Endothelial Injury
Warm Crystalloid			
Abbott[20]	Canine Jugular	Immersion 4 hr	4+
Gundry[22]	Human Saphenous	Immersion 1 hr <100 mmHg	4+
Cambria[11]	Canine Jugular	–	1+
Cold Crystalloid			
Abbott[20]	Canine Jugular	Immersion 4 hr	
Bouchek[21]	Human Saphenous		0–1+
Gundry[22]	Human Saphenous	Immersion 1 hr <100 mmHg	0–1+
Baumann[2]	Canine Cephalic	<100 mmHg	2+
Malone[13]	Canine Jugular	<100 mmHg	0–1+
Warm Saline-Distension			
Ramos[4]	Canine Cephalic	NS	3+
Gundry[22]	Human Saphenous	Immersion 1 hr 300 mmHg	4+
Cambria[11]	Canine Jugular	500 mmHg	4+
Cold Saline-Distension			
Abbott[20]	Canine Jugular	1000 mmHg	4+
Ramos[4]	Canine Jugular	600 mmHg	3–4+
Bouchek[21]	Human Saphenous	400 to 700 mmHg	4+
Gundry[22]	Human Saphenous	Immersion 1 hr 300 mmHg	4+
Malone[13]	Canine Jugular	300 to 700 mmHg	3–4+
Bush[10]	Canine Jugular	200 mmHg	3–4+
Bush[9]	Human Saphenous	200 mmHg	2+
Sottiurai[6,25]			
Blood-Distended			
Abbott[20]	Canine Jugular	1000 mmHg	
Ramos[4]	Canine Cephalic	600 mmHg	1–2+
Gundry[22]	Human Saphenous	Immersion 1 hr 300 mmHg	2–3+
Sottiurai[6,25]			0–1+
Cold Blood			
Gundry[22]	Human Saphenous	Immersion 1 hr <100 mmHg	0–1+
Baumann[2]	Canine Cephalic	<100 mmHg	4+
Warm Blood			
Ramos[4]	Canine Cephalic	NS	1–2+
Gundry[22]	Human Saphenous	Immersion 1 hr <100 mmHg	1–2+
Bush[9]	Human Saphenous	–	0–1+
Sottiurai[6,25]			
Papaverine Solutions			
Baumann[2]	Canine Cephalic		0–1+
Sottiurai[6,25]	Canine Jugular		0–1+

A literature analysis of the published studies on saphenous vein preparation, specifying the model utilized and any qualifying factors. The categories are grouped sequentially from most to least severe injury. NS = not stated.

90

In Situ versus Nonreversed or Reversed Vein Grafts

In situ utilization of the saphenous vein as a conduit has produced a better size match of the vein to the artery both proximally and distally. It is presumed that improved preservation of vein graft endothelium is to be expected. This can be attributed to the lesser degree of circumferential dissection and protection of the investing vasa vasorum. Endothelial sloughing, however, is probably more a factor of the induction of vein wall contraction and a secondary phenomenon of mechanical forces applied to the endothelium after implantation. Vasa vasorum disruption per se would not result in an endothelial ischemia but would cause a medial injury.

Preservation versus destruction of the endothelia is intrinsically a function of the choice of preservative solution. The more physiological distention of the vein graft by the heparinized autologous blood at ambient temperature in the in situ and nonreversed vein grafts has been demonstrated to be less injurious to the vein. Therefore, theoretically, an in situ graft should have less endothelial injury and medial myoblast stretching. An *appropriately* harvested, preserved, and prepared vein should be nearly equivalent, however, to the in situ vein in terms of endothelial and smooth muscle cell protection. Logerfo, Silver, and Sottiurai have independently supported this concept. Based on their experimental data, properly harvested and preserved veins do indeed maintain their endothelium as well as an in situ vein.[24]

The hormonal and secretory function of the endothelium may not have a similar reponse to injury as the vein morphology. The superior biochemical function of the in situ graft suggests that a subtle enzymatic dysfunction can occur despite a histologically intact endothelium. Malone's studies on fibrinolytic assays of in situ and reversed veins are apropos. The fibrinolytic activity was significantly ($P < .004$) decreased in all distended veins as opposed to control segments.[13] Bush studied the thromboxane and prostacylin production of arterialized in situ and reversed grafts. In an initial study in 1984, the harvested human saphenous vein segments subjected to 200 mmHg distention for 90 minutes with cold saline solution showed a basal production of 6-keto-prostaglandin-alpha-1 was 9.4 ± 1.6 ng/cm^2/25 min for in situ and 0.63 $\pm$ 0.19 ng/cm^2/25 min ($P < .05$) for reversed veins. On scanning electron microscopy, there was more endothelial injury to the saline prepared reversed saphenous vein than nonreversed vein prepared with balanced electrolyte solution and papaverine or in situ vein. In 1986,

Bush investigated whether the initial endothelial preservation persisted after implantation using normothermic blood versus cold saline for vein preparation. Blood storage resulted in an endothelial preservation similar to that of in situ vein while saline with distention demonstrated a significant injury. All grafts, however, developed an abnormal luminal surface within 24 hours with endothelial loss and heavy leukocyte adherence. Platelet adherence occurred only at denuded sites and was particularly true of the reversed grafts irrespective of their storage solution.

Pertinent clinical studies have also been reported. Taylor et al. demonstrated an equivalent 5-year patency rate to below-knee femoropopliteal bypass in reversed saphenous veins as to those reported for in situ revascularization.[27] Sottiurai has also noted results with translocated nonreversed veins that are slightly superior to the best reported results by those authors investigating in situ veins (Table 2).[24]

One possible theoretical advantage to the reversed saphenous vein graft has been reported by Sottiurai. He notes that there is a unique anatomical orientation of endothelial cells with reference to the direction of blood flow. The distal border of the proximal cell overlaps the proximal border of the adjacent cell much like shingles on a roof; the direction of blood flow is then analogous to rainwater flowing down the shingles. Blood flow in either in situ or nonreversed translocated vein grafts is therefore at a *reversed* direction to the orientation of the endothelial cells. Striking morphological changes in reorientation of endothelial cells overlapping then occur in response to the reverse direction of blood flow. Such a process takes place in a gradual and orderly fashion that is completed in 8 to 14 days.[26]

Saphenous vein injury during the valvulotomy that is integral to in situ vein bypass is also somewhat inevitable. Every precaution must be exercised to avert undue injuries because of the potential for acute graft thrombosis. Furthermore, overenthusiastic usage of the valvulotome can inflict substantial injury to the media. This will create a vast thrombogenic surface that predisposes the grafts to occlusion. Disruption of the vein at a side branch with the valvulotome also may occur. All of these are technical details of the operation that must be carefully attended to in order to prevent additional endothelial injuries.

Table 2.
Life Table Analysis of Translocated vs.
in Situ Infrainguinal Vein Bypass Grafts

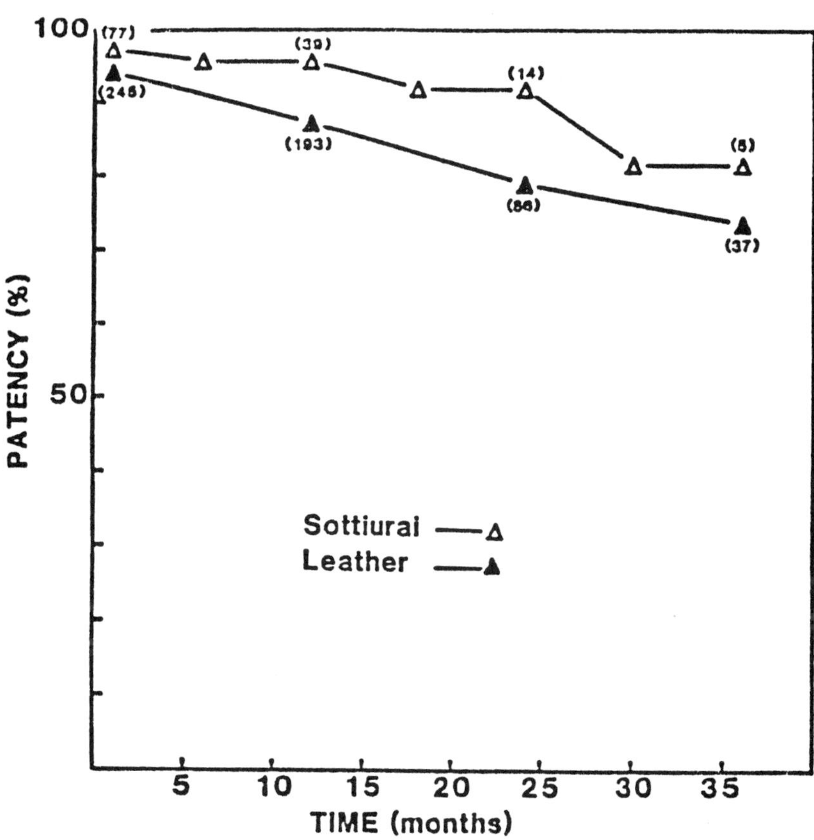

Life table analysis of the author's series of translocated nonreversed vein grafts compared to a preeminent published series of in situ grafts.

Detrimental Effects

There is a paucity of information in the literature denoting the prevalence and/or severity of the injuries to the vein and how these might relate to long-term patency.[8,9,21,28–39] Szilagyi in 1972 performed serial angiograms on 260 patients of a total 377 who had undergone below-knee or distal reversed saphenous vein bypasses. In addition, 21 grafts were recovered for comparison of histologic examination and angiographic findings. The study was remarkable for the fact that 33% of grafts revealed certain lesions, of which nearly half were potentially remediable defects. Several types of defects were recognized, *intimal thickening* (21/260, 9%), which was described as wavy narrowing of the lumen over an extensive area, was consistent with fibrointimal hyperplasia on microscopic analysis. Two thirds of such histologic findings progressed to either thrombosis or a graft failure. *Atherosclerosis* (20/260, 8%) in vein grafts were characterized by irregular plaques. *Fibrotic valves* (15/260, 6%) occurred in short segments at mid-graft; 73% of these segmental stenosis progressed to graft failure or thrombosis. *Fibrotic stenosis* (11/260, 4%) was defined as post-traumatic stenosis at para-anastomotic areas. Such lesions may be attributed to clamp injury or injuries from dissection. A high percentage of this pathological lesion progressed to graft failure. *Suture stenosis* (8/260, 3%) manifested as a sharp annular stenosis anywhere within the graft. This was attributed to flush ligation of a side branch. Graft failure related to this pathology was almost 75%. *Aneurysmal change* (10/260, 4%) was usually fusiform and nonprogressive.[40]

Similar findings have recently been recorded by Wittemore and then by Sladen. In analyzing early graft failure in femoropopliteal bypasses using reversed vein, Wittemore attributed local stenosis as the responsible pathology in 82% of cases. Sladen in a study of 173 reversed saphenous vein femoropoliteal bypass grafts, indicated that local stenosis occurred in 19% of cases and was recognized in half within the first year and nearly all within the first two years. Other pertinent cases of failure were fibrotic vein (9 of 46) and fibrotic valves (2 of 46); fully 40% (17/46) were due to anastomotic stenosis.[23]

Andros reviewed 46 angiographs of the 160 implanted basilic or cephalic vein grafts. He noted that a size differential between grafts and host arteries was a common pathology due to the intrinsic large arm vein and the fusiform dilatation of the grafts.[42]

It is implicit to all of these authors' findings that a high proportion of the failures of vein grafts in the first 12–18 months are directly the responsibility of the implanting surgeon, and early failures are directly related to the appropriateness or inappropriateness of his/her harvesting and handling techniques.

Summary

Venous contraction, endothelial disruption, and herniation that resulted from vein harvesting are commonly encountered pathology. The detrimental contraction per se can be reversed/prevented by the addition of papaverine to the preparation fluids or by local perivenous infiltration. Vein dissection must therefore be performed gently with minimal direct handling of the vein to minimize contraction and endothelial and medial injury.

Vein distention is better accomplished by arterial pressure after the proximal anastomosis; the proximal anastomosis should be performed first to allow vein distention to be obtained with autologous blood at arterial pressure. Autologous heparinized warm blood or blood derivatives containing papaverine are preferred solutions for vein irrigation and preparation. To avoid ischemia, veins should be left in situ after ligation of side branches. All vein grafts should be exposed to papaverine to render smooth muscle cell relaxation and avert mechanical stimulation of the myoblasts. The latter is known to enhance fibrocollagen production. The effects of preparation technique on venous endothelial injury are summarized in Table 1.

Arterialization of a vein graft can be obtained following the cascade events of cellular reactivity, adaptability, and histologic morphogenesis that occur in the vein graft. Preservation of cellular structures in the vein at the time of harvesting and avoidance of mechanical stimulation of the myoblast during vein preparation are prerequisites to producing an adequate myofibrous conduit that closely resembles an artery. In contradistinction, cellular damage and mechanical injury to the vein graft will produce a fibrocollagenous graft. In high flow state; such as hemodialysis access, aortomesenteric grafting, or aortorenal grafting, patency of the noncompliant fibrocollagenous tube may not differ from the more compliant myofibrous tube. However, in low flow states with high peripheral resistance (as is usually true of infrainguinal bypass) a more compliant conduit should have a superior long-term patency rate. Therefore, vein preparation is an important and integral step in achieving a vein graft that most closely resembles an artery and will produce superior patency rates (Table 3). Every precaution should be exercised to avoid undue injury to the vein graft during harvesting and preparation.

Table 3.
Recommendations for Optimal
Handling of the Saphenous Vein

Technique	Result
Gentle dissection	Avoids contraction
One incision	Avoids traction injuries
Do not mark with pen	Avoids alcohol injury
Side branch ligation away from vein	Avoids luminal compromise
Minimize ex vivo time	Avoids ischemia → medial fibrosis
Do not manually distend	Avoids injury → fibrointimal hyperplasia
Heparinized blood with papaverine	Optimal preservation of endothelial *and* media

General recommendations for optimal saphenous vein harvesting with the reason for each recommendation.

References

1. Sottiurai, VS, Lim Sue, S, Breaux, JR, et al: Arterial and venous vasa vasorum in canine and human saphenous vein (Submitted).
2. Baumann, FG, Catinella, FR, Cunningham, JN, et al: Vein contraction and smooth muscle cell extensions as causes of endothelial damage during graft preparation. *Ann Surg* 194:199–211, 1981.
3. Fuchs, JCA, Mitchener, JS, Hagen, PO: Postoperative changes in autologous vein grafts. *Ann Surg* 188:1–14, 1978.
4. Ramos, JR, Berger, K, Manfield, PB, et al: Histologic fate and endothelial changes of distended and nondistended vein grafts. *Ann Surg* 183:205–28, 1976.
5. Sottiurai, VS, Batson, RC: Autogenous vein grafts: Experimental studies. In JC Stanley (ed): *Biologic and Synthetic Vascular Prostheses.* New York, Grune and Stratton, Inc., 1982, pp 311–31.
6. Sottiurai, VS, Lim Sue, S: Comparative histocytology of proximal and distal human saphenous vein. (Personal data).
7. Nicolas, GG, Temuth, WE, Graham, WP: Preservation of venous tissue. *J Surg Res* 20:221–3, 1976.

8. Lawrie, GM, Lie, JT, Morris GC, et al: Vein graft patency and intimal proliferation after aortocoronary bypass: Early and late angiopathic correlations. *Am J Cardiol* 38:856–62, 1976.

9. Bush, HL, Jakubowski, JA, Cure, GR, et al: The natural history of endothelial structure and function in arterialized vein grafts. *J Vasc Surg* 3:204–15, 1986.

10. Bush, HL, Graber, JN, Jakubowski, JA, et al: Favorable balance of prostacyclin and thromboxane A_2 improves early patency of human *in situ* vein grafts. *J Vasc Surg* 1:149–58, 1984.

11. Cambria, RP, Megermann, J, Abbott, WM: Endothelial preservation in reversed and *in situ* autogenous vein grafts: A quantitative experimental study. *Ann Surg* 202:50–5, 1985.

12. Clowes, AW, Karnovsky, J: Suppression by heparin of smooth muscle cell proliferation in injured arteries. *Nature* 265:625–6, 1977.

13. Malone, JM, Kischer, CW, Moore, WS: Changes in venous endothelial fibrinolytic activity and histology with in vitro venous distention and arterial implantation. *Am J Surg* 142:178–82, 1981.

14. Sottiurai, VS, Stanley, JC, Fry, WJ: Ultrastructure of human and transplanted canine veins: Effects of different preparation media. *Surgery* 93:28–38, 1983.

15. Sottiurai, VS, Lim Sue, S, Batson, RC, et al: Effects of papaverine on smooth muscle cell morphology and vein graft preparation. *J Vasc Surg* 2:834–42, 1985.

16. Sottiurai, VS, Kollros, P, Glagov, S, et al: Morphologic alterations of cultured arterial smooth muscle cells by cyclic stretching. *J Surg Res* 35:490–7, 1983.

16a. Leung, DYM, Glagov, S, Matthews, MB: Cyclic stretching stimulates synthesis of matrix components by arterial smooth muscle cells *in vitro*. *Science* 181:415, 1976.

16b. Morinaga, K, Okadome, K, Kuroki, M, et al: Effect of wall shear stress on intimal thickening of arterially transplanted autogenous veins in dogs. *J Vasc Surg* 2:430–4, 1985.

17. Wyatt, AP, Taylor, GGW: Vein grafts: Changes in the endothelium of autogenous free vein grafts used as arterial replacements. *Br J Surg* 53:943–6, 1966.

18. Reichle, FA, Stewart, GL, Essa, N: A transmission and scanning electron microscopic study of luminal surfaces in dacron and autogenous vein bypasses in man and dog. *Surgery* 74:6945–60, 1973.

19. Brody, WR, Kosek, JC, Angell, WW: Changes in vein grafts following aortocoronary bypass induced by pressure and ischemia. *J Thorac Cardiovasc Surg* 64:847–51, 1972.

20. Abbott, WM, Mundth, ED, Austen, WG: Autogenous vein grafts: Effects of simple storage on structural properties. *Surg Forum* 24:260–2, 1973.

20a. Abbott, EM, Wieland, S, Austen, WG: Structural changes during preparation of autogenous venous grafts. *Surgery* 76:1030–40, 1974.

21. Bouchek, L: Prevention of endothelial damage during preparation of saphenous veins for bypass grafting. *J Thorac Cardiovasc Surg* 79:911–15, 1980.

22. Gundry, SR, Jones, M, Ishihara, T, et al: Optimal preparation technique for human saphenous vein grafts. *Surgery* 88:785–94, 1980.

22a. Stewart, GJ, Reichle, WG, Lynch, PR: Venous endothelial damage produced by massive sticking and emigration of leukocytes. *Am J Path* 74:507–32, 1974.

23. Sladen, JG, Gilmour, JL: Vein graft stenosis: Characteristics and effect of treatment. *Am J Surg* 141:549–53, 1981.

24. Sottiurai, VS, Batson, RC, Panetta, T, et al: Nonreversed translocated saphenous vein bypass: Clinical and experimental studies. (J Vasc Surg, Submitted).

25. Sottiurai, VS, Lim Sue, S, Feinberg, EL, et al: Distal anastomotic intimal hyperplasia: Biogenesis and etiology. *Eur J Vasc Surg* 2:245–56, 1988.

26. Sottiurai, VS, Lim Sue, S, Breaux, JR, et al: Adaptability of endothelial orientation to blood flow dynamics. *Eur J Vasc Surg* 3:145–151, 1989.

27. Taylor, LM, Phinney, ES, Porter, JM: Present status of reversed vein bypass for lower extremity revascularization. *J Vasc Surg* 3:288–91, 1986.

28. Bical, D, Bachet, J, Laurian, C, et al: Aortocoronary bypass with homologous saphenous vein: Long term results. *Ann Thor Surg* 30:550–7, 1980.

29. Bulkley, BH, Hutchins, GM: "Accelerated atherosclerosis"; A morphologic study of 97 saphenous coronary artery bypass grafts. *Circulation* 55:163–8, 1977.

30. Deweese, JA, Rob, CG: Autogenous venous grafts ten years later. *Surgery* 82:775–84, 1977.

31. Kurusz, M, Christmann, EW, Derrick, JR, et al: Use of cold cardioplegic solution for vein graft distention and preservation: A light and scanning electron microscopic study. *Ann Thorac Surg* 32:70–3, 1981.

32. Licalzi, LK, Stansel, HC: Failure of autogenous reversed saphenous vein femoropopliteal grafting: Pathophysiology and prevention. *Surgery* 91:352–8, 1982.

33. Lindenauer, SM, Ladin, D, Burkee, WE, et al: Unpublished data.

34. Lye, CR, Summer, DS, Hokanson, DE, et al: The transcutaneous measurement of the elastic properties of the human saphenous vein femoropopliteal bypass graft. *Surg Gynecol Obstet* 141:891–5, 1975.

35. Ochsner, JL, De Camp, PT, Leonard, GC: Experience with fresh venous allografts as an arterial substitute. *Ann Surg* 173:933–9, 1971.

36. Roberts, AJ, Hay, DA, Mehta, JL, et al: Biochemical and ultrastructural integrity of the saphenous vein during coronary artery bypass grafting. *J Thorac Cardiovasc Surg* 88:39–48, 1984.

37. Stanely, JC, Ernst, CB, Fry, WJ: Fate of 100 aortorenal vein grafts: Characteristics of late graft expansion, aneurysmal dilatation, and stenosis. *Surgery* 74:931–44, 1973.

38. Stanely, JC, Sottiurai, VS, Fry, WJ, et al: Comparative evaluation of vein graft preparation media: Electron and light microscopic studies. *J Surg Res* 18:235–46, 1975.

39. Vinni, KK, Kottke, BA, Titus, JL, et al: Pathologic changes in aortocoronary saphenous vein grafts. *Am J Cardiol* 34:526–32, 1974.

40. Szilagyi, DE, Elliott, JP, Hageman, JH, et al: Biologic fate of autologous vein implants as arterial substitutes. *Ann Surg* 178:232–46, 1973.

41. Wittemore, AD, Clowes, AW, Couch, NP, et al: Secondary femoropopliteal reconstruction. *Ann Surg* 193:42, 1981.
42. Andros, G, Harris, RW, Salles-Cunha, SX, et al: Arm veins for arterial revascularization of the leg: Arteriographic and clinical observations. *J Vasc Surg* 4:416–27, 1986.
43. Leather, RP, Powers, SR, Karmody, AM: A reappraisal of the *in situ* saphenous vein arterial bypass: Its use in limb salvage. *Surgery* 86:453–61, 1979.

Chapter 4

Arterial Injuries Caused by Balloon Catheter Embolectomy: Causes and Prevention

Philip B. Dobrin and Frederick N. Littooy

Prior to 1963, emboli and thrombi were extracted by direct surgical intervention.[1] This required general anesthesia, often involved extensive dissection, and inevitably caused some narrowing of the incised vessels following closure of the necessary linear incision arteriotomies. Moreover, direct surgical intervention was limited as to the vessels that could be explored due to vessel size and interposed anatomical structures. Various techniques were developed to extract emboli from small vessels and to dislodge residual thrombus adherent to the wall. These included retrograde flushing,[2] the application of compression bandages,[3] and the insertion of corkscrew-shaped wires.[4] However, none of these methods were particularly satisfactory. In 1963, Fogarty and coworkers[5] described the use of the inflatable balloon embolectomy catheter. This apparatus revolutionized the treatment of emboli and thrombi as it permitted their extraction by means of a small transverse incision in an accessible large vessel, often under local anesthesia.

The use of embolectomy catheters is effective and generally is safe. However, embolectomy occasionally may cause arterial injuries such as that illustrated in Figure 1. There appear to be six mechanisms of injury, as summarized schematically in Figure 2 and listed as follows:

From *Iatrogenic Vascular Injury: A Discourse on Surgical Technique*, edited by T.J. Bunt, M.D. © 1990, Futura Publishing Inc., Mount Kisco, NY.

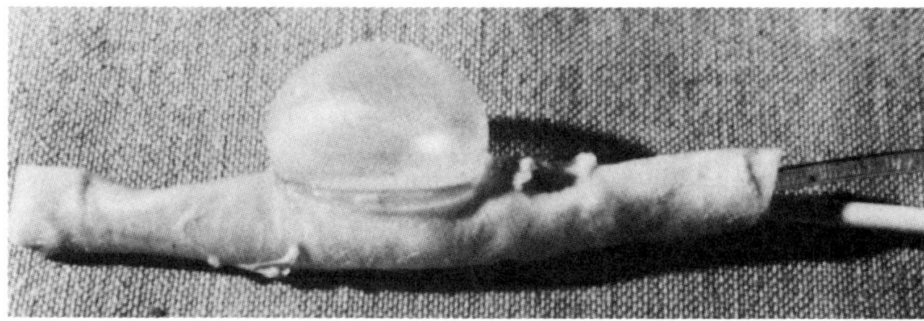

Figure 1. *Overinflated embolectomy balloon perforating artery in the dog. (From O'Donnell, JA, Hobson, RW II,[44] with permission.)*

A. puncture of the vessel by the catheter tip;
B. bursting of the vessel by an overdistended balloon;
C. dissection of an atherosclerotic plaque;
D. raising of an intimal flap;
E. bursting of the balloon with obstruction of peripheral vessels with balloon fragments; and
F. detachment and embolization of the balloon or catheter tip.

While some of these injuries are immediately apparent, others may progress insidiously. For example, raising of an intimal flap or dissection of an atherosclerotic plaque usually causes early postoperative thrombosis, whereas denudation of the intima may permit accelerated atherogenesis with delayed clinical manifestations. The initima is known to be a barrier to the transfer of lipoproteins from the blood into the vessel wall, and stripping of the intima in experimental animals has been demonstrated to cause atherogenesis.[6]

Many unrecognized vessel injuries can also occur due to balloon embolectomy, but may not be attributed to the procedure. Table 1 lists published arterial injuries caused by balloon embolectomy. Some of these injuries were treated successfully, whereas others resulted in compartment syndrome, limb loss, and death. The incidence of complications is unknown, but it probably is greater than generally is appreciated because most injuries are not currently reported. Moreover, some consequences such as accelerated atherosclerosis may not become clinically symptomatic until some time after embolectomy.[7]

In reviewing the literature up to 1976, Schweitzer and coworkers[8] computed that arterial perforation with the catheter tip accounted for 25.7% of reported acute injuries; rupture of the artery by the balloon

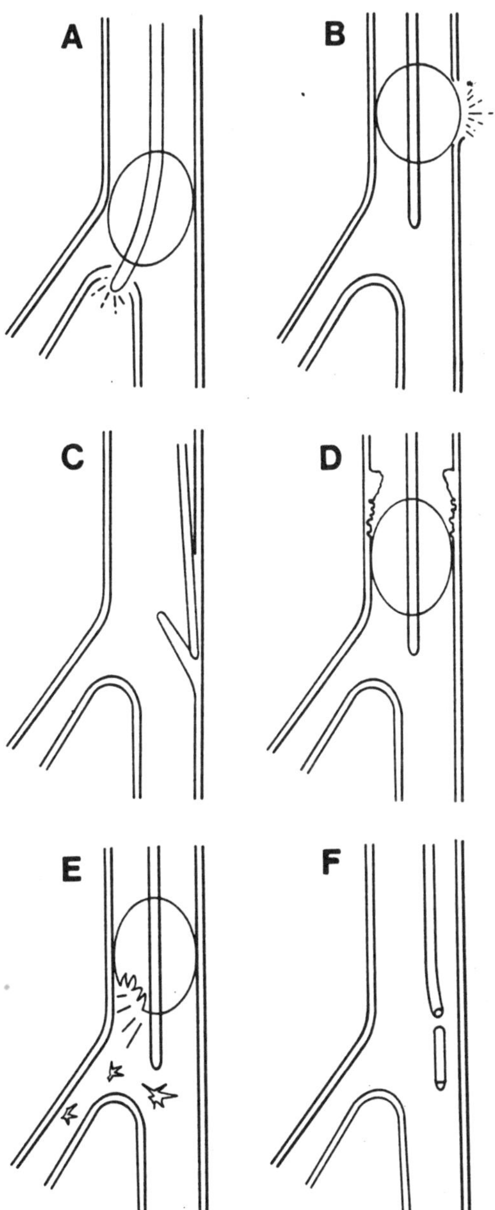

Figure 2. *Six mechanisms of arterial injury caused by embolectomy catheters and balloons. (Expanded from Foster, JH, et al.[9] reproduced from Dobrin, PB,[57] with permission.)*

Table 1.
Clinical Injuries Caused by Balloon Embolectomy

Injury	References
Arteriovenous fistula	6, 10, 11, 13, 18, 20, 26, 28, 29, 34, 47
Intimal dissection	9, 22, 24, 25, 33, 34, 48, 49
Perforation of artery with catheter tip	9, 14, 15, 41, 43, 49
Dissection of a plaque	3, 34, 43
Rupture of artery by balloon	6, 9, 12, 48
Bursting of balloon leaving fragments	8, 9, 15, 43
Separation of catheter tip and/or balloon	8, 15, 29, 49, 50
Accelerated atherosclerosis	

accounted for 13.5% of such injuries; dissection or disruption of the intima accounted for 12.2%; rupture of the balloon with embolization of fragments accounted for 4.1%; and formation of arteriovenous fistula and compartment syndrome together accounted for 13.6% of complications. There is no way to know the frequency of arterial injuries relative to the total number of embolectomies performed.

The only way to be certain that adequate embolectomy has been accomplished and that the vessels have not been injured is to obtain an intraoperative postembolectomy arteriogram. We strongly recommend this. It is less certain what should be done if the arteriogram demonstrates an injury. Small rents in the vessel may not need repair,[9] but large ones usually do. Major perforations, intimal flaps, and arteriovenous fistulas should be repaired at the time of recognition before extremity ischemia or chronic changes ensue. Rupture of the balloon requires immediate retrieval of balloon fragments. Patients who develop compartment syndrome should have that complication corrected by fasciotomy to prevent the development of nerve or muscle injuries.[6,8-35]

Mechanics of Balloon Embolectomy

Experimental studies have been performed in order to understand the mechanical basis of embolectomy-related injuries. The following principles and concepts have derived from that work and provide the basis for techniques used in the clinical setting.

Lateral Wall Pressure

When an embolectomy balloon is inflated within an artery, and that inflation is sufficient to distend the vessel, the balloon exerts a force or pressure against the wall. This distending force may be termed *lateral wall pressure* (LWP) and is comparable to the distending force exerted by blood pressure. If a balloon is inflated to just barely fill the lumen, then the balloon exerts approximately 0 mmHg LWP. During surgical embolectomy, however, the balloon is filled sufficiently to distend the artery in order to extract thrombus adherent to the wall. Under these conditions LWP is inevitably elevated to more than 0 mmHg. Although obvious in concept, LWP is elusive experimentally because it cannot be measured directly by a gauge squeezed between the balloon and the artery wall. No matter how slender the gauge, it will be subjected to artifactually high compressive forces. This will cause it to record unrealistically high pressures. In order to circumvent this problem, an in vitro technique was developed to indirectly measure LWP by using the elastic properties of the artery as a reference system.[36] The principles of this method are illustrated in Figures 3A through 3C. An artery is excised from an experimental animal just before sacrifice. The vessel is catheterized at both ends and mounted in a tissue bath at in situ length (Fig. 3A). One end of the vessel is sealed and the other end is suspended from a force gauge. The external and internal diameters are measured with a linear displacement transducer. The mounted vessel is pressurized in steps up to 300 mmHg. After several stepwise cycles, highly reproducible pressure-diameter curves are obtained (Fig. 3B). These curves are a manifestation of the elastic properties of the artery. An arteriotomy is then made near one end of the vessel and an embolectomy catheter is introduced. Fluid is injected into the balloon while vessel diameter is measured. The previously obtained pressure-diameter curve (Fig. 3B) is examined in order to determine the pressure associated with each diameter recorded for the vessel distended by the balloon; this corresponds to the LWP exerted by the balloon at each level of injected volume. Figure 3C illustrates one such estimate. In the case illustrated, the balloon exerted a LWP of 70 mmHg. The example given in Figures 3A through 3C demonstrates how the recorded diameter and elastic properties of the intact vessel can be used to determine LWP. This method requires measurement of the pressure-diameter curve for each individual vessel, but it does facilitate laboratory analysis of the mechanics of embolectomy from which general principles may be elucidated.

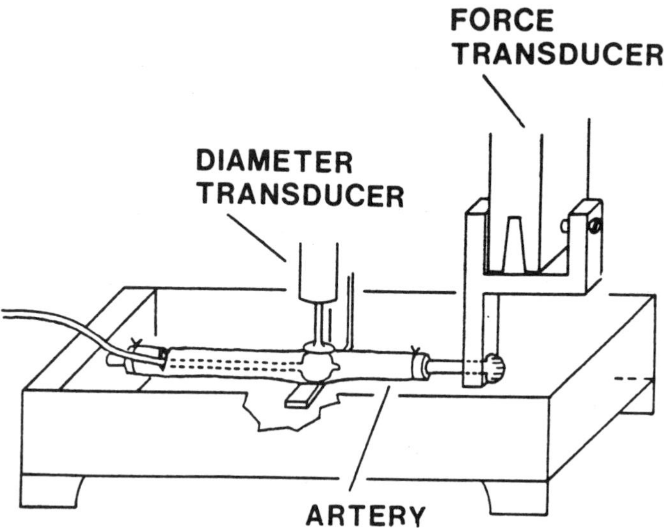

Figure 3A. *Apparatus used for studying lateral wall pressure and shear forces in excised arteries in vitro. Vessel is bathed in physiological salt solution at pH 7.4 and 37°C. (From Dobrin, PB,[36] with permission.)*

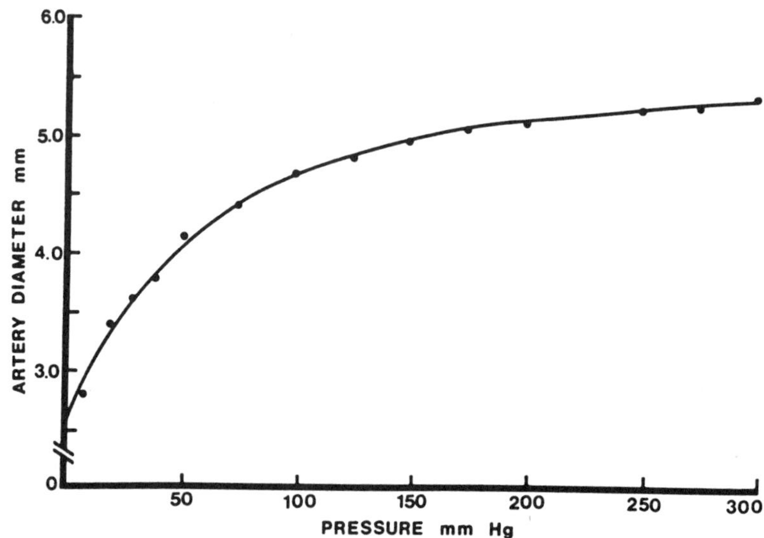

Figure 3B. *Pressure-diameter curve obtained for intact vessel in apparatus shown in Figure 3A. (From Dobrin, PB,[36] with permission.)*

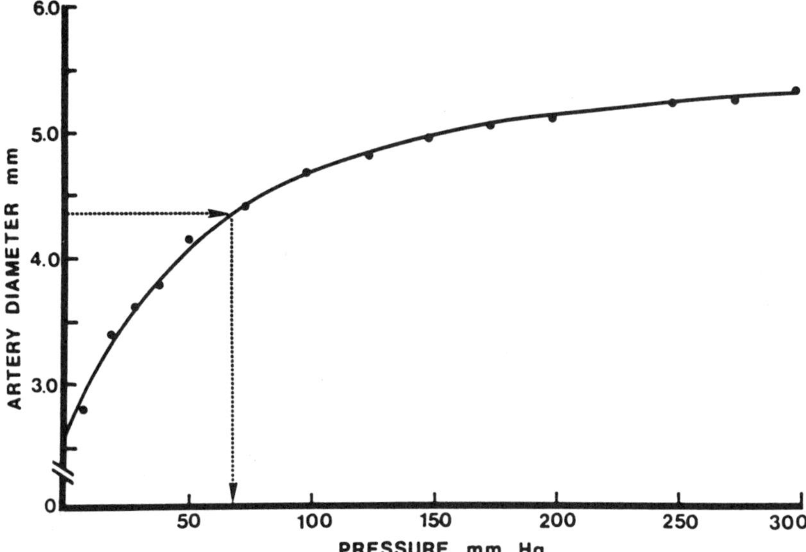

Figure 3C. *Diameter recorded after catheter has been inserted and balloon distended (horizontal broken line). Pressure-diameter curve reveals that this level of balloon inflation exerts about 70 mmHg lateral wall pressure (LWP) (vertical broken line).*

Balloon Pressure Versus Lateral Wall Pressure

Distention of an embolectomy balloon within an artery causes the pressure within the balloon to rise well before the balloon has come in contact with the wall; this is due to the innate stiffness of the balloon itself. After the balloon has filled, the lumen and the vessel is subjected to distention and the pressure within the balloon may rise still further due to the resistance of the vessel to deformation. This is in turn a function of the vessel's elastic modulus. However, this rise may be so subtle that it is obscured by the very high pressure and stiffness of the balloon. The important conclusion to these laboratory observations is that balloon pressure is a poor indicator of LWP and is therefore an unreliable method by which to clinically judge the adequacy of balloon dimensions,[36] e.g., whether it is filling the lumen. The LWP produced by balloon distention depends upon the size of the balloon relative to the size of the surrounding artery. In the operating room, adequacy of balloon volume is determined largely by "feel" as the surgeon injects volume and subjectively tests the drag upon catheter withdrawal. Experimental studies demonstrate that when balloons are filled sufficiently to give subjectively satisfactory levels of drag the balloons are distended to LWPs of 50-60 mmHg.[36] We have found, however, that if, after inflation to apparently satisfactory levels, one slightly deflates the balloon, remarkably lower LWPs can be obtained while still retaining satisfactory contact with the wall.[37] This entails a lower potential for injury with equivalent therapeutic advantage.

Balloon-artery Shear Forces

Withdrawal of an embolectomy catheter with the balloon distended produces a shearing force between the balloon and the artery wall. When this shear force is divided by the area of contact between the balloon and the artery one obtains *shear stress*. This stress tends to denude the intima, and if excessive, can disrupt the internal elastic lamella.[21,38] Shear forces have been measured using the method shown in Figure 3A in vitro or by attaching a force gauge to the catheter and performing embolectomy in vivo.[38,39] Figure 4 shows shear force recordings obtained with an embolectomy balloon distended to 25, 75, 175, and 200 mmHg of LWP. Examination also shows that there are two phases to the shear force. As catheter motion is begun there is a high force as the balloon overcomes static friction. After motion has begun, the force falls to a lower value as the balloon overcomes dynamic friction. This is analogous to what is experienced subjectively when

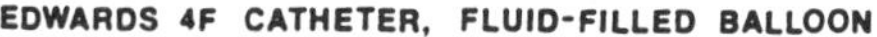
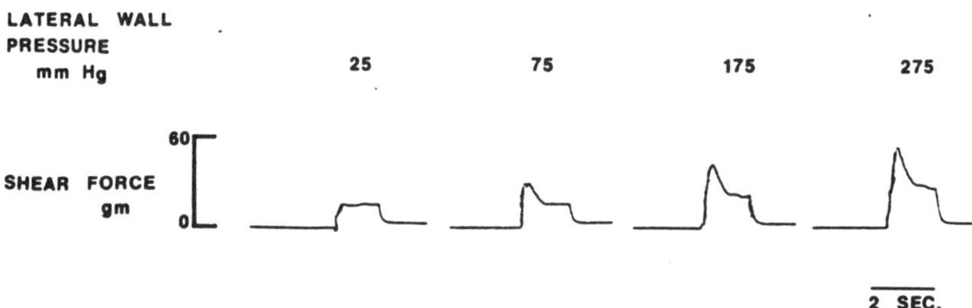

Figure 4. *Shear forces recorded with embolectomy balloons inflated to LWPs of 25, 75, 175, and 275 mmHg. Shear force has an initial high value as the balloon overcomes static friction, then a lower plateau as the balloon overcomes dynamic friction. Shear force rises with increased LWP. (From Dobrin, PB,[36] with permission.)*

one pulls a child on a sled over snow. The initial, high shear force may be termed "initial shear force," while the subsequent lower shear force may be termed "dynamic shear force."[36] Although probably not necessary in most circumstances, shear forces could be measured in the operating room by attaching the proximal end of balloon catheters to force gauges.[39] Similarly, shear forces could be regulated by attaching the catheter to a device that would slip whenever critical shear forces were exceeded. But the effectiveness of such a device would be limited by the fact that higher shear forces are generated as balloons are pulled through large vessels than when they are pulled through small ones. A higher force results from the greater area of contact and, therefore, frictional drag in large vessels. As a result, it may not be possible to define a single "optimum" shear force for all size vessels.

Long-term complications of catheter thromboembolectomy vascular injury have been reported. Bowles et al.[35] noted five female patients who presented with progressive lower extremity ischemia from 2 to 4 months following embolectomy. None had significant prior disease, and all had essentially normal vessels at time of prior embolectomy; yet they presented with diffuse severe smooth stenoses in that portion of the arterial tree in which embolectomy had been performed. Pathological examination of the involved vessels was obtained in two patients and revealed marked intimal cellular proliferation.[35]

Dobrin has correlated the development of myointimal hyperplasia after catheter embolectomy with both repeated withdrawals and the application of shear forces to the vessel. Low shear force (50 g) elicited less hyperplasia than did high (100 or 200 g) shear force ($P < .05$), and at all levels of shear force, multiple withdrawals were significantly ($P < .05$) more deleterious than single withdrawals.[40]

Histologic Reactions to Embolectomy

The histologic responses to embolectomy have been documented and are illustrated in Figures 5A through 5E for vessels subjected to single catheter withdrawals.[41] Catheter passage without balloon inflation causes no discernible injury (Fig. 5A). At 2 days following catheter passage with the balloon inflated, the intima is denuded of endothelium and is covered with platelets (Fig. 5B). By 7 and 14 days, the intima is hypercellular and may be up to four myointimal cell layers in thickness (Fig. 5D). This histologic sequence is typical of the response of arterial walls when exposed to shear forces of greater than 60 g, but

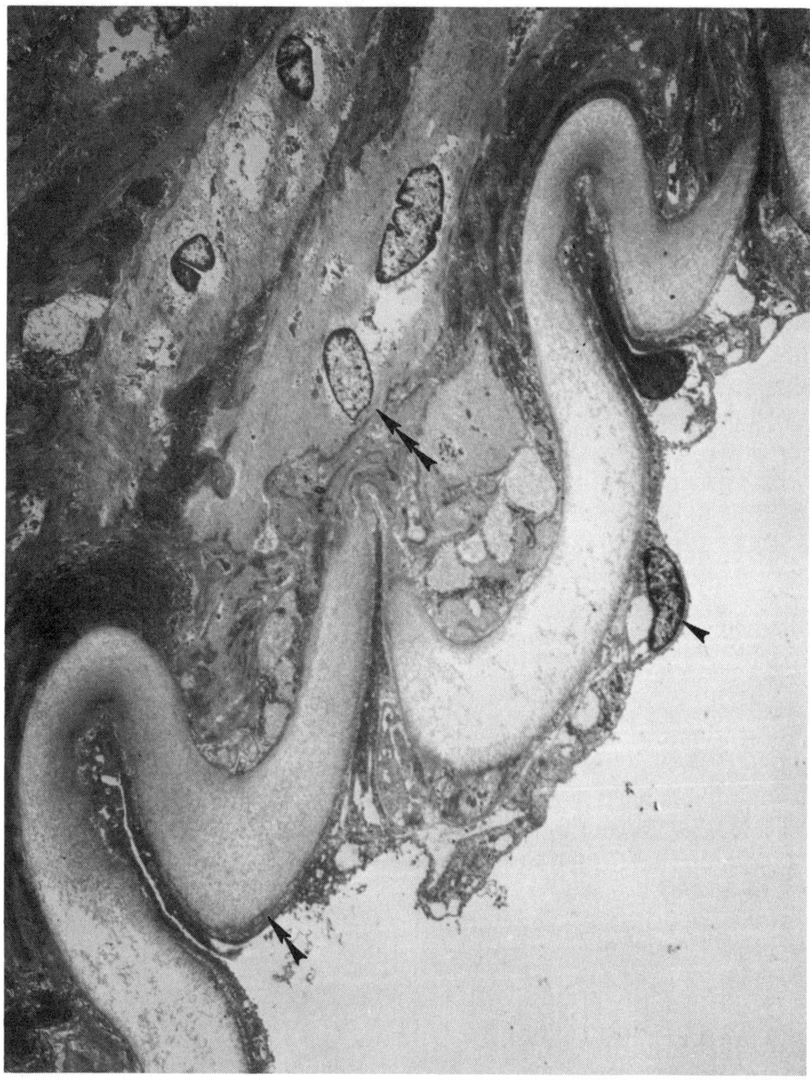

Figure 5A. *Electronmicroscope section of vessel after arteriotomy but without catheter insertion of a catheter. Endothelium is one cell thick (single arrow). Internal elastic lamella is intact (double arrow), as are medial smooth muscle cells (triple arrow). (From Jorgensen, RA, Dobrin, PB, [38] with permission.)*

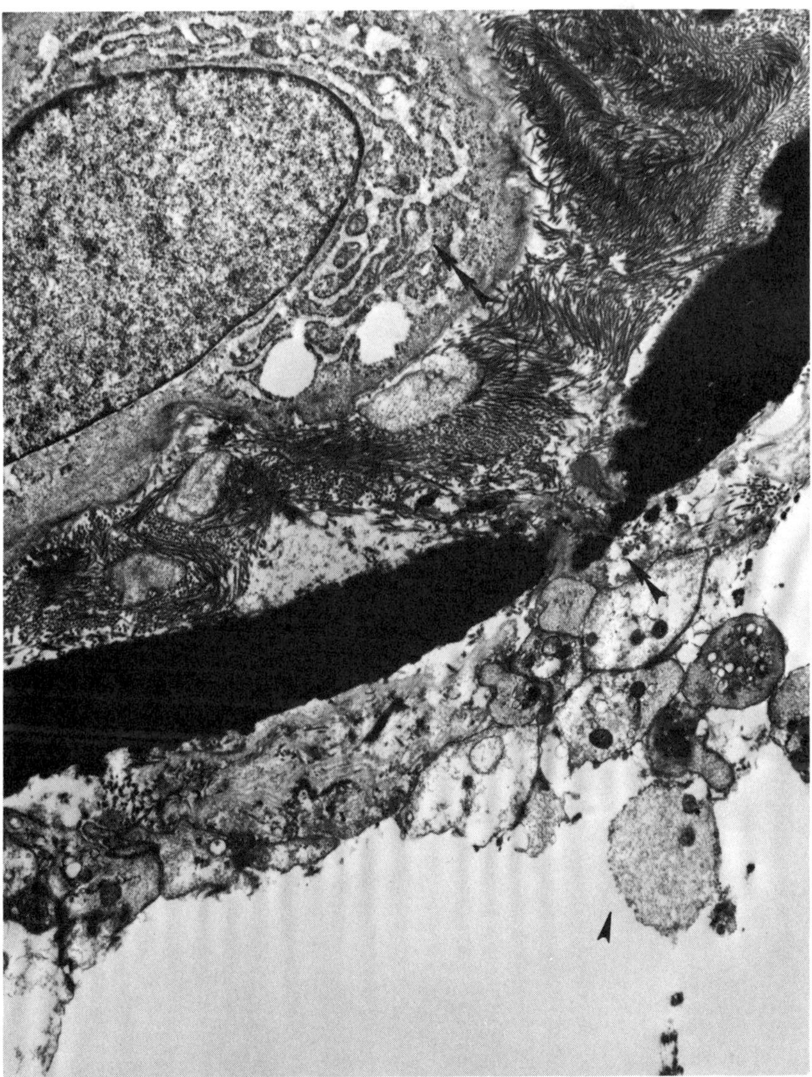

Figure 5B. *Dog carotid artery exposed to 60 g shear force and excised 2 days after embolectomy. Endothelial cells have been removed and are replaced by platelets (single arrow). Internal elastic lamella possesses normal fenestration (double arrow). Smooth muscle cells exhibit increased amounts of ribosomes (triple arrow). This suggests increased repair activity. (From Jorgensen, RA, Dobrin, PB,[38] with permission.)*

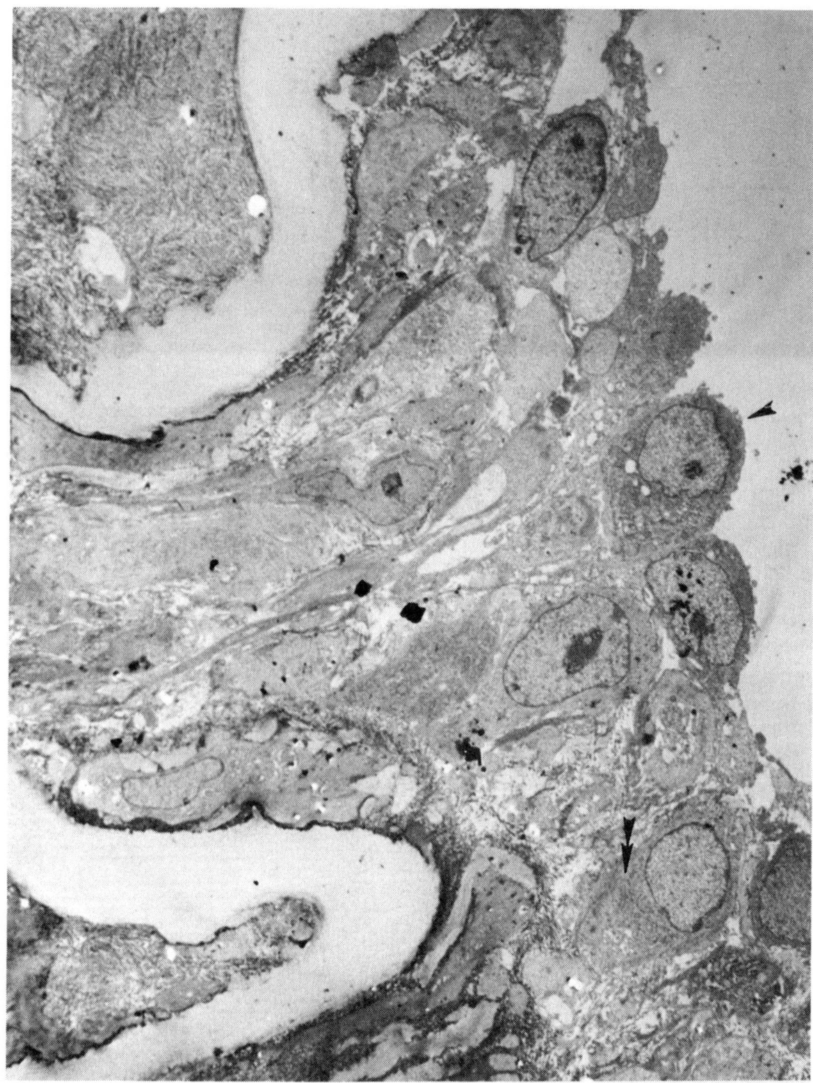

Figure 5C. *Dog carotid artery after exposure to 90 g shear force and excised 14 days after embolectomy. Intima is 3 to 4 cells in thickness (single arrow). Some of these cells exhibit increased amounts of ribosomes (double arrow). (From Jorgensen, RA, Dobrin, PB,[38] with permission.)*

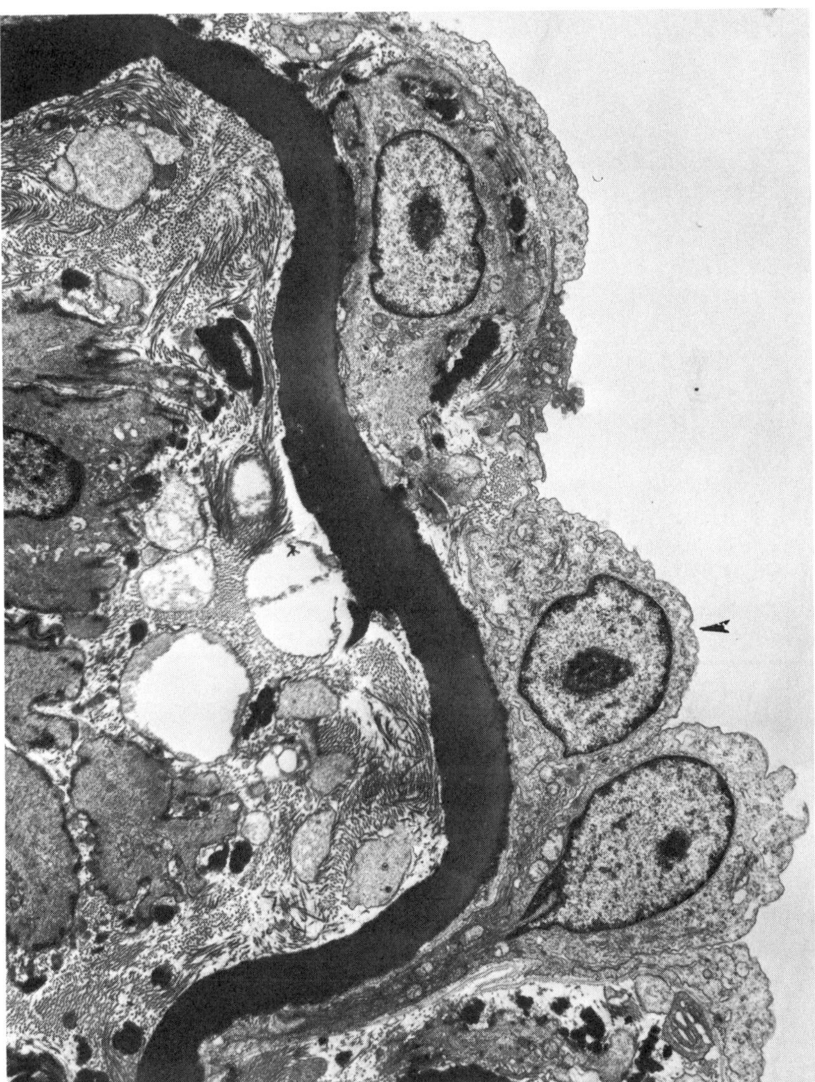

Figure 5D. *Dog carotid artery exposed to 90 g shear force and excised 28 days after embolectomy. Intima has returned to one cell thickness (arrow). Elastic lamella and media are normal in appearance. (From Jorgensen, RA, Dobrin, PB,[38] with permission.)*

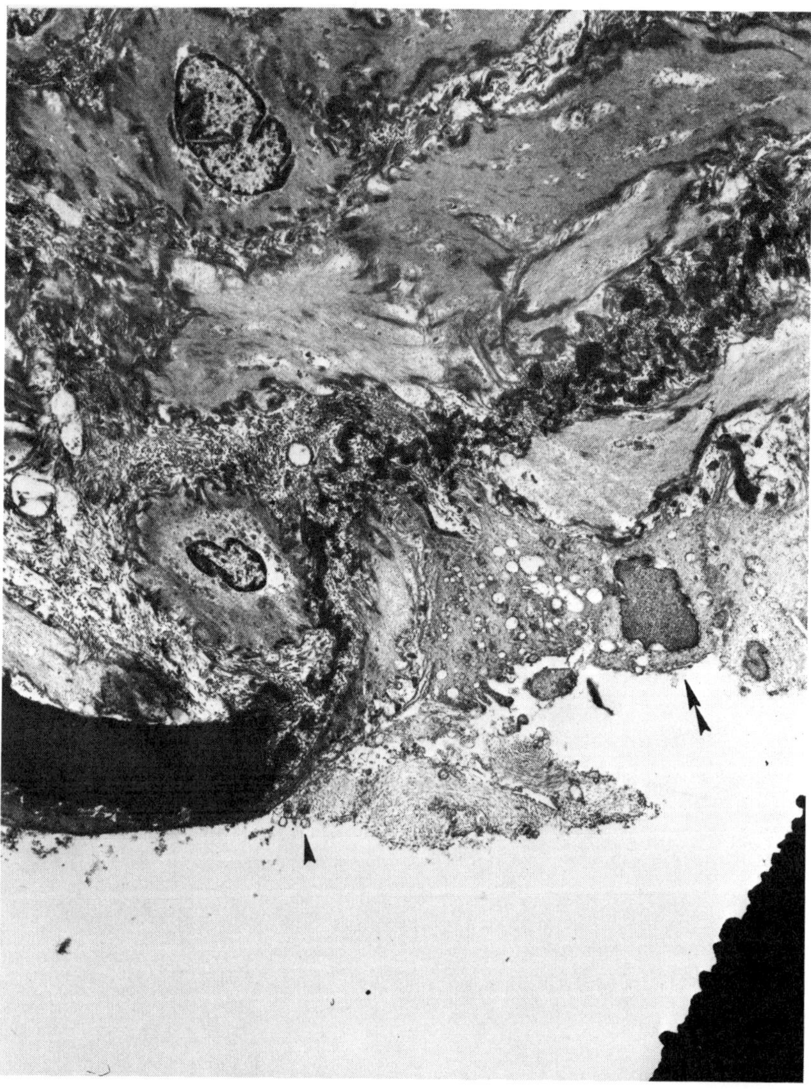

Figure 5E.   *Dog femoral artery exposed to 200 g shear force and excised 6 months after embolectomy. The vessel exhibits fractured elastic lamella which terminates abruptly (single arrow). Elastic fibers, collagen and smooth muscle cells are covered with a layer of myointimal cells (double arrow). (From Jorgensen, RA, Dobrin, PB,[38] with permission.)*

less than 200 g. Exposure to less than 60 g shear forces incurs intimal injury to a lesser degree with incomplete denudation. Although these responses are entirely intimal, during the recovery period, the smooth muscle cells in the media exhibit increased numbers of ribosomes and increased amounts of rough endoplasmic reticulum reflecting increased cellular metabolic activity. The internal elastic lamellae and media in these vessels show no immediate evidence of direct injury unless 200-g shear force or greater is applied (Fig. 5E). A recent histologic study,[21] however, has reported that disruption of the elastic lamellae may not appear until relatively late after embolectomy so that there may be an interval between injury and effect.

The histologic reaction to passage of a balloon depends upon the cumulative application of shear force. Vessels subjected to four successive catheter withdrawals at moderate force exhibit greater intimal hyperplasia than vessels exposed to a single catheter withdrawal.[42] This has obvious import to the surgeon performing the embolectomy.

Summary of Experimental Findings

Laboratory studies have provided some important principles. First, LWP is determined by the size of the balloon relative to that of the surrounding vessel; LWP is not reliably related to the pressure within the balloon. Second, when the catheter is withdrawn with the balloon distended, a shear force is developed between the balloon and the artery wall. As LWP is increased, shear force rises in an approximately linear fashion. This is important because shear force is related to arterial injury; as shear force rises so does arterial injury. Thus, it is essential to control and limit LWP and shear force.

Clinical Application of Laboratory Findings

The technique of balloon embolectomy seems so straightforward[5,19,43] that there appears to be little reason to dwell on it. Yet the severity and frequency of the complications listed in Table 1 attest to the hazards of the procedure. Table 2 and the following text consider details of technique derived from experimental studies. Application of these findings should decrease the likelihood of clinical injuries caused by embolectomy.

Table 2.
**Summary of Recommendations for the Clinical Use
of Embolectomy Catheters**

1. Use the smallest size catheter that will be effective.
2. Use a small bore, long stroke syringe such as a tuberculin syringe.
3. Fill the balloon with fluid before insertion to check for leaks.
4. Reject balloons that are markedly eccentric.
5. Insert the catheter with the balloon deflated, being careful to enter the true lumen and not a false subintimal lumen
6. Begin slowly withdrawing the catheter and, while the catheter is in motion, fill the balloon with fluid, not with air.
7. Withdraw until all thrombus has been removed and the lumen appears to be clear.
8. Repeat until all thrombus has been removed and the lumen appears to be clear.
9. Obtain an intraoperative postembolectomy arteriogram.

What Brand of Catheter Should Be Used?

There are several important differences in the design of catheters. Most manufacturers use a balloon fabricated of latex rubber; one manufacturer utilizes silicone rubber. Some balloons are more eccentric than others. Similarly, some balloons deflate more slowly than others. As a result, they are less responsive to an unsuspected narrowing of the vessel encountered during catheter withdrawal and may inflict locally excessive lateral wall pressures at that point.

When the histologic response to balloon passage was examined at comparable levels of shear force (50, 100, and 200 g) in healthy, nonstenotic vessels, there were no significant histologic differences elicited by commercially available brands of catheters.[40] This suggests that catheter selection may be made largely on the basis of the surgeon's preference, ease of handling, and cost. However additional studies are required to determine whether all brands of catheters perform equally in diseased, irregular, and stenotic vessels.

What Size Diameter Catheters Should Be Used?

When distended to a given LWP, large catheters exert significantly *more* shear force against the wall than small ones, i.e., 5F>4F>3F.[36]

This was true for several brands of catheters in both small and moderate size arteries,[36] as well as for catheters studied in rigid plastic tubes.[44] This reflects the greater drag exerted by the large surface area of large balloons. These data strongly support the use of small, rather than large, catheters for clinical embolectomy. The smallest balloon that may be expected to fill the lumen should be utilized. In addition, balloon size must be constantly adjusted to the changing luminal size as one progresses distal.

Should Eccentric Balloons Be Used?

When balloons are filled they may distend eccentrically, bulging more to one side than to the other (Fig. 6). Radiological studies show that if a balloon is eccentric when distended in air, it will remain so after it has been inserted into a vessel and has been distended out of direct vision.[45] If eccentricity is slight, i.e., less than 3:1, then this seems to be of little biological significance. However, if eccentricity is great,

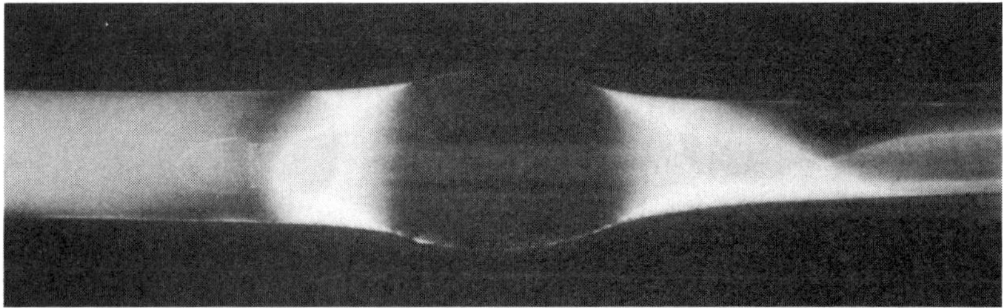

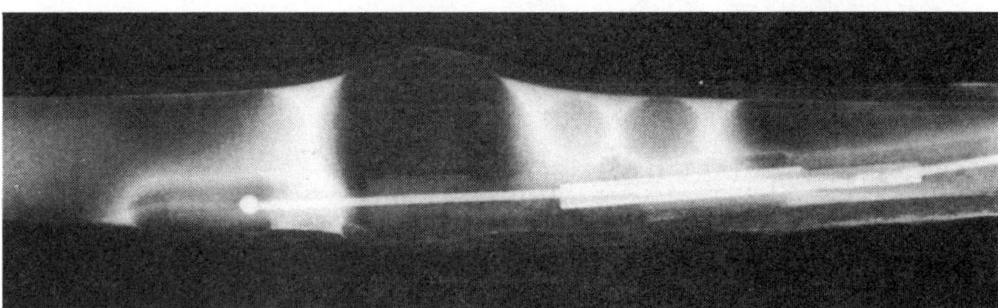

Figure 6. *Radiograms demonstrating an embolectomy balloon which distends symmetrically (top) and another which distends eccentrically (bottom). Eccentric balloon pushes the catheter into the vessel gouging a trough in the wall. (From Dobrin, PB, Jorgensen, RA,[45] with permission.)*

i.e., 8:1, then significant histologic injury can result. This occurs as the bulging side of the balloon pushes the less distended side and the catheter into the wall. This gouges a linear tear down the length of the vessel.[45] Therefore one should not accept or use an embolectomy catheter in the operating room if the balloon is markedly eccentric when it is distended in air to the diameter that will be used during operation. It should be noted that *all* balloons become eccentric when *overdistended*.

Should Balloons Be Filled With Fluid or Air?

Gas is compressible, whereas fluid is negligibly so. Therefore it might seem logical to use gas in preference to fluid as a substance for filling balloons. The compressibility of gas is not the only consideration, however, because the properties of the injected material must interact with the elastic characteristics of the balloon. As fluid is injected into a latex or silicone balloon the pressure in the balloon rises to a peak, then falls (Fig. 7). Although not shown in this figure, the curve rises again at very large injected volumes. This rising and falling pressure behavior is typical of many elastomeric materials and is familiar subjectively to anyone who has inflated a child's balloon by mouth. At first it is difficult to inflate (rising slopes in Fig. 7); then it becomes much easier (falling slopes in Fig. 7). The slope of the volume-pressure curve is proportional to the stiffness of the balloon. Because compressible gases follow Boyle's Law, the volume of gas present in a balloon must decrease as the pressure rises. As a result, the volume associated with the peak pressures shown in Figure 7 is unstable. At this diameter a gas-filled balloon tends to collapse, becoming ineffective, or expand to maximum dimensions lodging itself in the vessel lumen.[45] Most important is the fact that these changes are not under the control of the surgeon. They occur spontaneously with the catheter at rest or as the catheter is withdrawn through the vessel. The benefits of the compressibility are slight. Passage of a gas-filled balloon through an experimental 50% stenosis reduces shear force by an average of only 9%.[44] Clearly, fluid-filled balloons are more controllable than gas-filled balloons with little penalty in terms of shear force. Use of fluid-filled balloons also avoids concerns regarding air emboli in the event the balloon ruptures. All of these data strongly support filling balloons with fluid rather than gas.

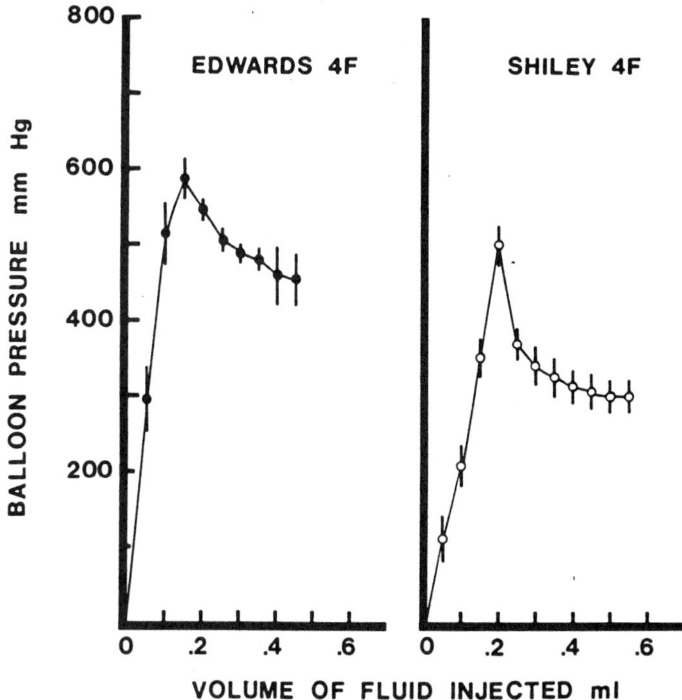

Figure 7. *Balloon pressure recorded as fluid is injected into the balloon. Slopes of curves are directly related to stiffness. At small injected volumes balloons are very stiff. At larger volumes they become compliant. (From Dobrin, PB,[37] with permission.)*

What Size Syringe Should Be Used?

Some authors[9] have suggested that large bore syringes should be used to avoid producing too great a pressure in the balloon. However, because the pressure *is* so high, the surgeon cannot accurately sense the size of the balloon by pressure. Instead, the surgeon perceives the drag between the balloon and the vessel wall. Since this depends upon the size of the balloon relative to the caliber of the lumen, it is imperative that the surgeon be able to *rapidly* adjust the volume injected. This is best accomplished by using a small bore syringe with a relatively long stroke. In laboratory studies the most precise control of 3F and 4F catheters withdrawn through uneven vessels was achieved by using a tuberculin syringe (unpublished observations). Larger catheters may require the use of slightly larger syringes.

Should Catheters Be Withdrawn Slowly or Rapidly?

Rapid motion decreases shearing forces. This is exemplified by the spinning of automobile tires on wet pavement. The reduction of shear force occurs only to the *dynamic* shear force; rapid motion negligibly reduces the *initial* shear force.[36] Initial shear force is by far the higher (Fig. 4) and potentially more injurious force involved. Therefore, little is gained by moving the catheter rapidly. Moreover, rapid catheter withdrawal risks the encountering of an unsuspected stenosis or of dislodging an atherosclerotic plaque without sufficient time for corrective deflations of the balloon. As a result, there is negligible benefit and much hazard to withdrawing an embolectomy catheter rapidly. These data support the *slow* and, if possible, *continuous* withdrawal of embolectomy catheters, deflating and inflating as necessary to correct for luminal changes.

Should There Be Concern For the Presence of Blood in the Vessel Lumen?

During the course of embolectomy back bleeding often occurs from collateral vessels. The filling of the lumen with blood could alter frictional characteristics and the force transmitted to the wall with passage of the balloon. Experimental studies show that heparinized blood in the lumen actually *decreases* the shear force recorded as compared with heparinized saline (Fig. 8). This is due to the thickness of the blood layer as well as the biphasic composition of blood (cells and plasma). Therefore, one need not be concerned with the presence of blood in lumen provided adequate heparinization has been achieved.

Should Balloons Be Filled With the Catheters At Rest or During Motion?

Experimental studies have shown that dynamic shear forces are lower than initial shear forces (Fig. 4). As a result, one may predict that distention of the balloon *during* catheter motion should obviate the high static friction that must be overcome when a fully distended balloon is set into motion. Figure 9 shows polygraph recordings of shear forces obtained in a vessel with a balloon distended to a given volume at rest before withdrawal (left), and distended to the same extent after motion had been initiated (right). These data clearly dem-

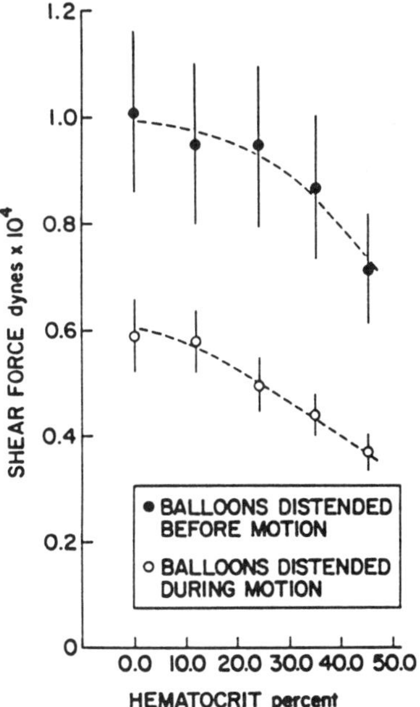

Figure 8. *Shear forces recorded with balloons held at constant LWP and blood inserted into vessel lumen. Shear force declines with increasing hematocrit. (From Dobrin, PB, Jorgensen, RA,[46] with permission.)*

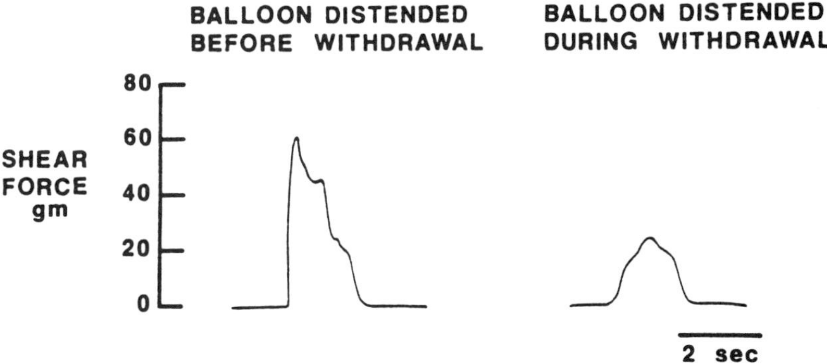

Figure 9. *Technique to avoid excessive shear force. Distending balloon during catheter motion avoids initial shear force. Withdrawal elicits only dynamic shear force. (From Dobrin, PB, Jorgensen, RA,[46] with permission.)*

onstrate that shear forces are decreased when the balloon is distended during motion.[45] This is comparable to a child's running with a sled to initiate motion before leaping on it. The observed reduction in shear force is greatest at high LWP so that filling the balloon during motion is most advantageous when shear forces are high and the risk of injury is greatest. Shear forces were reduced 23% at 25 mmHg LWP and 53% at 125 mmHg LWP.[46] These data strongly support filling the balloon during catheter motion.

Conclusions

This chapter has discussed some mechanical and histologic aspects of balloon embolectomy. Published accounts of injuries due to balloon embolectomy were reviewed, and the basic mechanics underlying embolectomy were examined. Histologic studies demonstrate that morphological injury correlates with the shear force imposed by the moving balloon. Finally, experimental observations were applied to clinical embolectomy giving specific clinical recommendations (Table 2). Use of these methods to avoid excessive shear forces should reduce the frequency of clinically significant arterial injuries.

References

1. Barker, WF: Arterial embolism: Acute arterial occlusion. In WF Barker (ed): *Surgical Treatment of Peripheral Vascular Disease*. New York, McGraw-Hill, 1961, pp 235–49.
2. Lerman, J, Miller, FR, Lund, CC: Arterial embolism and embolectomy retrograde flushing. *JAMA* 94:1128–113, 1980.
3. Keeley, JL, Rooney, JA: Retrograde milking: An adjunct in technique of embolectomy. *Ann Surg* 134:1022–26, 1951.
4. Shaw, RS: A method for the removal of the adherent distal thrombus. *Surg Gynecol Obstet* 110:255–56, 1960.
5. Fogarty, TJ, Cranely, JJ, Krause, RJ, et al: A method for extraction of arterial emboli and thrombi. *Surg Gynecol Obstet* 116:241–44, 1963.
6. Shifrin, EG, Anner, H, Levy, P, et al: Arteriovenous fistula in the lower limb in consequence of Fogarty balloon catheter embolectomy. *J Cardiovasc Surg* 26:310–13, 1985.
7. Chidi, CC, DePalma, RG: Atherogenic potential of the embolectomy catheter. *Surgery* 83:549–57, 1978.
8. Schweitzer, DL, Aguam, AS, Wilde, JR: Complications encountered dur-

ing arterial embolectomy with the Fogarty balloon catheter. *Vasc Surg* 10:144–56, 1976.

9. Foster, JH, Carter, HW, Graham, CP, et al: Arterial injuries secondary to the use of the Fogarty catheter. *Ann Surg* 171:971–78, 1970.

10. Barker, WF, Stern, WE, Krayenbuchl, H, et al: Carotid endarterectomy complicated by carotid cavernous sinus fistula. *J Cardiovasc Surg* 169:568–72, 1968.

11. Bradley, EL, III, Salam, AD: Peroneal arteriovenous fistula: An unusual iatrogenic complication of Fogarty catheter thromboendarterectomy. *Vasc Surg* 9:63–66, 1975.

12. Byrnes, G, MacGowan, WAL: The injury potential of Fogarty balloon catheters. *J Cardiovasc Surg* 16:590–93, 1975.

13. Colas, JL, Castonguay, Y, Grondin, P: Faux aneurisme arterial tibial anterieur apres thrombo-embolectomie an catheter de Fogarty. *Union Med Can* 99:1294–1276, 1970.

14. Cranley, JJ, Krause, RJ, Strasser, ES, et al: Complication with the use of the Fogarty balloon catheter for arterial embolectomy. *J Cardiovasc Surg* 10:407–09, 1969.

15. Dainko, E: Complications of the use of the Fogarty balloon catheter. *Arch Surg* 105:79–82, 1972.

16. Dale, WA: Endovascular suction catheters. *J Thorac Cardiovasc Surg* 44:557–58, 1962.

17. Dujovny, M, Laha, RK, Barriouneuvo, P: Endothelial changes secondary to use of Fogarty catheter. *Surg Neurol* 7:39–41, 1977.

18. Eggers, F, Lukin, R, Chambers, AA, et al: Iatrogenic carotid-cavernous fistula following Fogarty catheter thromboendarterectomy. *J Neurosurg* 51:543–45, 1979.

19. Fogarty, TJ: Complications of arterial embolectomy. In HG Beebe (ed): *Complications in Vascular Surgery*. Philadelphia, JB Lippincott, 1973, pp 95–102.

20. Gaspar, DJ, Gaspar, MR: Arteriovenous fistula after Fogarty catheter thrombectomy. *Arch Surg* 105:90–92, 1972.

21. Goldberg, EM, Goldberg, MC, Choudhury, LN, et al: The effects of embolectomy-thrombectomy catheters on vascular architecture. *J Cardiovasc Surg* 24:74–80, 1983.

22. Goldberg, L, Ricci, MT, Sauvage, LR, et al: Thrombolytic therapy for delayed occlusion of knitted dacron bypass grafts in the axillofemoral, femoropopliteal and femorotibial positions. *Surg Gynec Obstet* 160:491–98, 1985.

23. Hogg, GR, MacDougall, JT: An accident of embolectomy associated with the use of the Fogarty catheter. *Surgery* 61:716–18, 1967.

24. Holm, J, Schersten, T: Subintimal dissection secondary to the use of the Fogarty catheter. *J Cardiovasc Surg* 15:684–86, 1974.

25. Lord, RSA, Ehrenfeld, WK, Wylie, EJ: Arterial injuries from the Fogarty catheter. *Med J Australia* 2:70–71, 1968.

26. Love, L, Marson, R: Carotid cavernous fistula. *Angiology* 25:231–36, 1974.

27. Lucas, JF, III, Makhoul, RG, Cole, CW, et al: Mononuclear cells adhere to sites of vascular balloon catheter injury. *Curr Surg* 43:112–15, 1986.

28. Mavor, GE, Walker, MG, Dahl, DP, et al: Damage from the Fogarty balloon catheter. *Br J Surg* 59:389–91, 1972.
29. Ochlert, WH: A complication of the Fogarty arterial embolectomy catheter. *Am Heart J* 84:484–86, 1972.
30. Parsa, F, Owens, ML, Wilson, SE: Arteriovenous fistula following use of Fogarty catheter. *Vasc Surg* 105:90–92, 1972.
31. Rob, C, Battler, S: Arteriovenous fistula following use of Fogarty balloon catheter. *Arch Surg* 102:144–45, 1971.
32. Spaet, TH, Stemerman, MB, Veith, FJ, et al: Intimal injury and regrowth in rabbit aorta. Medial smooth muscle cells as a source of neointima. *Circ Res* 36:58–70, 1975.
33. Stoney, RJ, Ehrenfeld, WK, Wylie, EJ: Arterial rupture insertion of a Fogarty catheter. *Am J Surg* 115:830–31, 1968.
34. Tringaud, R, Masse, C, Boissieras, P, et al: Les traumatismes vasculaires consectufs a l'utilization de sonde de Fogarty. *Lyon Chir* 58:369–74, 1974.
35. Bowles, CR, Olcott, C, Pakter, RL, et al: Diffuse arterial narrowing as a result of intimal proliferation: A delayed complication of embolectomy with the Fogarty balloon catheter. *J Vasc Surg* 7:4:487–94, 1988.
36. Dobrin, PB: Balloon embolectomy catheters in small arteries I. Lateral wall pressures and shear forces. *Surgery* 90:177–85, 1981.
37. Dobrin, PB: Balloon embolectomy catheters in small arteries II. Comparison of fluid-filled and gas-filled balloons. *Surgery* 91:671–79, 1982.
38. Jorgensen, RA, Dobrin, PB: Balloon embolectomy catheters in small arteries IV. *Surgery* 93:798–810, 1983.
39. Burdick, JF, Williams, GM: A study of the lateral wall pressure exerted by balloon-tipped catheters. *Surgery* 87:638–44, 1980.
40. Schwarcz, TH, Dobrin, PB, Mrkvicka, R, et al: Balloon embolectomy catheter induced arterial injury: A comparison of four catheters. *J Cardiovasc Surg* (In press).
41. Inberg, MV, Scheinen, TM, Vanttinen, EA: Surgical experiences in acute peripheral ischemia. *J Cardiovasc Surg* 11:114–21, 1970.
42. Schwarcz, TH, Dobrin, PB, Mrkvicka, R, et al: Early myointimal hyperplasia following balloon catheter embolectomy: Effect of shear forces and multiple withdrawals. *J Vasc Surg* 7:4:495–99, 1988.
43. Fogarty, TJ, Cranley, JJ: Catheter technique for arterial embolectomy. *Ann Surg* 161:325–30, 1965.
44. O'Donnell, JA, Hobson, RW, II: Balloon and lateral wall pressures during use of balloon embolectomy catheters. *Surgery* 84:583–87, 1978.
45. Dobrin, PB, Jorgensen, RA: Balloon embolectomy catheters in small arteries III. Surgical significance of eccentric balloons. *Surgery* 93:402–08, 1983.
46. Dobrin, PB, Jorgensen, RA: Balloon embolectomy catheters in small arteries. A technique to prevent excessive shear forces. *J Vasc Surg* 2:692–96, 1985.
47. Davie, JC, Richardson, R: Distal internal carotid thromboendarterectomy using a Fogarty catheter in total occlusion. *J Neurosurg* 27:171–77, 1971.
48. Green, RM, De Weese, JA, Robb, CG: Arterial embolectomy before and after the Fogarty catheter. *Surgery* 77:24–33, 1975.

49. Krause, RJ, Cranley, JJ, Strasser, ES, et al: Further experience with a new embolectomy catheter. *Surgery* 59:81–87, 1966.
50. Proven, JL, Ransford, AO: The role of the Fogarty embolectomy catheter in the treatment of arterial embolism in the limbs. *Br J Surg* 57:59–62, 1970.
51. Dobrin, PB: Mechanisms and prevention of arterial injuries caused by balloon embolectomy. *Surgery* 106:457–466, 1989.

Chapter 5

Neointimal Hyperplasia

T.J. Bunt

Neointimal hyperplasia (NIH) can be defined as the production of an overly exuberant luminal lining tissue within the proximate graft and the host artery to which it is attached in response to an anastomosis. It is seen most frequently with synthetic grafts, but has also been noted with reversed saphenous venous grafts. As such, it has been recognized as a major cause of intermediate or late failure (6–18 months) of otherwise functional bypasses.

Neointimal hyperplasia is considered within the broad subject of iatrogenic vascular injury because it is a negative event occurring within the artery as a result of surgical intervention. It has great importance in determining long-term patency and is theoretically preventable, or at least may be ameliorated, by specific technical efforts aimed at prevention.

The cause of NIH are controversial. There are some close similarities in the pathogenesis and the pathology of neointimal hyperplasia with fibrointimal hyperplasia of implanted vein grafts, which has been discussed in Chapter 3. This chapter seeks to summarize what is known about its varied causes and discusses methods that should theoretically decrease its incidence.

Pathology

Neointimal hyperplasia occurs grossly as a thick shelf of grey, white, or yellow tissue usually just distal to the anastomosis on the

From *Iatrogenic Vascular Injury: A Discourse on Surgical Technique,* edited by T.J. Bunt, M.D. © 1990, Futura Publishing Inc., Mount Kisco, NY.

arterial side and extending back up onto the graft surface for 1–2 cm. The result is a fairly circumferential stenosis of the distal anastomosis; however maximal deposition is at distinct areas, as characterized by Sottiurai. Distal anastomoses were harvested from thrombosed, reversed saphenous vein,[1] bovine,[2] Dacron,[3] and PTFE[4] femoropopliteal or femoral distal grafts that were removed end block at reoperation or amputation. Each anastomosis was immediately fixed and analyzed for the distribution and degree of neonintimal hyperplasia. Regardless of the type of graft that was implanted, most NIH occurred at the heel and toe of the graft and on the floor of the artery to which it was anastomosed. NIH analysis by scanning and transmission electron microscopy was essentially the same for all types of implanted grafts. All of the synthetic grafts had significant NIH at the distal anastomosis as did 6 of 11 of the implanted veins.[5] There may be associated overt fresh thrombus, particularly if recent occlusion of the graft was the reason for finding the problem. Histologically, the mature lesion is rich in mucopolysaccharides and collagen, but has very few smooth muscle cells and only scattered elastin fibrils.

The development of NIH is insidious and seems to be related to progressive endothelial injury with recurrent cycles of injury and reconstitution of the endothelium; medial changes are also noted. Initially, there are changes in the orientation of medial and subintimal smooth muscle cells such that the long axes are no longer parallel, but instead become perpendicular to the lumen. Transmigration then occurs as well as hypertrophy of smooth muscle cells, with evidence of increased endoplasmic reticulum formation and other cytoplasmic activity. This is followed by expansion of the subintimal media. Collagen and elastin fibers appear after several days and steadily increase in amount, while the population of smooth muscle cells appears to remain constant. By 2 months the lesion has become more fibrous and less cellular. Scanning and transmission electron microscopy demonstrate that the overlying endothelial morphology appears normal. Functional studies, however, suggest a changed hormonal secretory status. The underlying subintimal smooth muscle cells are variably transformed into myofibroblasts, characterized by a decrease in monofilaments and an increase in the rough endoplasmic reticulum, which parallels their change in function from one of contractility to one of secretion. These characteristic smooth muscle cell changes are felt to be the sine qua non for the diagnosis of neointimal hyperplasia. In addition, bundles of elastin and fibers are interspersed among the abundant collagen fibrils and ground substance and maintain a pattern that is oriented in parallel to the external contours of the plaque.[1,3,5–11]

Wall stresses from cyclical pulsation, conformational stress, or compliance mismatch all have a common denominator in the induction of smooth muscle cell-mediated increase in arterial wall diameter. Thoma, in 1983, suggested that arterial wall thickness was governed by tension at the arterial wall as expressed by LaPlace's Law.[12] Rodbard noted that pressures could be correlated with muscle hypertrophy and increased fibroblast activity with subsequent ground substance production.[13] Leung noted that induced wall stresses from cyclic stretching stimulated the production of matrix components from arterial smooth muscle cells in tissue cultures and an experimental rabbit model.[7,14] Wolinsky demonstrated that only the portion of the circuit under increased tension developed actual NIH.[15] The natural conclusion of these many experiments is that the response of the arterial wall to increased wall tension is smooth muscle cell hypertrophy, conversion to myofibroblasts, production of collagen and ground substance, and resultant increase in wall thickness. NIH can, therefore, be considered a pathological variant of this process that is localized to the para-anastomotic area by the localization at that anatomical area of the various abnormal biomechanical forces. FIH is a pathological variant that is encountered throughout the venous graft, but concentrated at areas of additional medial injury (as described in Chapter 3).

Etiology

The possible etiologies of NIH are manifold—most relate to the detrimental effects of either mechanical/engineering mismatches between the host and implant or to stresses incurred by abnormal flow patterns. This is of theoretical importance, not only for graft design, but for study of methods that might ameliorate the observed responses pharmacologically (immunosuppression, platelet agents, etc.) and in terms of the potential for possible alteration of basic vascular surgical techniques that would minimize the mechanical disadvantages engendered. This discussion is confined to the latter aspect.

The mechanical factors that have been associated with NIH by various authors include:

1. compliance mismatch;
2. conformational stress at the anastomosis;
3. para-anastomotic hypercompliance zones;
4. shear stresses related to aberrant flow patterns.

Each of these is discussed in detail. It should be *clearly* stated at the outset that the role of each mechanical concept in the evolution of NIH is speculative and controversial.

Pathophysiology: Mechanical Factors

I. Compliance Mismatch

Compliance is a measure of the distensibility or pliability of a vessel. It is defined as the change in luminal diameter per unit change in the distending pressure. Compliance appears to be a factor of vessel wall thickness and is inversely proportionate to the modulus of elasticity. The impedance of a vessel or its resistance to flow is a factor of fluid inertness, distal resistance, diameter, and compliance of the conduit. Since resistance and inertness are essentially constant, differences in flow between conduits are most directly related to diameter changes and/or changes in compliance; major compliance differences, increases in wall thickness, or decreasing luminal diameter will invoke progressively greater influences on flow.

A graft that is equal in diameter and equal in compliance to its host theoretically transmits a pulse wave without alteration; compliance mismatches or diameter changes cause a change in the pulse wave velocity, shape, or amplitude. The effect is bimodal, with increased pulse amplitude at the proximal and decreased pulse amplitudes at the distal end of the noncompliant conduit. The effect of this change for a noncompliant vessel is usually an increase in the amplitude of the pressure wave, which results in a local increased wall tensile stress. Thus, compliance mismatch is a statement of the difference in compliances between two conduits that are anastomosed, and is a relative statement of the degree of resultant wall tensile stresses that is placed on both conduits.[16–22] A diameter mistmatch is equally problematic since impedance is also dependent on the diameter of the conduit. Sudden changes in diameter entail conversion of flow energies to wall shear energies.

Wall tensile stresses are a function of the elastic modulus and are directly dependent on wall thickness and on luminal diameter. Theoretically, there would not be any wall stress to a luminally matched, end-to-end anastomosis of similar tissues. However, any other variance, including end-to-side anastomosis, a marked luminal change, or a change in the tissue elastic modulus or compliance of each component, would result in significant wall stress.

All grafts currently used as arterial substitutes have compliances that are different from that of an autologous artery; that is, all have compliance mismatches. In addition, theoretically there could be further changes in graft compliance with increasing time of implantation as a result of fibrous incorporation. By extension of this, resultant increased stiffness from fibroplasia might induce a further graft compliance mismatch. Interestingly enough, the only studies that directly address this issue are not conclusive, but do suggest that there is little significant change in the compliance of implanted grafts over time. Thus, Walden and Lye in independent studies have noted no significant change in the compliance of vein or synthetic femoropoliteal grafts despite a gross histologic thickening due to incorporation. This was true for vein grafts in Lye's study and for Dacron, PTFE and vein over a short follow-up of three months in Walden's study (Fig. 1).[16–24]

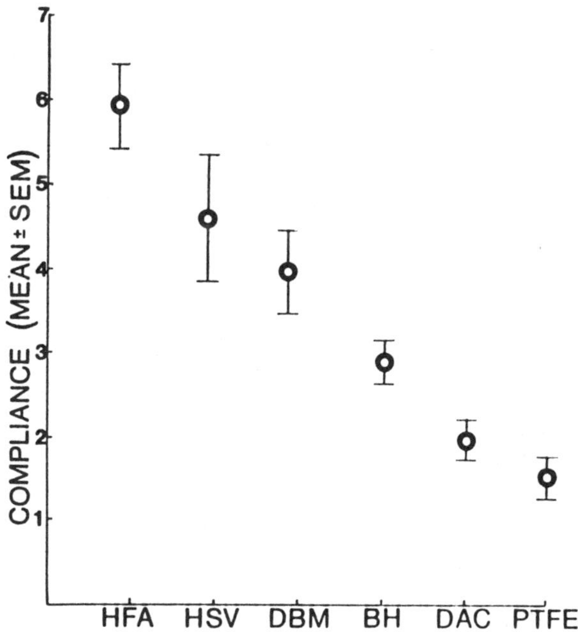

Figure 1. *Compliance (percent radial change per mmHg $\times$ 10^{-2}) of various arterial conduits: HFA = human femoral artery; HSV = human saphenous vein; DBM = glutaraldehyde treated umbilical cord grafts; BH = bovine heterograft; DAC = Dacron; PTFE = polytetrafluorethylene. (From Walden et al: Matched elastic properties and successful arterial grafting. Arch Surg 115:1166–69, 1980, with permission.)*

Literature Review of Compliance

The possible deleterious influence of compliance mismatch on small graft patency was first illuminated by Clark in 1976. Clark noted that normal arteries are anisotropic with elastic moduli that are slightly greater in the longitudinal axis than in the circular axis. In a study of canine implanted grafts, he noted that only 3 of 12 isotropic 5-mm grafts remained patent at 1 year versus 8 of 12 anisotropic grafts varying in diameter from 2–8 mm. His study initially raised the concept of compliance mismatch based on isotropism as a significant etiologic factor in the early thrombosis of small diameter grafts.[17]

White studied the compliance of femoral interposition grafts with in vivo electromagnetic real-time angiometry, noting that canine artery has a compliance index of 7.7% $\pm$ 0.6% radial changes/mmHg $\times$ 10^{-2}. This compliance value is similar to that of a human artery at 9.1% $\pm$ 1.6% (radial changes/mmHg 10^{-2}). Canine veins, however, were less compliant at 3.3% $\pm$ 0.7% (radial changes/mmHg 10^{-2}), but were far more compliant than PTFE grafts at 1.4% $\pm$ 0.6% radial changes.[25] Abbott has noted similar baseline measurements and added the notation that a canine vein measured at 3 months implantation had undergone little change in its initial compliance. The initial value was 2.52% $\pm$ 0.16% radial changes and the 3-month value was 2.2% $\pm$ 0.5%.[16] A complete summary of the reported compliances of various grafts is indicated in Table 1, listing from top to bottom as a function of declining relative compliance relative to native artery.

Rodgers et al. in 1986 utilized an in vitro methodology to study the biomechanics of anastomosed vessels, employing a pulse duplicator apparatus designed to impose realistic pulsatile hemodynamics on anastomosed vessels. Excised canine carotid arteries serve as the host vessel to which a number of biological and synthetic vascular prostheses were anastomosed end to end. Each host artery-graft segment was studied under two hemodynamic conditions: normotension (perfusion pressure of 120/80 mmHg/flow rate of 110 mL/min) and hypertension (180/110 mmHg/200 mL/min). In vitro hemodynamic measurements were taken of intraluminal and transmural pressure, flow rate, and the outer diameter of the anastomosed segment both proximal and distal to the anastomosis. From these measurements, calculations were made of the incremental modulus of elasticity (which can be thought of as the inverse of compliance) at and adjacent to the anastomosis. Calculations were also made of biomechanical bending stresses

Table 1.
Mechanical Measurements of Various Conduits

Material	Compliance	Reference
Human		
Artery—Normal	9.1% ± 1.6%	35
Artery—Diseased	5.9% ± 1.5%	21
Vein—Early	4.4% ± 1.8%	21
Vein—Long-term	3.4% ± 0.36%	23
Umbilical vein	3.7% ± 0.5%	21
Bovine heterograft	2.6% ± 0.3%	21
Dacron	1.9% ± 0.3%	21
PTFE 4 mm Early	1.4% ± 0.6%	35
PTFE 4 mm Early	1.19% ± 0.1%	16
PTFE 4 mm Long-term	1.03% ± 0.39%	29
PTFE 4 mm Long-term	0.8%	35
PTFE 6 mm Early	1.2% ± 0.3%	16
PTFE 6 mm Long-term	1.6% ± 0.2%	21
Canine		
Artery	8.7% ± 3.1%	20
Artery	7.7% ± 0.6%	35
Artery	5.86% ± 0.26%	16
Vein—Early	4.09% ± 1.65%	29
Vein—Early	3.3% ± 0.7%	35
Vein—Early	2.52% ± 0.16%	16
Vein—Late	1.5%	35
Vein—Late	2.2% ± 0.16%	16

Published measurements of relative compliance for various conduits in both human and canine models.

associated with the construction of an end-to-end anastomosis (Fig. 2). The results of their work indicates that compliance and diameter mismatch are most pronounced when umbilical vein and/or 6-mm thin-walled e-PTFE substitutes are anastomosed to the canine carotids (Fig. 2). Regarding suture line bending stresses, their data demonstrate that these stresses propagate up to 2 cm proximal and distal to the anastomosis and are most pronounced in a narrow region extending 2 mm from the anastomosis. The magnitude of these suture line stresses is dependent upon hemodynamics and the vascular substitute used. Thus, an anastomosis between compliant and noncompliant conduits is seen to induce wall shearing stresses over the usual distance from the anastomosis in which NIH is shown to occur.[21,22] An

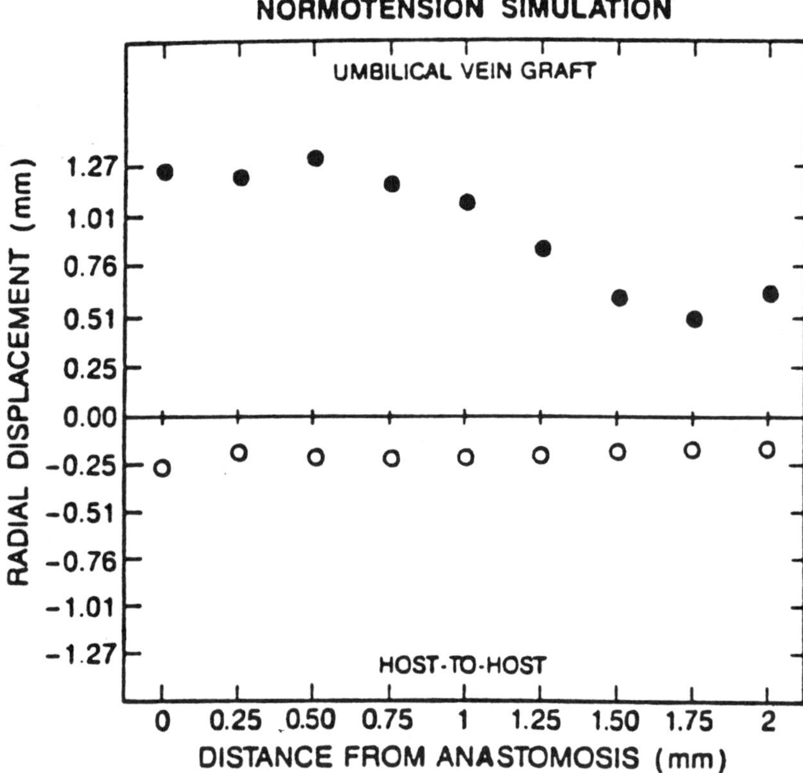

Figure 2. *The contour of radial wall displacement for typical host carotid artery anatomosed to either umbilical vein graft (closed circles) or to itself (open circles) over a distance of 2 mm to either side of an end-to-end anastomosis. (From Rodgers et al: Characterization* in vitro *of the biomechanical properties of anastomosed host-artery-graft combination.* J Vasc Surg 4:396–402, 1986, *with permission.)*

interesting adjunct of this work is their finding that traditional linear elasticity models of the blood vessel wall fail to adequately describe the magnitude and longitudinal propagation of anastomotic induced bending, which suggests that models containing viscoelastic and anisotropic parameters might better serve to describe the biomechanics at such interfaces (Fig. 3).

Hasson et al. had earlier provided similar evidence. They studied the compliances of longitudinal sections of arteries at their anastomoses after completion of end-to-end and end-to-side constructions. They noted that the compliance changes serially along the artery in both directions extending away from the anastomosis. He therefore

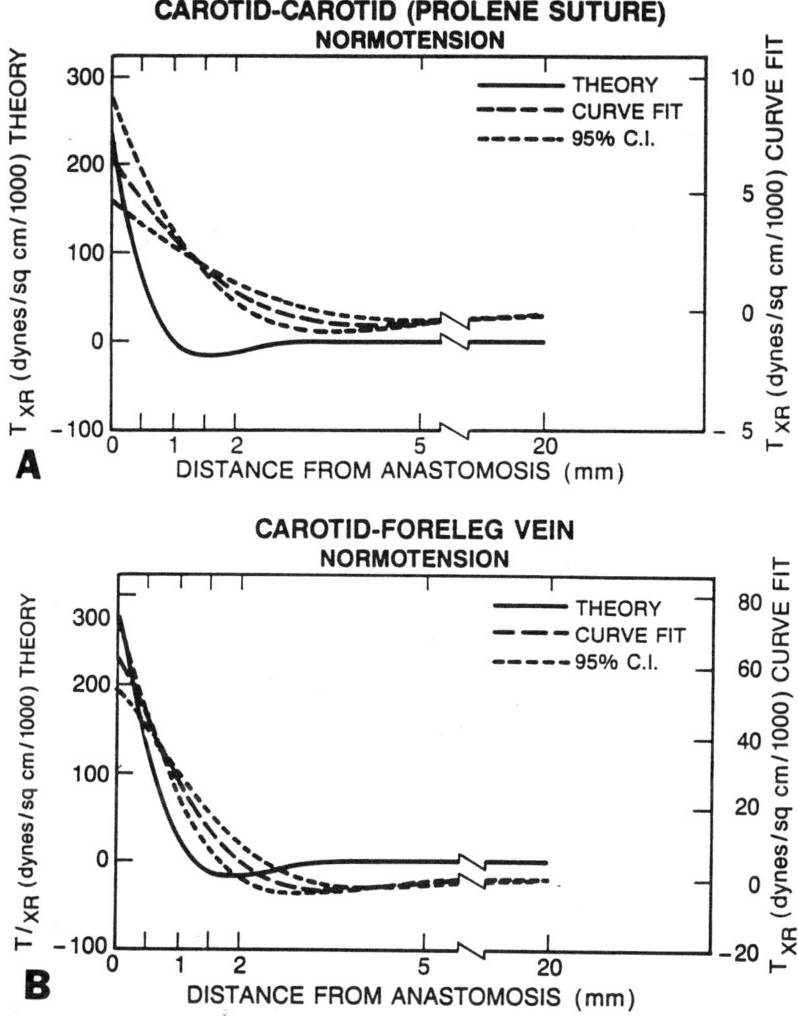

Figures 3A–D: *Demonstrates the poor correlation between measured and calculated anastomotic-induced bending stresses (Txr) at diastole for a host artery anastomosed to itself (A), to canine vein (B), to a human umbilical vein graft (C, p. 136), and to PTFE (D, p. 136). Solid line curves are theoretical calculations of fit. Broken line curves are actual measured stresses with 95‰ to confidence intervals. The left ordinate axis should be used to interpret values on the solid curve (elastic model calculation) and the dashed curves should be reviewed using the right ordinate axis. Despite prediction of a return to baseline beyond 2 mm from the anastomosis, all measured curves show persistent bending stresses at 2 cm and beyond. The absolute value of induced stress is dependent on the compliance of the anastomosed graft. (Modified from Rodgers, VJR et al: Experimental determination of biomechanical shear stress about an anastomotic junction. J Biomech Eng 20:795–803, 1987.)*

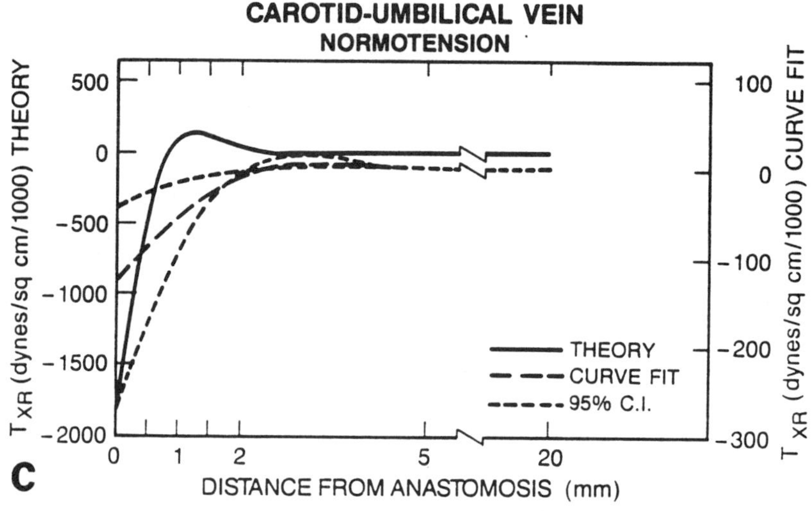

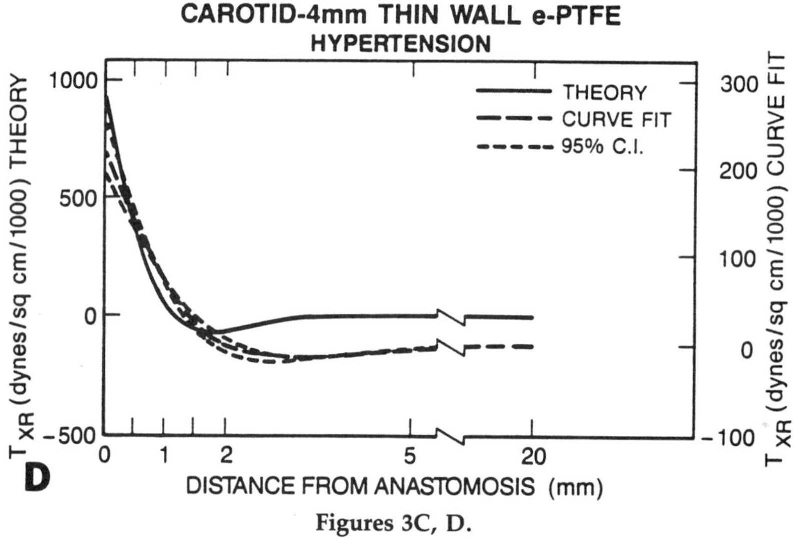

Figures 3C, D.

described a zone of changing compliance and, in particular, a zone of *increased* compliance that was seen frequently (70%–80% of cases), but not invariably, with *all* varieties of anatomoses; thus indicating that a suture line could exert effects on the artery distant to its actual site. They termed this zone the para-anastomotic hypercompliant zone (PHZ), which typically occurred from 2 to 6 mm (average 3.6 mm) to either side of the anastomosis (Fig. 4). The PHZ resulted in an in-

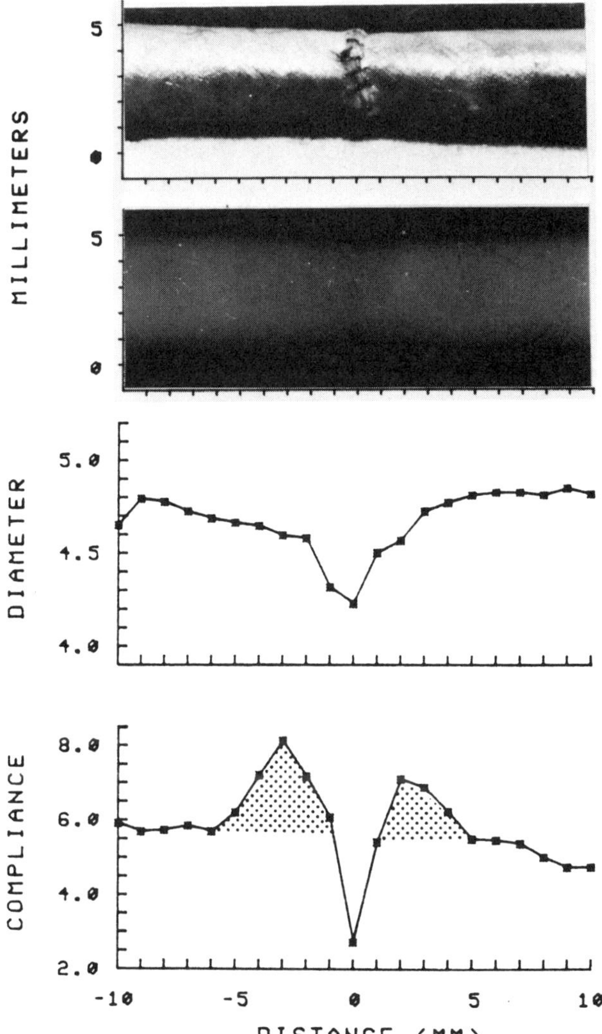

Figures 4A–D. *Detailed description of arterial anastomosis with: (A) photograph of anastomosis constructed with continuous suture; (B) angiogram illustrating control of luminal wall; (C) ultrasonically measured diameter versus distance from the anastomosis; and (D) compliance versus distance. Location of anastomosis is designated 0mm. Regions of PHZ in which values of compliance are greater than references are stippled for emphasis. Units of compliance are % radial change/mmHg × 10^{-2}, diameter is in mm. (From Hasson et al: Increased compliance near vascular anastomoses. J Vasc Surg 2:419–24, 1985, with permission.)*

creased compliance mismatch at precisely the approximate para-anastomotic anatomical area where neointimal hyperplasia ordinarily is seen. The effect of the PHZ is an increased cyclical stretch with resultant increased wall stresses applied to a very focal area in a fairly circumferential fashion. In addition, the fact that PHZ occurs *proximally* to the anastomosis helps to explain why NIH also occurs proximally as well as distal to an anastomosis. PHZ is, in part, a reflection of the transmission of longitudinal stress from the pulse wave across the anastomosis and the generation of reflected waves. Since this should be equal in both directions, but PHZ was more common distally, would indicate that it does not completely describe the phenomenon.[18]

Hasson, in a follow-up study, noted that PHZ occurred in end-to-end and end-to-side anastomoses and was independent of the exact suture technique. However, anastomotic diameter was better maintained by the interrupted technique. He also noted that a continuous suture induced a greater compliance mismatch (averaging 50%) at the anastomosis and that the compliance mismatch was further augmented if a PHZ was also generated. The implications of these studies for the choice of interrupted versus continuous suture in vascular anastomoses seems clear.[19]

Related information about the effect of an anastomosis on local compliance has been provided by Klein, who studied the effect of continuous and interrupted sutures in a canine femoral reanastomosis model. Compliance was measured before anastomosis and at 1 cm proximal and distal to the anastomosis after completion. Compliance was decreased in both models with a significantly (P <.01) *greater* decrease with a running suture as opposed to interrupted sutures. Thus, although the anastomosis of two mechanically and size matched conduits theoretically should *not* result in a compliance mismatch, the presence of an anastomosis per se, at least with synthetic suture, changes the mechanical characteristics of the conduit and induces a relative compliance mismatch.[20]

Clinical correlation of compliance mismatches with graft patency rates has also been noted. Walden, in 1980, compared ex vivo human femoral arteries to various implanted grafts and correlated their compliances with known patency rates when utilized as femoropopliteal bypass grafts (Fig. 1). He noted that increasing patency rates correlated well with a decreased disparity between the conduit compliance and that of the host femoral artery. All conduits were significantly (P <.05) less compliant than autologous artery (see Table 2).[24]

Table 2.
Ratios of Graft-to-Host Biomechanical Properties

Normotension Category	n	D_G/D_H*	E_G/E_H
Carotid—carotid (prolene suture)	6	0.99 ± 0.04	1
Carotid—umbilical vein	5	1.55 ± 0.12	1.98
Carotid—carotid (Gore-Tex suture)	6	1.00 ± .01	1
Carotid—4mm thin wall e-PTFE	6	1.01 ± .03	5.05
Carotid—6mm thin wall e-PTFE	6	2.05 ± 0.06	26.7
Carotid—foreleg vein	4	0.98 ± .01	6.16
Hypertension Category	n	D_G/D_H*	E_G/E_H
Carotid-Carotid (Prolene suture)	8	0.95 ± .02	1
Carotid—umbilical vein	6	1.44 ± .12	0.94
Carotid—carotid (Gore-Tex suture)	6	0.99 ± .01	1
Carotid—4mm thin wall e-PTFE	6	0.93 ± .04	2.04
Carotid—6mm thin wall e-PTFE	6	1.66 ± .07	16.1
Carotid—foreleg vein	5	1.05 ± .08	6.27

*Mean ± SEM

Describes the ratios of graft-to-host biomechanical properties under conditions of normotension (top) and hypertension (bottom) for various conduits anastomosed end-to-end to canine carotid artery. D = diameter; E = elastic modulus. D_G/D_H is the ratio of values at host vessel at 2 cm, and graft vessel at 2 cm. E_G/E_H represents the ratio of elastic modulus of graft to that of host. (Modified from Rodgers et al.: Characterization *In vitro* of the Biomechanical Properties of Anastomosed Host Artery-Graft Combinations. J Vasc Surg 4:396–402, 1986.)

II. Conformational Stresses

Anastomoses may be constructed in end-to-end or end-to-side configurations. The routine end-to-end anastomosis is done with spatulation of the two ends to allow luminal matching, or even some increased luminal diameter at the anastomosis, in an effort to avoid constriction. However, the match has to be quite exact; overzealous spatulation will result in a wall shear stress as outlined below.

Alternatively, the anastomosis may be constructed with interrupted sutures rather than with continuous sutures. This not only allows a more exact matching of the two ends but may result in a decreased wall stress.

Literature Review

Pomposelli has noted interesting information regarding the possible role of conformational stress, particular as it regards the aberrant flow characteristics of cobra head anastomoses. When an arteriotomy is sutured to the graft cobra head, the artery must open up to accommodate the graft, which effectively increases its local radius of the curvature (Fig. 5)—LaPlace's Law relates wall tension to the product of pressure and the radius of curvature and dictates that there will be an increased wall tension at the splayed out anastomotic area. Pomposelli placed plastic inserts into the thoracic aortas of rabbits to induce a conformational change from circular to ellipsoidal without altering flow characteristics or introducing compliance changes that might be incurred by a suture line (Fig. 6). The inserts were calculated

Cross-section of Anastomosis

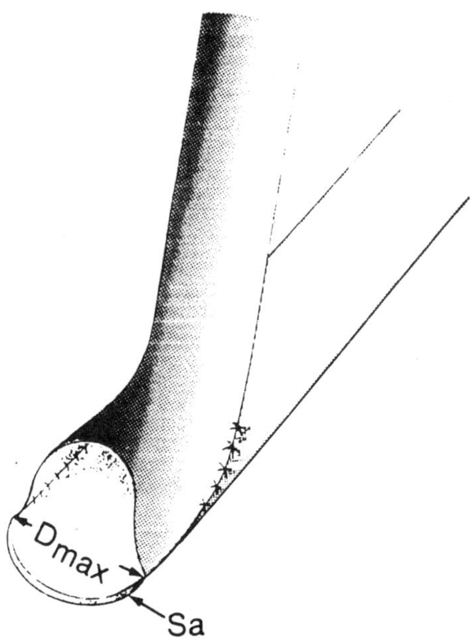

Figure 5. *A cross-section through a typical cobra head end-to-side distal anastomosis showing the effective increase in arterial diameter at the anastomosis. D max = maximal diameter; Sa = arterial segment. (From Pomposelli et al: Conformational stress and anastomotic hyperplasia. J Vasc Surg 1:525–34, 1984, with permission.)*

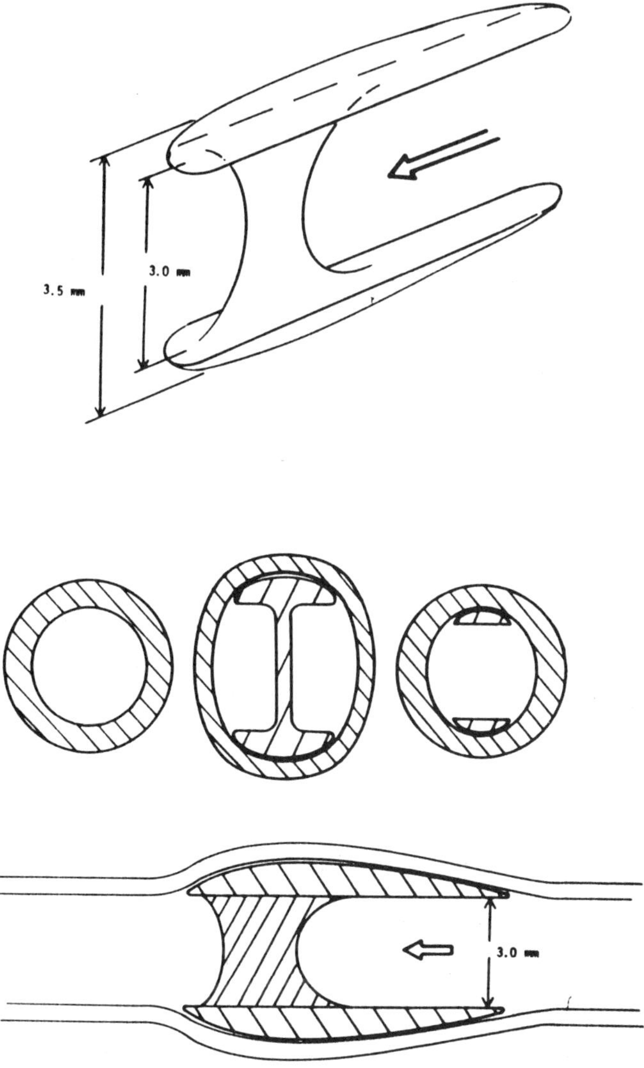

Figure 6. *Three-dimensional and cross-sectional views of an insert placed in rabbit aortas to cause a local increased conformational stress equivalent to that induced in a 4-mm artery by an end-to-side anastomosis. Heavy arrows demonstrate directions of flow. (From Pomposelli et al: Conformational stress and anastomotic hyperplasia. J Vasc Surg 1:525–34, 1984, with permission.)*

to increase wall tension by 80%–100%. This was the calculated theoretical wall stress that would be induced by an anastomosis of a 4- to 6-mm synthetic graft to an artery ranging in size from 3 to 5 mm.

There were several findings from the study. Harvest of the aortas at 3 days to 6 months revealed a progressive development of a subintimal lesion that was histologically compatible with NIH, was reliably produced in all models, and varied from 150–800 microns in thickness (normal intimal thickness being 200 microns). There was no plaque in two controls who had inserts placed and then immediately removed after several minutes.

Pomposelli also calculated the theoretical stresses that would be incurred by anastomosis of variably sized grafts and variably sized arteries and noted that there was a direct correlation in the amount of wall shear stress created by the anastomosis and the subsequent development of NIH. The critical size of the artery did not scale linearly with the size of the attached prosthesis, but had a precipitous increase at critical diameters that averaged 4-mm artery sizes for 4-mm prostheses and 4- to 4.5-mm artery size for 6-mm prosthesis (Fig. 7).[26]

Madras has emphasized the importance of diameter matching as being equally important as compliance matching, noting that impedance varies with the length of the diameter raised to the power of 2.5, and the square root of the elasticity. He notes that there is a finite limit to size matching of conduits to very small arteries and that the cobra head configuration of anastomoses places undue conformational stress on the artery with an average 200%–300% increase in wall tension. This far exceeds calculated stresses from mismatched elastic noduli. Thus, the mere performance of a cobra head variety of anastomosis, as is standardly performed, must inevitably increase the effective arterial diameter at the anastomosis and, thereby, cause a wall shear stress due to increased wall tension. Although it was designed to improve flow at a distal anastomosis, the cobra head may actually be detrimental due to the wall stresses it imposes, and these may be the critical determinants of patency in small vessels.[27]

Zarins, using a high cholesterol diet-induced atherogenic baboon model, has noted the effect of chronic cyclic stretching as a major etiologic factor in the development of atherosclerosis. The theoretics of that data seem applicable to the development of NIH. Cyclic stretching causes local wall shear stresses and an effective local endothelial injury that is associated with increased intimal collagen synthesis and an

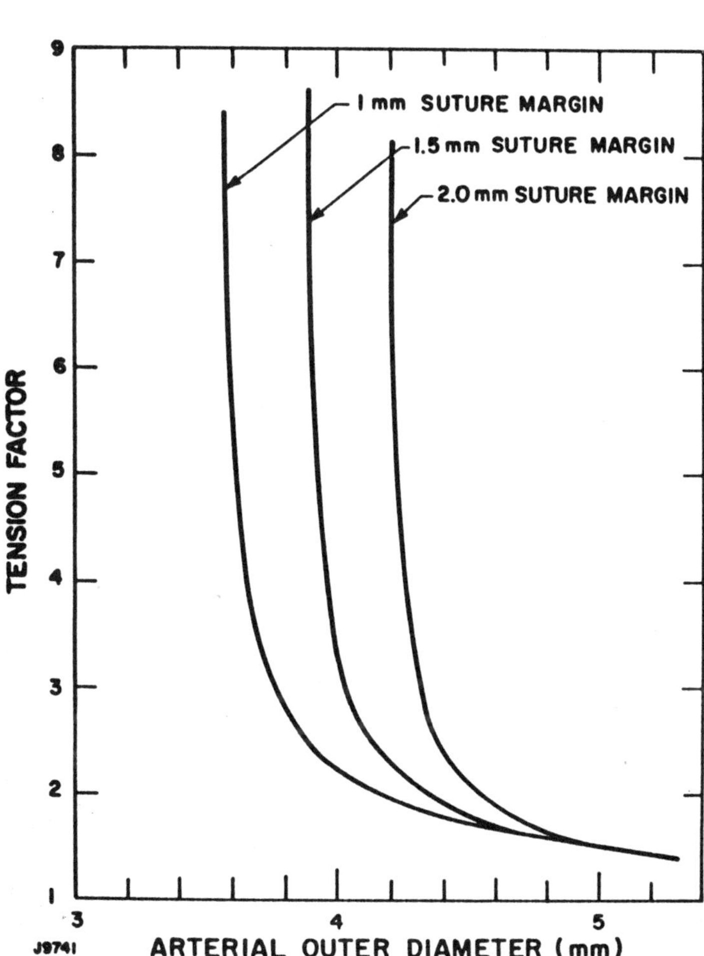

Figure 7. *Demonstrates tension curves for arterial walls of vessels with a diameter 3 to 5 mm at end-to-side anastomosis with a 6-mm synthetic graft, utilizing three different suture margins. Wall tension does not correlate linearly with the arterial outside diameter, but reaches a threshold at 4 to 4.5 mm. More tension is applied by a suture line of deeper (2 mm) bites than by one with smaller bites. (From Pomposelli et al: Conformational stress and anastomotic hyperplasia. J Vasc Surg 1:525–34, 1984, with permission.)*

increased permeability of the endothelium. Reduction in aortic wall motion by either external constricting bands or surgical coarctation of the thoracic aorta resulted in a markedly decreased intimal injury distal to the coarctations and, therefore, a decreased formation of atherosclerotic plaque despite the high cholesterol diet. Aortic wall motion decreased from 0.42 ± 0.02 mm to 0.23 ± 0.03 mm (P <.001): this correlated with a decrease in normal systolic/diastolic aortic diameter change from $6.4\% \pm 0.5\%$ to $3.1\% \pm 0.5\%$.[28]

Cyclic wall stretching may be a component mechanical problem in NIH formation when a conduit is exposed to new stresses. Examples include an arterialized vein graft, or the vein just distal to a newly formed arteriovenous dialysis fistula; situations in which the distal vessel previously protected from pulsatile flow by proximal occlusive disease is newly re-exposed to arterial pressures by newly established graft flow; and in locally endarterectomized segments with decreased wall tensile strengths due to the endarterectomy.

III. Flow Shear Stresses

Flow through a nonbranched, uniform diameter artery follows concentric laminae with fast central velocities and serially slower velocities with increasing exterior radius. Laminar flow is disrupted by subsequent branches or by abrupt changes in diameter. Arterial bifurcations are, therefore, associated with an increased atherogenesis based on disruptions of laminar flow. The same theorems can be applied to the effects of anastomoses (which are essentially iatrogenic branches) and their effects on flow. Flow disturbances might theoretically produce an endothelial injury by high shear stresses or could induce areas of low shear stress due to stagnant flow associated with increased platelet deposition. High shear stresses have been dismissed by most authors as not being a significant factor since normal biological systems do not attain sufficiently high shear stress. However, low shear stresses *have* been demonstrated to be a significant factor.

Imparato, in 1972, noted that neointimal hyperplasia occurred at such disparate situations as the apex of a long patch used to close a superficial femoral artery endarterectomy, at vein patches for aortorenal bypass grafting, in branch renal vessels just distal to a renal endarterectomy, and in the common femoral artery distal to an aortobifemoral graft onlay anastomosis. He suggested that NIH could occur in either a high flow or low flow situation and suggested that this might be related to differential wall shear stress. Experimentally, he constructed several canine models, most notably a renal artery fistula into the inferior vena cava, and demonstrated predictable development of NIH at various points of the model that were uninvolved in the direct surgical dissection. These were above and below the right renal artery origin from the aorta and extending for approximately 0.5 cm at the proximal end and at the inferior vena cava anastomosis. He related this to the geometry of flow and suggested angulation-related flow stresses related to the surgical change in arterial position and resultant flow characteristics.[29]

Berguer in 1980 also implicated low flow as a cause of intimal hyperplasia, although the study related more indirectly to the formation of fibrointimal hyperplasia with vein grafts. He noted that the flows within coronary artery bypass graft saphenous veins averaged only 60 cc/min while flows in femorotibial grafts performed with the same material averaged 90–100 cc/min; the incidence of fibrointimal hyperplasia (FIH) is well recognized to be much higher in coronary artery bypass grafting than in distal revascularization. To prove his hypothesis that low flow was the predominant problem, he implanted veins in canine carotid arteries in a complex model that varied the velocity of flow and was able to correlate the development of FIH with the absolute velocity. In a low flow situation (14 $\pm$ 65 cc/min), FIH developed at an average of 94.2 $\pm$ 75.8 microns of intimal thickening, while high flow situations (200 $\pm$ 75 cc/min) developed an average 1.8 $\pm$ 19.9 microns of intimal thickening (P <.005). However, significantly, he could not specifically correlate the amount of flow with the degree of FIH that developed.[30] The findings have relevance to the more isolated development of NIH at anastomoses based on low flow shear stresses as will be discussed below.

Morinaga studied veins in a canine model, measuring wall shear stresses as they related to flow. He noted that changes in wall shear stress was the most important factor in determining subsequent FIH development and not the changes in flow rates per se. Wall shear stresses decreased as the flow rate decreased, which had led other authors to suggest that low flow alone was related to FIH. Their experiments, however, separated out both factors. In a low flow/high stress situation, defined as flow at 2.9 $\pm$ 1.8 cc/min and a wall tension of 178.8 $\pm$ 11 dynes/cm^2, there was only 31 $\pm$ 14 microns of intimal thickness that subsequently developed. In contrast, a high flow/low wall tension situation, defined as flow at 79.7 ± 3.2 cc/min and a shear stress of 33.1 ± 1.9 dynes/cm^2, developed 259 ± 36 microns of subsequent neointimal thickness (P <.005). Thus, they felt that wall shear stress was the important factor in the development of NIH and that low flow could be tolerated if there was a low wall shear stress and the endothelium was intact, thus preventing additional factors of platelet adherence.[31]

The relationship of relative low flow to the development of FIH and NIH are potentially interrelated. Low flow per se indicates a higher chance of local platelet deposition. In addition, low flow at anastomoses has been correlated with local platelet adherence.

Logerfo used a dye injection technique to photograph simulations of flow characteristics that occur at various angles and sizes of bifurcations (Fig. 8). Although his model was performed to simulate the carotid bifurcation and its resultant modes of atherogenic plaque formation, the findings are applicable to flow disturbances that might occur at anastomoses (Fig. 9A–F). He noted that at a 30° angle, there was a saddlelike flow separation causing areas of both high and low wall shear stresses. During diastole, retrograde eddy currents formed and there was formation of a stagnant boundary layer. The slower moving fluid of the flow disturbance is called a boundary layer. It is attached to the wall by frictional forces and also by the viscous action of the fluid. If there is a sudden change in luminal diameter or the direction of flow such that the fluid flows essentially against a local pressure gradient, there may be stagnation or actual reversal of flow. The boundary layer that becomes separated from the wall is called a *boundary separation zone.*

Logerfo noted that plaque formation in the carotid is highest over those areas that clinically correspond to areas of low flow shear stress and are not usually seen at the high shear stress area of the divider. Therefore, he felt that low flow shear stresses were the most significant factor in atherogenesis at the carotid bifurcation. However, he also noted that high shear forces might be a factor in activating platelets locally. These activated platelets then entered into the stagnant boundary separation zone and were more likely to participate in any endothelial injury processes at that level.[23]

Logerfo also studied the boundary layer separation in models of side-to-end anastomosis. He noted that fluid energy losses across the anastomoses were insignificant and that the only significant mechanical problems appear to be related to flow disturbances. Anastomoses

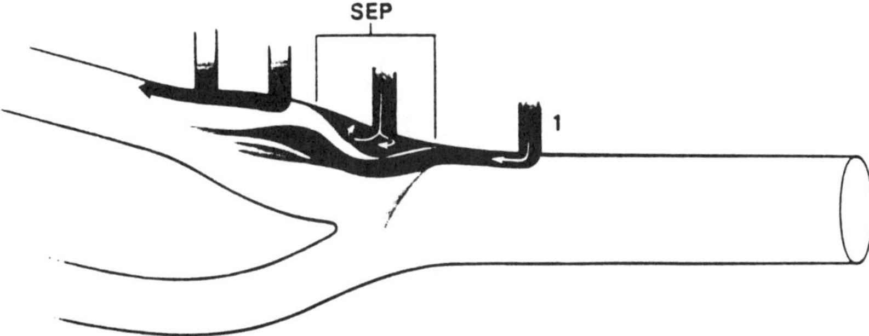

Figures 8A, B. *Shows systolic (A) and diastolic (B) flow patterns at a model of the carotid bifurcation, utilizing dye injection techniques during pulsatile luminal flow. (A, above) demonstrates near wall flow at peak systole. The upstream dye (1) flow along the wall is deflected around a boundary separation zone opposite the external carotid orifice (side graft analogue). A saddlelike region of separated fluid (SEP) exists at this area. A light region of dye is noted to circumferentially traverse the vessel wall into the external carotid artery.*

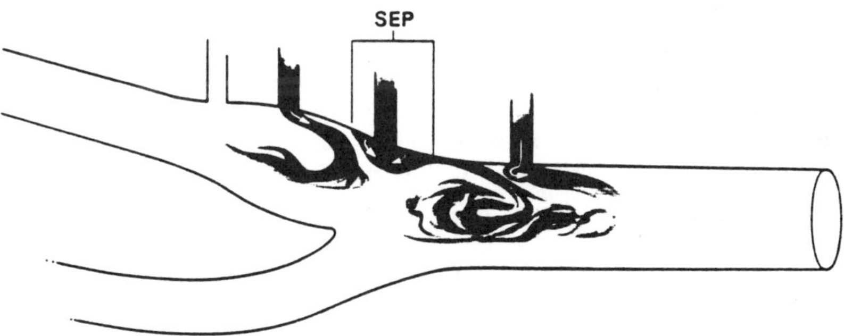

Figure 8B. *At peak diastole, dye from each part flows retrograde along the vessel wall and into the vessel curve in an unstable manner. The region of a separated boundary layer flow (SEP) is still present across from the external carotid origin. (Modified from Logerfo et al: Structural details of boundary layer separation in a model human carotid bifurcation under steady and pulsatile flow conditions. J Vasc Surg 2:263–6, 1985, with permission.)*

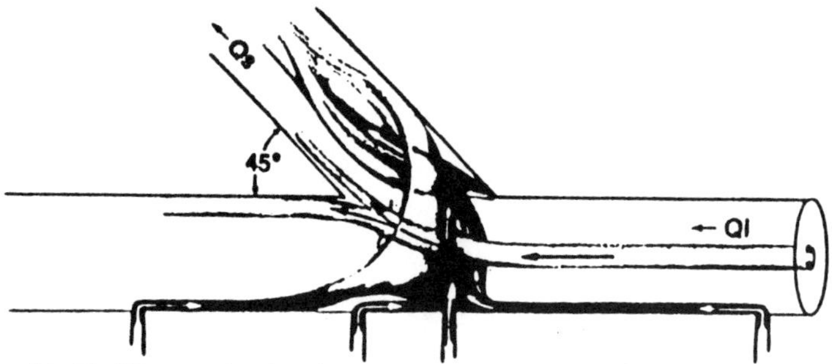

Figures 9A–E. *Five proximal and one distal anastomotic flow models to demonstrate the degree of flow separation incurred by various angles of anastomotic take-off. (A, above) 15° bifurcation at a flow split of Qs/Qi = .50. The separated zone forms a thick ring of slowly moving fluid encircling the main limb and then entering the graft side arm. Central core flow is deviated and impinges on the flow divider. No flow disturbances are noted.*

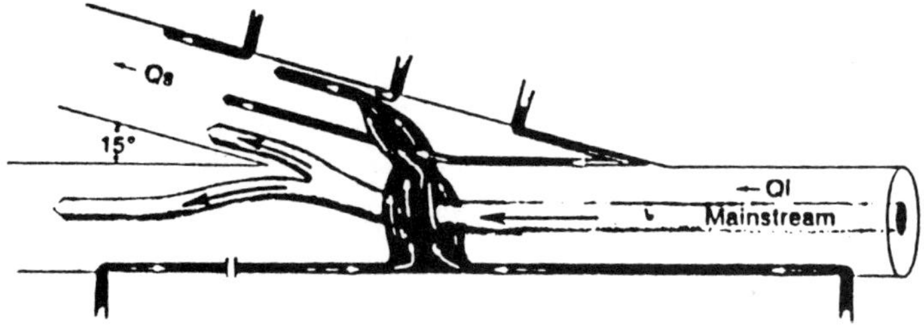

Figure 9B. *45° bifurcation at a flow split of Qs/Qi = .50. The only region of very slowly moving fluid adjacent to the vessel wall is a narrow ring forming at the proximal end of the separation zone. There is further disturbance of the boundary layer flow downstream from the divider in the main limb. Central core flow impinges on the flow divider, and some disturbance is noted downstream in the main limb.*

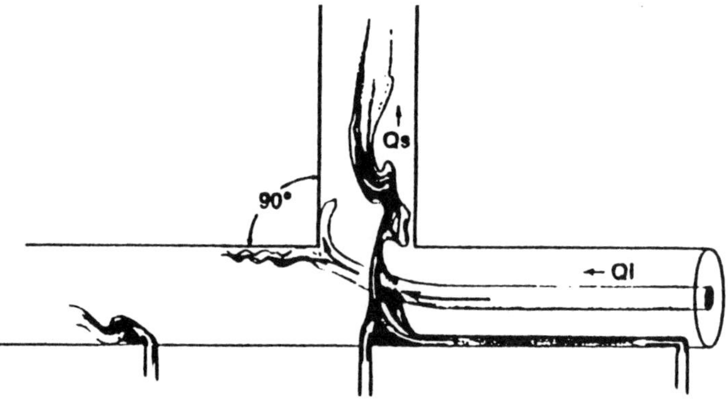

Figure 9C. *90° bifurcation at a flow split of Qs/Qi = .50. The separated fluid forms a thin ring in the main limb and a complex partially disturbed pattern in the graft. Core flow deflects to the flow divider, joins the complex flow within the graft, and becomes disturbed in the downstream main limb.*

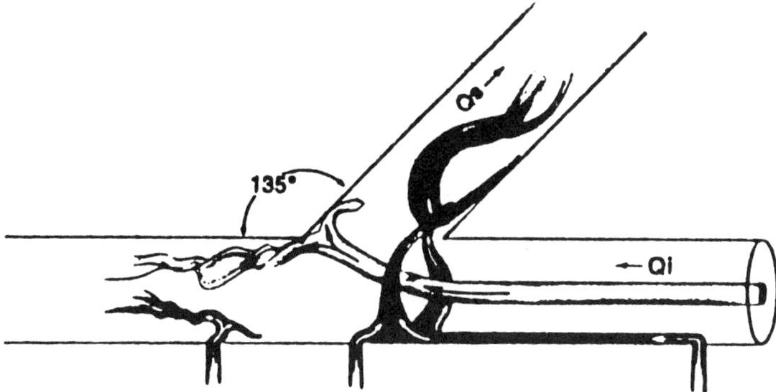

Figure 9D. *135° bifurcation at a flow split of Qs/Qi = .50. Separated near wall flow forms a thin ring and is disturbed at irregular intervals. Central core flow deviates into the graft but does not impinge on the hood. After deflection, there are downstream disturbances.*

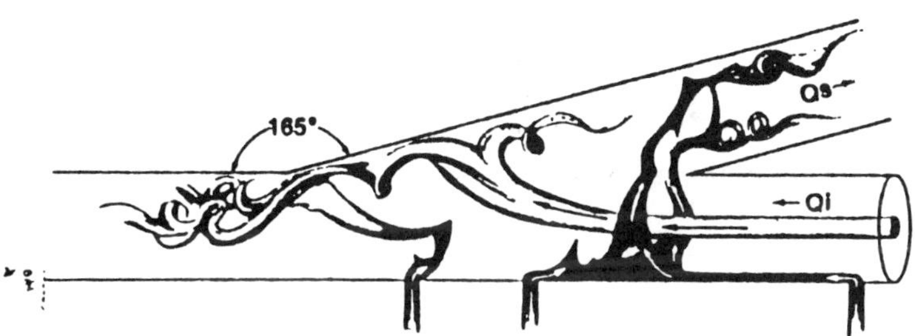

Figure 9E. *165° bifurcation at a flow split of Qs/Qi = .50. Strong disturbances are seen throughout the separated zone. Central flow impinges on the graft hood and is heavily disturbed in both the graft and main limb downstream.*

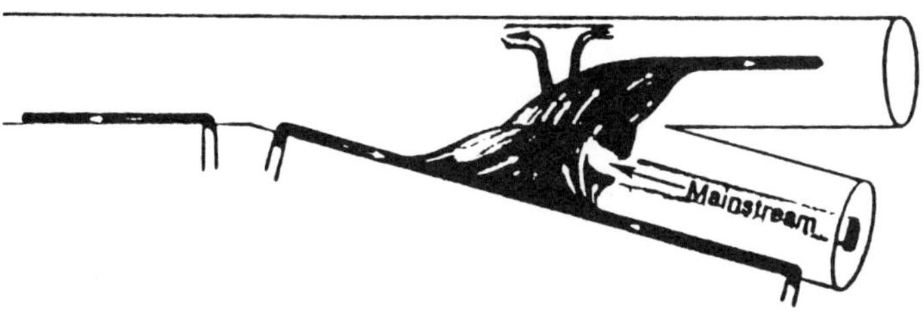

Figure 9F. *Distal anastomosis 45° with both outflow branches patent and equal flow. Separated flow forms a thick ring of slowly moving fluid within the graft hood; central core flow impinges on the recipient vessel wall. (Adapted from Nowak, MD, et al: Models of side-to-end anastomoses; effects of angle and flow split. J Surg Res 32:489– 98, 1982.)*

caused varying degrees of a ring of slow moving fluid that cut across the main stream of flow. The exact geometry of this slower moving fluid was highly influenced by the angle of the anastomosis. Fractionation of flow occurred secondary to adverse local pressure gradients that were formed and were augmented during diastole. Studies of the flow model demonstrated that the flow was unstable, but not turbulent at the usual Reynold's numbers that are consistent with the clinical situation. Flows within the separation area were consistent with low wall shear stresses.

A large portion of the side branch flow (i.e., a graft) was noted to be derived from the boundary separation layer. Thus, the blood entering into the graft has a higher potential for carrying activated platelets that have been displaced retrograde and circumferentially and have been derived from the slower moving outer shell of the main limb flows.[32]

Logerfo in 1983 analyzed a canine model in which crossover Dacron femoral grafts were fashioned as either bidirectional or unidirectional in flow and analyzed the resultant degree and/or localization of NIH at these anastomoses. His observations were that NIH was maximal at the distal or downstream anastomosis and occurred only to a lesser degree at the proximal or upstream anastomosis in both groups (P <.001); the NIH was progressive with time of implantation; and there was no increase in the formation of NIH with the greater flow separation that was caused by the bidirectional anastomosis. In that canine series, 6 of 28 grafts failed within 62–96 days due to the formation of an NIH plug at the distal anastomosis. Therefore, he noted although flow studies in the laboratory had demonstrated greater flow separations and, therefore, theoretically greater wall shear stresses if there was *bi*directional flow at a distal anastomosis, he could not confirm this in the canine model.[23,32–34]

Zarins has confirmed the association between low shear stress and the formation of plaque, using laser Doppler velocimeter analysis of a scale model of the carotid bifurcation. The inner wall of the carotid sinus, corresponding to the flow divider, had the highest wall stress at 41 dynes/cm^2 during systole and 10 dynes/cm^2 during diastole. Intimal thickening at this location on exactly corresponding human cadaveric carotid bifurcations was usually minimal. At the outer wall, where intimal plaques were maximal in the cadaveric specimens, shear stresses were 4 dynes/cm^2 at systole to -7 dynes/cm^2 during diastole. Intimal thickening, therefore, was highly correlated with the reciprocal of maximum shear stress (P <.0005) or the reciprocal of mean shear stress

(P <.0001). In addition, marked oscillations in the direction of wall shear were highly correlated with intimal thickening (P <.0001).[28]

These studies explain the incidence of NIH at distal and proximal anastomosis as being a problem of low wall shear stresses that activate platelets. There may also be an associated endothelial injury; adherent platelets release platelet-derived mitogens and cause resultant smooth muscle cell hypertrophy that results in the end-stage lesion referred to as NIH. There may also be shear stress-dependent impairment of mass transfer, with detrimental effects on the transport of cholesterol in and out of the area as well as an impaired transport of oxygen to the intima at that point.

Clowes has noted that there is a *chronic* endothelial injury associated with ongoing recurrent endothelial regeneration at anastomoses. Smooth muscle cells proliferate under this endothelium and continue to migrate to the subintima even after complete endothelial regeneration. This would indicate a continued platelet deposition and mitogen release stimulating this smooth muscle transmigration. In repair of a normal vessel, smooth muscle cells proliferate until the endothelium has undergone complete regeneration. The proliferation ceases at that point. This does not appear to be the case at anastomoses where that proliferation and transmigration continue. The source of the mitogens may be from adherent platelets or, he theorized, they might be emanating from the endothelial cells themselves due to the chronic injury state or even a possible paracrine stimulation of one smooth muscle cell to adjacent smooth muscle cells; or that the endothelial cells, because they were not quiescent, were unable to synthesize heparin-like inhibitors of smooth muscle cell hypertrophy as was normal.[2,6]

Further characterization of this paracrine stimulation of smooth muscle cells recently has been provided by Limmani et al. In a laboratory model, fourth passage adult human saphenous vein endothelial cells could be shown to secrete a PDGF-like substance that caused an elevenfold increase in tritiated thymidine uptake of PDGF receptor-labeled 3T3 cells. Their work indicates that endothelial cells may directly stimulate smooth muscle cell hypertrophy without intermediary platelet action.[8]

Summary of Pathogenesis

The sequence of events in the formation of neointimal hyperplasia (NIH) after construction of anastomosis involves both acute and chronic events. All of these can be modulated by the surgeon with theoretically positive effects.

The *acute* events relate heavily to topics covered in Chapters 3, 4, 6 and 7. There is local arterial ischemia at donor and recipient sites for anastomosis (proximal and distal anastomoses) as a result of periadventitial dissection with vaso vasorum disruption. This could be minimized by limiting circumferential dissection of the artery to sites of vascular control only. There is local ischemia of the arterial segment between vascular clamps during the formation of the anastomosis. This can be minimized by expeditious suturing and limiting occlusive times to that needed for the anastomosis. If the guidelines from other chapters are not studiously observed, there is the potential for local endothelial injury from injudicious dissection and handling of the arteriotomy, as well as injuries from physically passing the needles through its walls. Similarly, there are distinct perianastomotic injuries associated with the misuse of vascular occlusive devices. The end result of all of these is an endothelial and medial injury whose severity is the responsibility of the surgeon. The endothelial injury is probably transient and healed within days to weeks. However, the healed endothelium may not be as hormonally functional as noninjured endothelium, may not respond appropriately to continued mechanical stresses, and may, therefore, engender a continued endothelial injury. The process initiated during the period of injury with platelet adherence and mitogen release, therefore, may well be continuous despite histologic restitution of the endothelium.

Furthermore, all of these acute mechanisms are equally associated with medial injuries, particularly the production of ischemia and/or direct medial crush by instrumentation. Medial injury results in smooth muscle cell hypertrophy and proliferation of the fibrocollagenous ground substance. Although NIH by definition is a predominant intimal and/or subintimal change, it does extend to the underlying media and, therefore, associated medial injury and fibroplastic changes would be additive in nature.

Chronic changes relate to the increased wall stresses placed by anastomosis, including low flow shear stresses, formation of a boundary separation area with activation of platelets, cyclical stretch of the arterial wall, conformational stress placed on the recipient artery, and factors of wall stress secondary to compliance mismatches with modulation of amplitude of the transmitted pulse waves. The interplay of these varying mechanical stresses results in a chronic endothelial injury with recurrent platelet deposition, mitogenic factor release from platelets and/or injured endothelium, and resultant stimulation of smooth muscle cells to hypertrophy or transform to myofibroblasts. Modulation of the mechanical disadvantages incurred by an anastomosis is potentially available to the surgeon, although admittedly the effects of this modulation in terms of preventing NIH is, at this point, a matter of speculation.

NIH has come to be recognized as the second most common cause of failure of infrainguinal bypasses and the most common cause of failure of dialysis or other arteriovenous fistulae. It is associated with the distal, more than the proximal, anastomosis of arterial grafts and predominantly with the venous anastomosis of arteriovenous shunts. It is more likely to occur with synthetic grafts than with autologous veins. It seems to be more prevalent with end-to-side as opposed to end-to-end anastomoses and with continuous rather than interrupted sutures of end-to-end anastomoses. All of these can be explained as a combination of biomechanical factors.

The increased incidence of NIH with end-to-side versus end-to-end may be explained by invoking a number of mechanisms. First, utilization of the end-to-side configuration for bypass indicates the use of some conduit, be it vein or synthetic, that entails a compliance mismatch between host artery and the conduit. Second, there are greater flow disturbances incurred by an end-to-side as opposed to an end-to-end anastomosis, invoking flow shear stresses, formation of boundary separation zones, and secondary activation of platelets. Third, an end-to-side anastomosis, be it proximal or distal, entails the creation of a conformational stress at the arteriotomy. Conversely, an end-to-end anastomosis, particularly if luminally matched, invokes no conformational stress, no distinct flow disturbances or wall shear stresses, and only incurs a secondary para-anastomotic hypercompliant zone and the effects of direct compliance mismatch.

The increased incidence of NIH at the distal, as opposed to the proximal, anastomosis may also be explained by invocation of several mechanisms. With end-to-side anastomosis, the conformational stress presumably is greater at the smaller, distal artery since the arteriotomy is opened up a relatively greater amount than occurs with the larger, proximal artery unless a tapered graft has been used to better match proximal and distal luminal diameters. Flow disturbances may well be of similar severity, depending on the exact angle of take-off/insertion and the size disparity or flow division between the conduit and the native vessel. However, the activation of platelets by incorporation within the boundary separation zone of the proximal anastomosis may explain why there is an increased NIH incidence distally, this being a reflection of an increased tendency to aggregate distally after activation proximally. Compliance mismatches apply to either anastomosis, as does the formation of a para-anastomotic hypercompliance zone. End-to-end proximal and/or distal anastomoses presumably would have very low incidences of NIH since only factors of compliance mismatch and PHZ apply. Most of the negative inference of the distal anastomosis essentially accrues from the utilization of an end-to-side or bypass configuration.

The increased incidence of NIH associated with the use of synthetic as opposed to autologous vein conduits can also be explained by the interplay of several mechanisms. First is the recognized differential thrombotic threshold velocities for vein grafts as opposed to synthetic grafts; a vein tolerates a lower flow situation without subsequent thrombosis than a synthetic graft does. Second, compliances of all synthetic grafts are significantly decreased in reference to the autologous artery as opposed to the autologous vein conduit, even after correction for the incorporation of the vein and its subsequent fibroplasia after implantation. Beyond the negative effects of this relatively greater compliance mismatch is the fact that the secondary induction of a para-anastomotic hypercompliance zone at the peri-anastomotic area is also substantially increased. Theoretically, there should be a greater conformational stress exerted on an arteriotomy by a more rigid synthetic graft than by the more compliant vein graft. Thus, the differences in compliance multiply the negative effects from not only the compliance mismatch itself, but also an increased change of a PHZ being generated and a presumed increase in conformational stress. Third, the NIH probably relates to a differential reactivity of platelets to an endothelialized, as opposed to a nonendothelialized surface since it is well recognized that synthetic grafts rarely, if ever, form a complete luminal surface endothelium in opposition to the natural tendency of vein grafts to heal with endothelialization.

Although NIH occurs more commonly at the distal anastomosis, it does occur proximally as well. This would be a factor of the para-anastomotic hypercompliant zone that is engendered by any anastomosis, local boundary separation zones that are incurred by use of the bypass or end-to-side configuration, and local conformational stresses with the end-to-side anastomosis.

Detrimental Effects

Actual determination of the effects of neointimal hyperplasia can be obtained from a number of studies, particularly long-term follow-ups of grafts performed for lower extremity revascularization. The initial observations were made by a variety of authors in clinical and/or laboratory evaluation of grafts as new grafts were introduced and assessed for their patency rates. Thus, Rosenberg noted 30% (3 of 10) of bovine femoropopliteal grafts failed. All demonstrated a focal stenosis of neointimal hyperplasia at the distal anastomosis.[35] Similarly, Veith noted 28 failures of 187 infrainguinal bypass grafts to be due to the development of NIH that, in his series, occurred equally at proximal and distal anastomosis. In a later follow-up of 450 bypasses, he noted that 45 failed in the intermediate to late period; 49% of these failed due to progression of distal disease and 11% due to progression of proximal disease. However, 18% were felt to have failed due to the development of a neointimal hyperplastic stenosis.[36] Kelly noted routine failure of 2.8- to 5.4-mm PTFE grafts in a canine model within 2 to 4 weeks. All were the result of early development of NIH at the distal anastomosis.[37] Echave followed 250 patients for three years, all with implanted 6.5- to 4.5-mm tapered PTFE femoropopliteal grafts. Ten of these patients developed neointimal hyperplastic stenosis with subsequent graft thrombosis at 3 months to 1 year.[38] In an experimental study of canine femoral interposition grafts, Phillips noted that 50% (5 of 10) end-to-end and 60% (6 of 10) end-to-side anastomoses developed a proximal neointimal hyperplastic plug.[39] Weymen in a study of veins versus bovine glutaraldehyde tanned and dialdehyde tanned grafts in a canine model noted that the patency of the vein graft was 97% in early follow-up. The various bovine grafts, however, attained patency rates of only 13% and 50% with all failures being due to the early development of a marked fibrointimal hyperplasia.[40]

Walden correlated the clinical patency of various conduits for femoropopliteal bypass grafting with their elastic properties and was able to show an inverse relationship between compliance and patency. Compliant grafts (saphenous vein, umbilical vein) had 2-year patency rates greater than 80%, while noncompliant grafts (Dacron, PTFE) had less than 45% 2-year patencies[24] (Table 2).

Szilagyi noted on serial angiograms of Dacron grafts implanted as femoropopliteal grafts that 2.7% developed an anastomotic stenosis. Ten of these developed within the first year and all developed within the first 2 years.[41] Sladen in a follow-up of 173 reversed vein femoropopliteal bypasses noted 33 stenoses to occur. Seventeen of these were immediately perianastomotic and were felt to be due to neointimal hyperplasia.[43] O'Donnell followed 36 PTFE femoropopliteal grafts that had failed and noted that the most common factor in failure was progression of distal atherosclerosis in 64%, but that the next most common factor was formation of NIH anastomotic stenosis in 19%.[4]

Summary

In the absence of specifically directed laboratory research, recommendations for surgical technical maneuvers to decrease the incidence of neointimal hyperplasia must be made both tentatively and speculatively. Still, there is good reason to expect successful extrapolation of what is known in the clinical and laboratory situation to the surgical situation. One can look at the presumed etiologies and minimize the specific situations that seem to maximize injury potentials.

Neointimal hyperplasia has a high association with the distal rather than the proximal anastomosis; with synthetic grafts as opposed to autologous veins; and is associated with smaller diameter lower flow and, therefore, infrapopliteal conduits as opposed to larger diameter, higher flow, inflow conduits.

Construction of an anastomosis per se induces a degree of local compliance mismatch that can be minimized potentially by attention to technical details. End-to-end re-anastomosis of veins or arteries should be done carefully to preserve an *exact* luminal match, the anastomosis should be performed preferentially with interrupted sutures to decrease the development of a perianastomotic hypercompliance zone and any resultant compliance mismatch, and there should be no attempt to enlarge the area of anastomosis—constrictions and luminal enlargements are detrimental. As a matter of speculation, consideration should be given to utilization of an absorbable suture rather than synthetic sutures in *autologous* reanastomoses to minimize the subsequent development of a suture-induced para-anastomotic hypercompliant zone; realizing that the scar induced by anastomosis may well confer some degree of local mismatch that is, as yet, unstudied.

End-to-side anastomoses should minimize the angle of the anastomosis to optimize flow through the iatrogenic side branch and minimize subsequent flow disturbances with formation of boundary separation zones. In addition, the amount of flow diverted through the side branch should be carefully tailored to be greater than 50%, but not to exceed 100% so as to minimize the effect of flow division; realizing that the only clinical in vivo study performed in this regard was inconclusive of that particular point. In addition, consideration should be given to the use of interrupted sutures to decrease the development of a para-anastomotic hypercompliant zone. A Linton patch of autogenous vein interposed between a synthetic conduit and the autologous artery theoretically should result in a somewhat better compliance match at the more critical end-to-side anastomosis; although it inevitably involves additional and untested problems with changes in the interval venous segment as well. Preliminary data recently has been presented by Wolfe to show that such a segment protects the distal crural vessel at the expense of myointimal hyperplasia within the venous segment itself.[43]

Synthetic conduits universally have a compliance mismatch that is aggravated by a secondary induction of a PHZ with continuous suture. Obviously, a venous conduit should be used instead of a synthetic conduit as much as possible. When a synthetic graft is necessary, a conduit with a better compliance match might be preferable; however other factors/problems with biological versus synthetic grafts must be considered. Suture technique, again, is performed optimally in an interrupted or semi-interrupted fashion. The cobra head that is standardly used to maximize flow should be kept to a minimum to avoid unnecessary spraying out of the arterial walls and development of a conformational stress, particularly at the distal artery. Conduits should be closely matched in size to the vessels to which they are anastomosed to minimize additional flow disturbances. Finally, if possible, an end-to-end anastomosis should be considered to optimize the flow characteristics and minimize conformational stress problems. For example, if a bypass is being performed distally to an occluded vessel, an end-to-end anastomosis to the distal, patent vessel might be preferable to an end-to-side anastomosis performed just distal to the occlusion.

References

1. Imparato, AM, Baumann, FG, Pearson, J, et al: Electron microscopic studies of experimentally produced fibromuscular arterial lesions. *Surgery* 139:497–504, 1974.

2. Clowes, AW, Kirkman, TR, Clowes, MM: Mechanisms of arterial graft failure. II: Chronic endothelial and smooth muscle cell proliferation in healing polytectrafluoroethylene prostheses. *J Vasc Surg* 3:877–84, 1986.

3. DeWeese, J, Green, R: Anastomotic neointimal fibrous hyperplasia. In VM Bernard, JB Towne (eds): *Complications in Vascular Surgery*. New York, Grune and Stratton, 1980.

4. O'Donnell, TF, Mackey, W, McCullough, JC, et al: Correlation of operative findings with angiographic and non-invasive hemodynamic factors associated with failure of PTFE grafts. *J Vasc Surg* 1:136–42, 1984.

5. Sottiurai, VS, Yao, YST, Flinn, WR, et al: Intimal hyperplasia and neointima: An ultrastructural analysis of thrombosed grafts in humans. *Surgery* 936:809–17, 1983.

6. Clowes, AW, Gown, AM, Hanson, S R, et al: Mechanisms of arterial graft failure. I: Role of cellular proliferation in early healing of PTFE prostheses. *Am S Path* 118:43–54, 1985.

7. Leung, O, Glagov, S, Matthews, SM: Elastin and collagen accumulation in rabbit ascending aorta and pulmonary trunk during postnatal growth. *Circ Res* 41:316–23, 1977.

8. Limmani, A, Fleming, T, Molina, R, et al: Expression of genes for platelet derived growth factor in adult venous endothelium. *J Vasc Surg* 711:10–16, 1988.

9. Chien, S, Usami, S, Fan, FC, et al: Effects of mechanical disturbances on uptake of macromolecules by the arterial wall. In RM Nerem, J F Cornhill (eds): *The Role of Fluid Mechanics in Atherogenesis Proceedings* 1978, pp 16-1–16-4.

10. Lyon, RT, Runyon-Hass, A, Davis, HR, et al: Protection from atherosclerotic lesion formation by reduction of artery wall motion. *J Vasc Surg* 5:59–67, 1987.

11. Paasche, PE, Kinley, CE, Dolan, FG: Consideration of suture line stresses in the selection of synthetic grafts for implantation. *J Biomech* 6:253, 1973.

12. Thoma, R: *Untersuchen Uber Die Histolgenese Und Histomechanik Des Gefasgstem*. F Enke, Stuttgart, 1893.

13. Rodbard, S: Negative feedback mechanisms in the architecture and function of the connective and cardiovascular tissue. *Perspect Biomed* 12:507–27, 1970.

14. Leung, D, Glagov, S, Matthews, M: Cyclic stretching stimulates synthesis of matrix components of arterial smooth muscle in vitro. *Science* 191:475–77, 1976.

15. Wolinsky, H: Response of the rat aortic media to hypertension. *Circ Res* 26:507–22, 1970.

16. Abbott, WM, Bouchier-Hayes, DJ: The role of mechanical properties in graft design: In H Dardik (ed): *Graft Materials In Vascular Surgery*. Miami, Miami Symposia Specialists, Inc. 1978.

17. Clark, RE, Apostolov, S, Kordos, JL: Mismatch of mechanical properties as a cause of arterial prosthesis thrombosis. *Surg Forum* 27:208–10, 1976.

18. Hasson, JE, Megerman, J, Abbott, WM: Increased compliance near vascular anastomosis. *J Vasc Surg* 2:419–23, 1985.

19. Hasson, JE, Megerman, J, Abbott, WM: Suture technique and para-anastomotic compliance. *J Vasc Surg* 3:591–97, 1986.
20. Klein, SR, Goldberg, L, Miranda, RM, et al: Effect of suture technique on arterial anastomotic compliance. *Arch Surg* 117:45–47, 1982.
21. Rodgers, VGJ, Teodori, MF, Brant, AM, et al: Characterization *in vitro* of the biomechanical properties of anastomosed host artery-graft combinations. *J Vasc Surg* 4:396–402, 1986.
21a. Lye, LR, Sumner, DS, Hokanson, DE: The transcutaneous measurement of the elastic properties of the human saphenous vein femoropopliteal bypass graft. *Surg Gyn Obstet* 141:981, 1975.
22. Rodgers, VGJ, Teodori, MF, Borovetz, HS: Experimental determination of mechanical shear stress about an anastomotic junction. *J Biomech* 20:795–803, 1987.
23. Logerfo, FW, Nowak, MD, Quist, WC: Structural details of boundary layer separation in a model human carotid bifurcation under steady and pulsatile flow conditions. *J Vasc Surg* 2:263–69, 1985.
24. Walden, R, L'Italien, GJ, Megerman, J, et al: Matched elastic properties and successful arterial grafting. *Arch Surg* 115:1166–69, 1980.
25. White, RA, Klein, SR, Shors, EC: Preservation of compliance in a small diameter microporous silicone rubber vascular prosthesis. *J Cardiovasc Surg* 28:485–90, 1987.
26. Pomposelli, F, Schoen, F, Cohen, R, et al: Conformational stress and anastomotic hyperplasia. *J Vasc Surg* 1:4:525–34, 1984.
27. Madras, PN, Ward, CA, Johnson, WR, et al: Anastomotic hyperplasia. *Surgery* 90:922–23, 1981.
28. Zarins, CK, Bomberger, RA, Glagov, S: Local effects of stenoses: Increased flow velocity inhibits atherogenesis. *Circulation* 64(Suppl II):221–27, 1981.
29. Imparato, AM, Bracco, A, Kim, GE: Intimal and neointimal fibrous proliferation causing failure of arterial reconstructions. *Surgery* 72:1007–17, 1972.
30. Berguer, R, Higgins, RF, Reddy, DJ: Intimal hyperplasia, an experimental study. *Arch Surg* 115:3:332–35, 1980.
31. Morinaga, K, Okadome, K, Kuroki, M, et al: Effect of wall shear stress on intimal thickening of arterially transplanted autogenous veins in dogs. *J Vasc Surg* 2:430–34, 1985.
32. Logerfo, FW, Soncrant, T, Teel, T, et al: Boundary layer separation in models of side-to-end arterial anastomoses. *Arch Surg* 114:1369–73, 1979.
33. Logerfo, FW, Quist, WC, Nowak, MD, et al: Downstream anastomotic hyperplasia: A mechanism of failure in Dacron arterial grafts. *Annals Surg* 197:479–84, 1983.
34. Nowak, MD, Logerfo, FW, Quist, WC, et al: Models of side-to-end anastomoses; effects of angle and flow split. *J Surg Res* 32:489–98, 1982.
35. Rosenberg, N, Thompson, JE, Keshishnian, JM: The modified bovine heterograft. *Arch Surg* 111:222, 1976.
36. Veith, FL: In answer to Echave.
37. Kelly, GL: Discussion of Echave.

38. Echave, V, Koolnick, AD, Haimov, M: Intimal hyperplasia as a complication of the use of polytetrafluorethylene graft for femoropopliteal bypass. *Surgery* 86:791, 1979.
39. Philips, CE, Jr., DeWeese, JA, Campeti, L: Comparison of peripheral arterial grafts. *Arch Surg* 82:38, 1961.
40. Weyman, AK, Plume, SK, DeWeese, JA: Bovine heterografts and autogenous veins as canine arterial bypass grafts. *Arch Surg* 110:746–51, 1975.
41. Szilagyi, D, Smith, RF, Elliott, JP, et al: Long term behavior of Dacron arterial substitute: Clinical, roentgenologic, and histologic correlation. *Ann Surg* 162:453, 1965.
42. Sladen, JG, Gilmour, JL: Vein graft stenosis, characteristics and effect of treatment. *Am J Surg* 141:549–52, 1981.
43. Wolfe, JHN, Griggs, MJ, Nicolaide, NN: Enhanced distal compliance may improve prosthetic femorocrural graft patency. Presented at The International Society of Cadiovascular Surgeons Meeting, June, 1989, Chicago, Illinois.

Chapter 6

Injury Patterns from Small Technical Details: Sutures, Needles, Anastomoses

T.J. Bunt, William M. Moore, and Philip B. Dobrin

After all the complex judgments and decisions as to which operation with which graft; and after all the intricacies of the dissection, exposure, and control of the involved vessels, it would seem that the anastomosis itself, the mere joining together of two vessels/grafts, would be straightforward. Yet each apprentice surgeon must find amusingly noteworthy (if not frankly mind-boggling) the broad diversity of opinions as to how anastomoses should be constructed—no less the pedantic or dogmatic way in which such opinions are delivered. Each teacher has his/her own way and vociferously criticizes a student's attempts at some other method. It is indeed a microcosm of the "art" of current academic surgical teaching.

The salient questions one should always ask oneself and one's teacher: "Why? What is the evidence for it?" In terms of anastomoses, "What is too large a bite? Too small a bite? Too far apart? What *is* the standard way?" (as in the commonplace operative dictation, "end-to-side anastomosis was then performed in standard fashion!").

It is not our purpose to deliver another weighty opinion (to be henceforward vociferously defended), but rather to describe what little concrete evidence there might be for selecting suture, needle size, and/or curve, and how a suture line needs to be constructed.

It should first of all be realized that clumsy, repetitive, and/or overly vigorous handling of the suture/needle is likely to result in demonstrable injury to the needle or suture or both. Potential complications resulting from fracture or other injury of the *suture* are intellectually obvious; if the fractured segment is included in the suture line, there is real potential for suture disruption under stress, with resultant early anastomotic disruption or late pseudoaneurysm formation. Potential complications resulting from injuries to the *needle* are less evident. Certainly a chewed-up needle makes larger holes in synthetic graft matrices, resulting in leaky anastomoses and an increased potential for the graft tearing under stress. Whether or not the same chewed-up needle causes any significant injury when passed through a vessel may be a moot point. One would suspect that it does, and that the greater the local injury, the greater the potential for platelet aherence. Mason and Mohammad have demonstrated that there is a marked increase in platelet aggregation at the site of anastomosis, which is a function of endothelial injury at time of arteriotomy and due to the handling of the arteriotomy edge[1]; in addition they have noted that platelets preferentially adhere to the sites of suture insertion and to the sutures themselves (Fig. 1). Thus, realization of the results

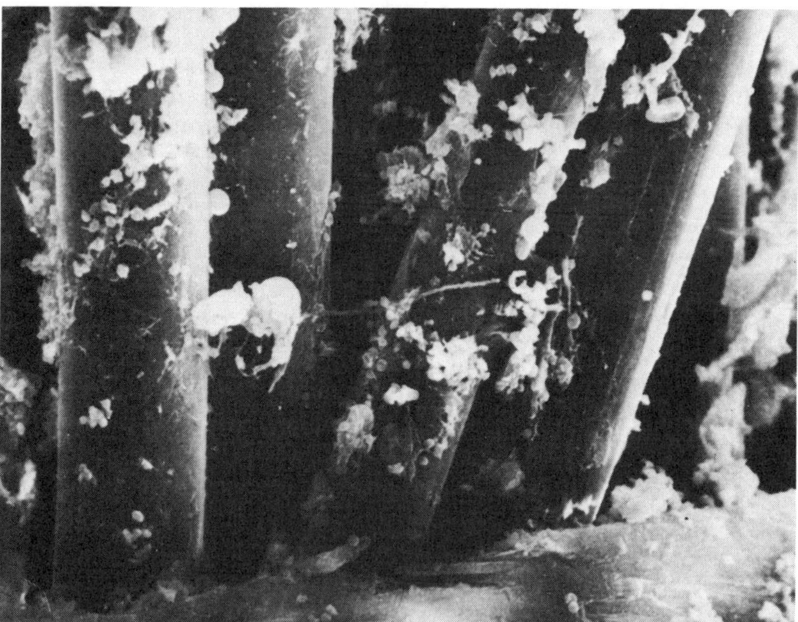

Figure 1. *View from luminal surface of umbilical vein segment at suture line; large fibrillar structures on sutures with numerous adherent platelets. (From Mason, RG, Mohammad, SF: A human model for study of blood vascular wall interactions. Arch Surg 115:955–60, 1980, with permission.)*

of these finer points of potential injury should lead to increased care in handling of the suture/needle. This should essentially obviate the potential for injury and/or its complication, and so is worthy of both examination and emphasis.

Needle Size

There is no intrinsic structural or strength differential to anastomoses constructed with varying needle size or radius of curvature; this is strictly a function of the suture size as related to tensile strength. Why then are there different sizes of needles, and which is optimal for which sort of work?

Needles may be described by various engineering terms (Figs. 2, 3).

Radius: the radius of needle curvature is the distance from the needle to the center of the circle that would be made by continuing its arc full circle. Radius therefore describes the "curve" of the needle.

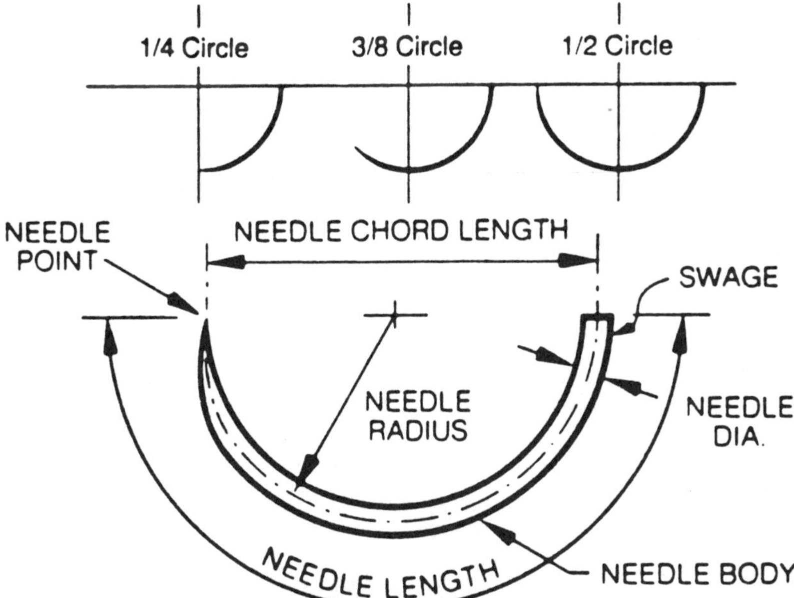

Figure 2. *Engineering terms used to describe a given needle.*

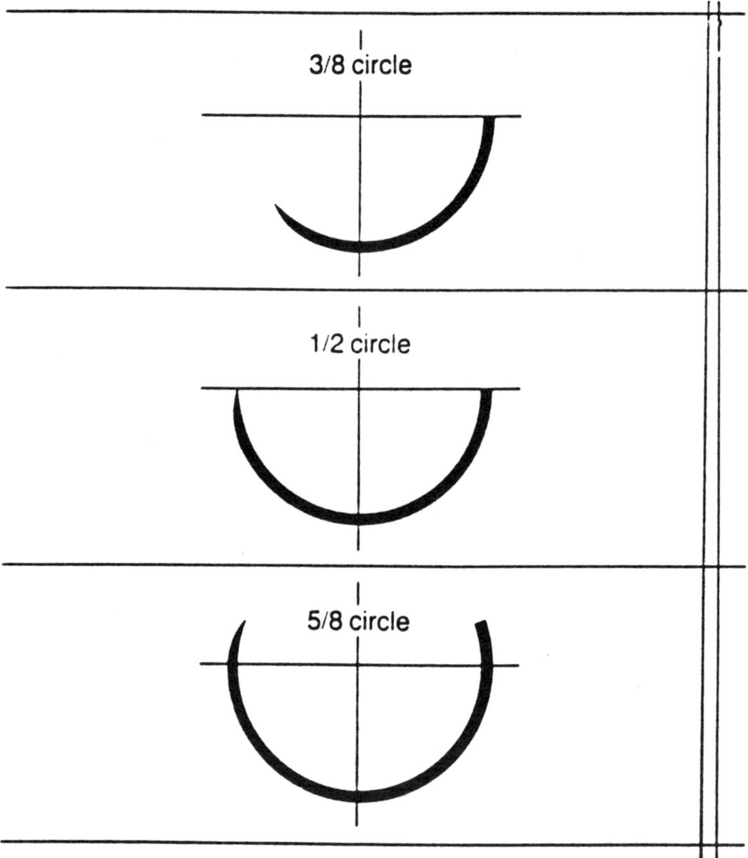

Figure 3. *The three most common needle types.*

Diameter: the gauge or thickness of the needle body. As such, it is an indicator of needle strength.

Chord: the shortest distance between the butt and the needle tip. Combined with needle radius, this describes *needle length,* which is the distance from needle butt to tip as measured on the needle circumference itself. Chord is a statement of the circle size of which the needle represents one segment: smaller chords indicate higher radii of curvatures.

Needle/Suture Ratio: most sutures utilize swaged-on needles that are crushed down over the end of the suture. The ratio describes the size difference between the encompassing needle butt and the encompassed suture; as such it describes how much larger a hole will be made by the needle than can be filled by the following suture.

The primary purpose of varied needle sizes is to facilitate mechanical passage of the needle through the vessel. This relates to the strength of the needle relative to the resistance (thickness, consistency) of the vessel and to the radius of the vessel lumen compared to the radius of curve of the needle. Table 1 lists one manufacturer's statistics

Table 1.
Engineering Statistics for a Variety of Commonly Utilized Cardiovascular Sutures

	UNITS = INCHES				SUT/NDL RATIO – PROLENE*						SUT/NDL RATIO – MERSILENE*					
TYPE	LENGTH	CHORD	RADIUS	DIAMTR	7/0	6/0	5/0	4/0	3/0	2/0	7/0	6/0	5/0	4/0	3/0	2/0
BV-1	0.37	0.29	0.16	0.008	0.3	0.4										
BV	0.44	0.35	0.19	0.008	0.3	0.4										
BB	0.66	0.52	0.28	0.014			0.4									
				0.017				0.4								
				0.020					0.4							
TF	0.49	0.31	0.16	0.014			0.4									
				0.017				0.4								
RB-2	0.52	0.34	0.17	0.010		0.3										
				0.012			0.4									
RB-1	0.69	0.44	0.22	0.014			0.4						0.4			
				0.017				0.4						0.4		
				0.022					0.4						0.4	
				0.026						0.5						0.5
SH-1	0.86	0.56	0.28	0.022					0.4							
SH	1.02	0.69	0.34	0.022				0.3								
				0.024					0.4						0.4	
				0.026						0.5						0.5
MH	1.43	0.94	0.47	0.024					0.4							
				0.026						0.5						
CT-2	1.05	0.69	0.34	0.039					0.2	0.3						
CT-1	1.43	0.94	0.47	0.039					0.2	0.3						
CT	1.57	1.11	0.56	0.044						0.3						
CTX	1.89	1.30	0.66	0.044						0.3						

*Information provided by Ethicon, Inc., Somerville, NJ.[9]
SUT/NDL ratio = suture-to-needle ratio.

for commonly used vascular suture needles. This information facilitates an understanding of the various concepts of optimal needle selection and use. Smaller needles have a decreased intrinsic strength and therefore bend more readily when used on thicker or more diseased (fibrotic, calcific) vessels. They are also more vulnerable to instrumental injury if used with heavier needle drivers. However, their decreased radius of curvature allows optimal positioning within the decreased radius of lumen of small vessels, thus facilitating anastomosis for such small caliber vessels. All of the converse characteristics are true for larger needles. They facilitate suturing in calcific, fibrotic vessels and the larger size allows more forceful handling by stronger needle drivers without needle fracture or bending. However, their larger size makes suturing within small vessels cumbersome.

Cutting or tapercut needles facilitate anastomosis in calcific vessels when used in conjunction with other techniques such as buttressing the needle with a Küttner cottonoid externally and using a rocking rather than a driving motion. Guidoin has studied the endothelial injury patterns of the cutting needle with scanning electron microscopy and notes that it causes less apparent intimal injury than the equivalently sized tapered needle.[2] Most sutures have large needle-to-suture ratios; put succinctly, the needle makes a much larger hole in the graft matrix/vessel than can be filled by the following suture. This entails a leaky anastomosis, particularly in the synthetic grafts; this is aggravated by instrument damage to the needle with further graft laceration, as discussed below.

Needle Injury

Application of needle drivers to the delicate needle of vascular sutures results in a defined injury to the needle that is dependent on the size of the needle (e.g., its strength), the size and type of needle driver, and how the needle driver is handled by the surgeon. Although a certain portion of this needle destruction is inevitable, it can be ameliorated by careful needle driver selection and handling. The tungsten carbide facing of standard needle drivers is much harder than the steel surface of the needles. Forceful closure of the driver of the needle and/or rotation of the needle within the clamp jaws will reliably excoriate the needle surface. The injured needle surface (Fig. 4) has jagged burrs that lacerate the graft/vessel, causing either larger suture line

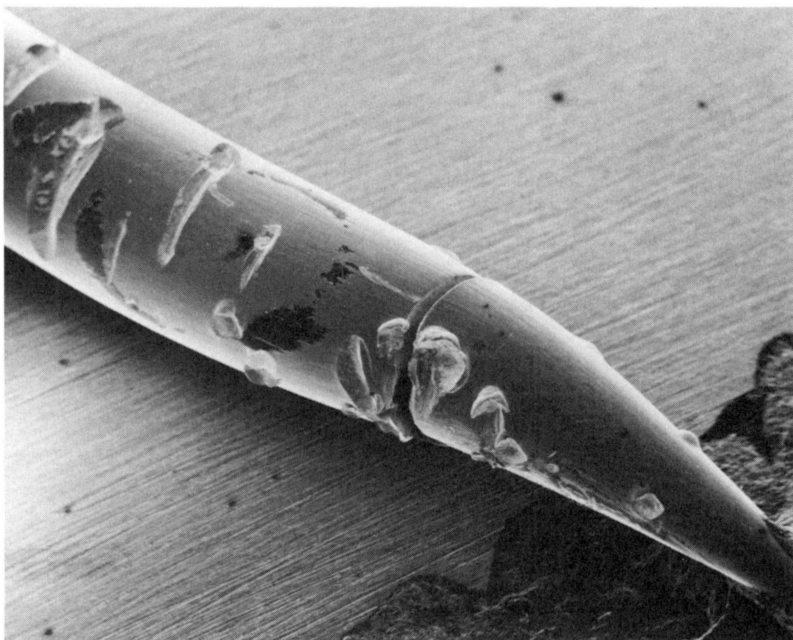

Figure 4. *Scanning microscopy of a needle after engagement with a standard needle driver showing large gouge marks from the teeth of the needle driver as well as jagged burrs of needle substance. The needle point has fractured at the site of three concurrent gouges. (Courtesy Ethicon, Inc., Somerville, NJ.[9])*

holes or increased local intimal injury at the anastomosis. Application of the needle driver jaws to the needle point may fracture same, leaving a blunter tip whose entry through tissue/graft requires great force and causes even greater local injury. Application to the suture at the butt end of the needle causes a fracture of the suture filaments with subsequent suture breakage (Fig. 5).

If the needle tip fracture is recognized, it can be remedied by selection of a new needle/suture rather than continuance with the injured one. Fracture of the suture itself at the needle butt would not pose a problem, but fracture of the suture in its midsection would lead to anastomotic disruption: Dobrin's work below is pertinent. Continued use of a badly excoriated needle or one with fracture of the tip entails a greater local endothelial injury and greater propensity for platelet adherence and should be avoided.

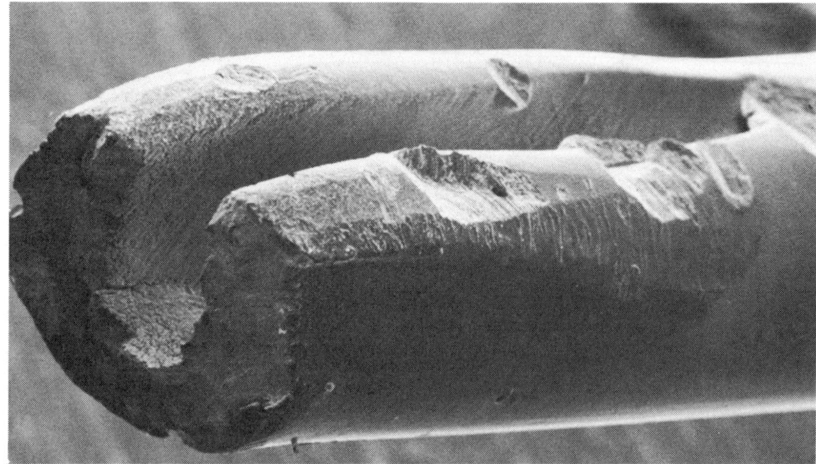

Figure 5. *Scanning microscopy of a needle after engagement of the butt end with a needle driver showing gouges from the teeth of the needle driver and a fracture of the crystalline matrix of the suture. (Courtesy Ethicon, Inc., Somerville, NJ.[9])*

Suture Choice

Selection of a suture size is based on the need for smaller or larger needle size for handling and on a somewhat empiric concept that a larger suture with presumed greater tensile strength should be used in larger vessels. However, Dobrin has studied the tensile strength characteristics of monofilament suture and noted an apparently paradoxically *increased* strength to smaller radius sutures. He examined 50 segments of 3-0, 4-0, 5-0, 6-0, and 7-0 polypropylene sutures under stepwise elongation stress. The elastic nodulus (suture stiffness) and tensile strength of the sutures were directly related to the circumference of the suture and varied inversely with the cross-sectional area (Figs. 6–8). This suggests that for monofilament extruded sutures such as polypropylene, the primary strength of the suture resides in its outer skin and that smaller diameter sutures therefore have greater *relative* tensile strength than larger sutures. The presumed mechanism is that the outer skin crystalizes rapidly as the filament is being extruded under pressure, and the crystals align in the direction of the extrusion stress. Central core crystallization occurs secondarily as the filament cools, is not under extrusion stress, and therefore is not aligned. Thus, large sutures can bear more absolute force than small

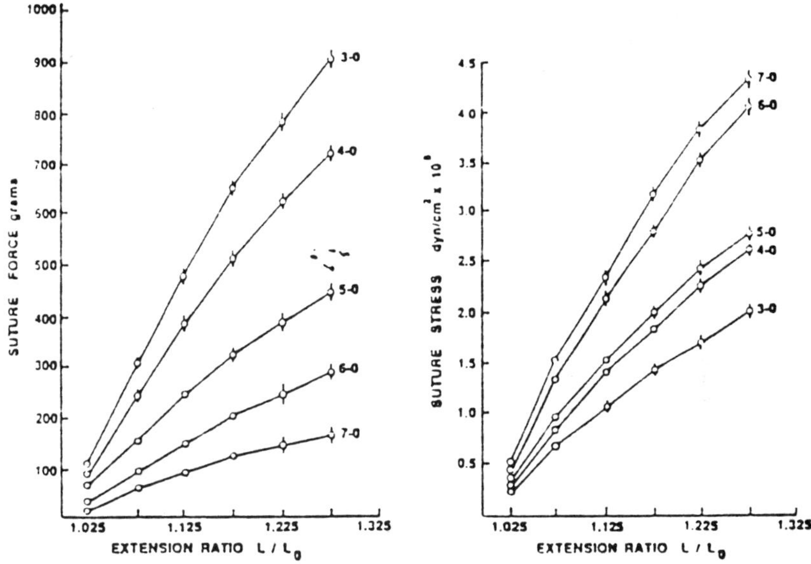

Figure 6. *The extension-force curves (left) and extension-stress (right) curves for 50 polyprolene sutures of varying size. Large sutures exert more force but less stress than small sutures. (From Dobrin, P: Some mechanical properties of polypropylene sutures. J Surg Res, in press, with permission.)*

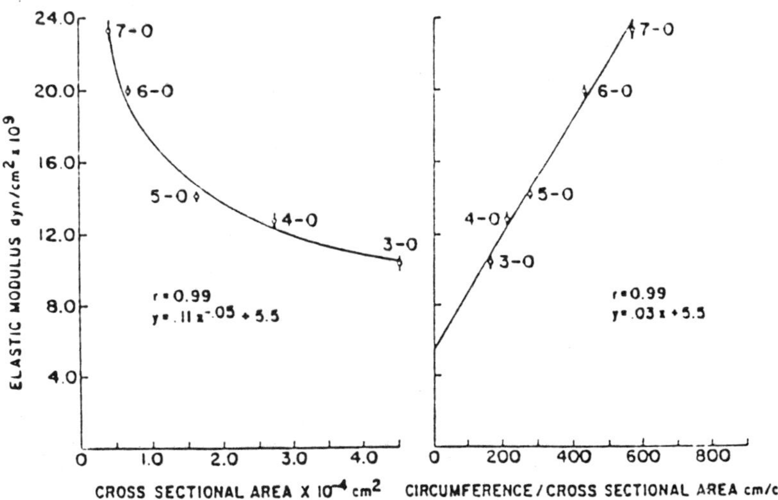

Figure 7. *The relationship of elastic modulus of various polypropylene sutures to their circumference and cross-sectional area; the EM decreases with increasing cross-sectional area (left) but increases with increasing circumference to cross-sectional area ratios (right). (From Dobrin, P: Effects of surgical manipulation on the breaking strength of polypropylene sutures. Arch Surg 124:665–669, 1989, with permission.)*

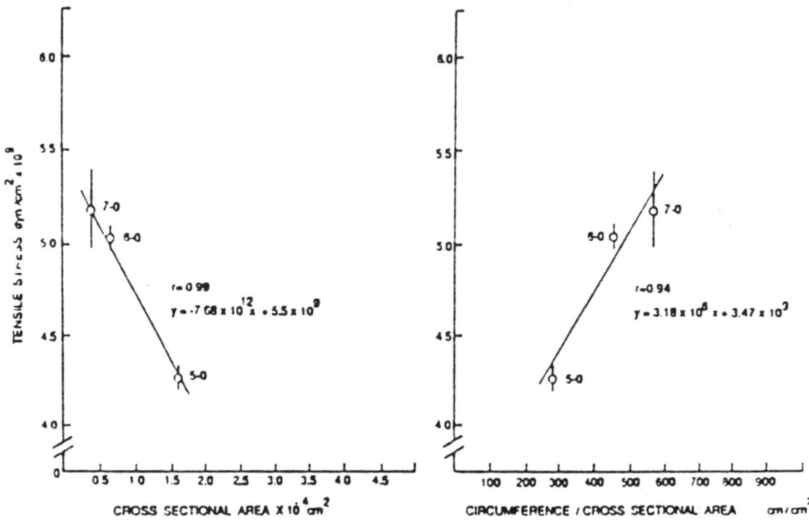

Figure 8. *The relationship between tensile strength and cross-sectional area for various sized polypropylene sutures, demonstrating that the tensile strength decreases with increasing cross-sectional area (left) but rises with increasing circumference to cross-sectional area ratio (right). (From Dobrin, P: Effects of surgical manipulation on the breaking strength of polypropylene sutures. Arch Surg 124:665–69, 1989, with permission.)*

sutures, but the tensile strength per cross-sectional area is greater for the smaller suture.[3]

In engineering terms, a safety factor is a term describing the ability of a structure to withstand applied forces. Acceptable safety factors for structural steel average 1.65 to 2.0. Dobrin calculated the safety factors for monofilament polypropylene sutures before and after anastomotic loading (Table 2): although there was a significant decrease in the safety factor (4.45 to 1.96 for 5-0, 3.12 to 1.92 for 6-0, and 2.41 to 1.32 for 7-0), the margins were still acceptable for 5-0 and 6-0 in a carotid arteriotomy; the 7-0 was low enough to warrant concern about its use in anastomoses.

Ninety-five percent of the total load placed on a suture during anastomosis is imparted by the knot itself, and all sutures in Dobrin's study broke at the entry of the suture into the knot. This certainly emphasizes the necessity for careful, gentle knot tying without undue additional stress being imparted to the suture (Table 3).

Table 2.

A.* Suture Size	Safety Factor	Load Ratio
5-0	4.45	22%
6-0	3.12	32%
7-0	2.41	41%

*Safety factors and load ratios for polypropylene sutures used to close a longitudinal arteriotomy in a 5-mm radius carotid artery at 100 mmHg and constant in situ length.

B† Suture Size	Safety Factor	Load Ratio
5-0	1.96	51%
6-0	1.92	52%
7-0	1.33	75%

†Safety factors and load ratios for polypropylene sutures used to close a longitudinal arteriotomy in a 5-mm radius carotid artery at 100 mmHg and 6% extension beyond in situ length.

Depicts the relative safety factors for three sizes of polypropylene carotid arteriotomy closures at in situ length and after extension simulating normal neck extension. There is significant reduction in the safety factor for a 7-0 suture. (From Dobrin, P: Polypropylene suture stresses following closure of longitudinal arteriotomy. *J Vasc Surg* 7:423–28, 1988, with permission.)

Factors in suture fracture include too much load, possible manufacturing defects, and acquired iatrogenic weaknesses. Increased intraluminal pressure, e.g., hypertension, is an additional factor, but in Dobrin's calculations is responsible for only 1% to 2% of added loads and is unimportant. The primary reasons for suture fracture/disruption thus are fully the responsibility of the surgeon.[3-5]

Suture Injury

Inappropriate handling of the suture, particularly of monofilament crystalline sutures, may result in subtle disruptions of the crystalline matrix of monofilament sutures or subtle fraying of the fabric in braided sutures. If the injured segment is included within the suture line and thereby exposed to constant expansile and tension stresses, it may later break, resulting in (early) anastomotic disruption or (late) pseudoaneurysm formation.

Figure 9 shows the effect of suture engagement with a needle driver or hemostat. Figure 10 shows the less readily apparent fracture induced by grasping the suture with vascular forceps. All demonstrate

Table 3.

Suture Size	Cross-sectional Area* cm^2	Knot Force F_k grams	Knot Stress σ_k dyne/cm$^2 \times 10^9$	Pressure Stress σ_p dyne/cm$^2 \times 10^9$	Total Suture Stress dyne/cm$^2 \times 10^9$	Tensile Strength dyne/cm$^2 \times 10$
5-0	1.59×10^{-4}	151.8 ± 10.06	0.94 ± 0.07	0.02	0.96	4.27 ± 0.08
6-0	6.82×10^{-5}	108.0 ± 19.6	1.56 ± 0.29	0.05	1.61	5.03 ± 0.06
7-0	3.89×10^{-5}	81.9 ± 13.0	2.07 ± 0.30	0.08	2.15	5.19 ± 0.21

*Cross-sectional area values provided by Ethicon, Inc., Somerville, NJ.

Depicts the engineering statistics for 3 polypropylene sutures subjected to standard knots as would be performed after completion of an anastomosis. (From Dobrin, P: Polypropylene suture stresses following closure of longitudinal arteriotomy. *J Vasc. Surg* 7:423–28, 1988, with permission.)

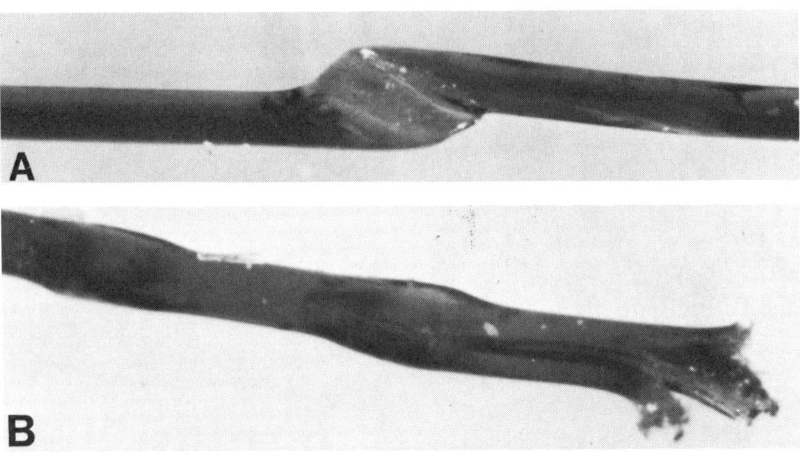

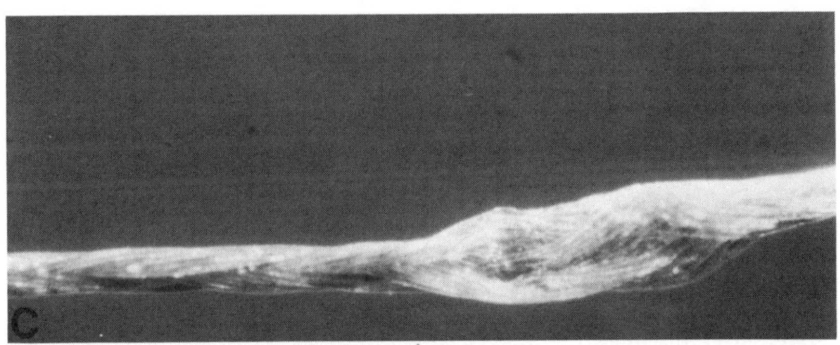

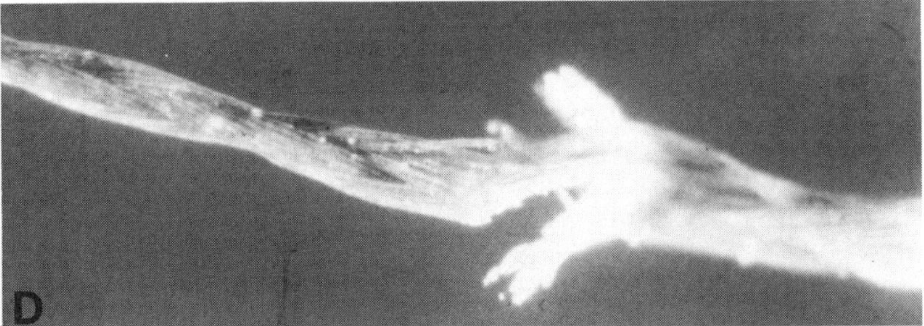

Figures 9C, D. *When subsequently exposed to stretch, both sutures break at the site of the crush injury. (Figures 9A, B, C, D courtesy of Ethicon, Inc., Somerville, NJ.[9])*

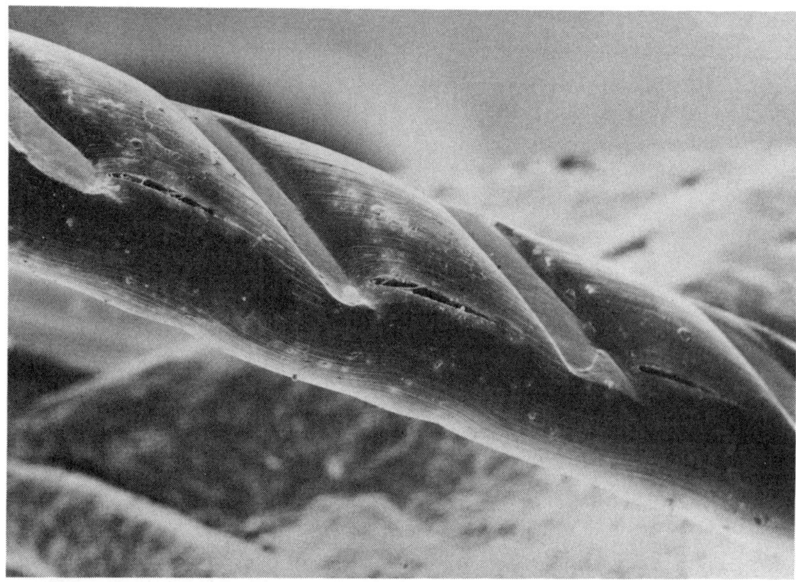

Figure 10. *The longitudinal crush or crystalline matrix fractures induced by vascular forceps application. The gouges represent the teeth. There are longitudinal fractures of the suture skin as well. (Courtesy Ethicon, Inc., Somerville, N.J.[9])*

distraction of the suture structure with fraying or laceration of the exterior surface and frank crystalline fracture. Dobrin's work would indicate that damage to the external surface of monofilament sutures is of particular importance; any external surface injury may result in sigificant reduction in tensile strength of the suture, which resides predominantly in its external surface. Thus, it should be apparent that the suture itself needs to be treated with gentleness and should never be engaged with any instrument in an area that will be used in the final anastomosis (needle driver, forceps, hemostat, or "atraumatic" microvascular clamp). Dobrin has also looked at the force applied to a suture by experienced surgeons when handling the suture with DeBakey forceps (Fig. 11). Gentle application results in an average 278 g of applied force; significant reduction in tensile strength, however, did not occur until forces over 1,000 g were applied. This would suggest that gentle occasional handling of a suture with forceps may be tolerated, although forceful application will result in later suture breakage.

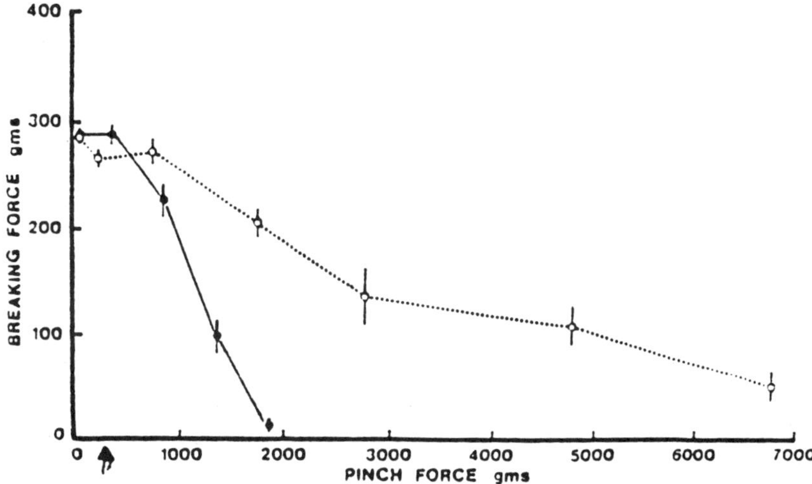

Figure 11. *The effect of grasping a polypropylene suture with vascular forceps on subsequent breaking strength of the suture. Two manufacturers of an identical forceps are presented; 167 6-0 polypropylene sutures were tested. The arrow depicts the average force exerted by a surgeon lightly grasping a suture with forceps; this is considerably less than the threshold level of 1,000 g. (From Dobrin, P: Effects of surgical manipulation on the breaking strength of polypropylene sutures. Arch Surg 124:665–69, 1989, with permission.)*

Dobrin has also studied other surgical manipulations of sutures that may result in decreased suture strength. Sutures are prepared by the manufacturer as strands coiled around a cardboard insert. This results in a twist or kink. It might be inferred that the suture would be weakened at the kink, however, Dobrin has tested such sutures and found no difference in tensile strength (Table 4). Similarly, when a suture line is constructed, there are rotational forces applied to the suture, resulting in axial twists. Dobrin has demonstrated that up to four axial twists can be tolerated without demonstrable decrease in strength (Table 5).[3–5]

On the other hand, Dobrin has demonstrated a significant 71% (P <.05) reduction in tensile strength if a random or stray knot occurs in a suture line during handling: breakage may occur at the knot where stresses are maximally imparted to the suture. Thus, a suture with a stray knot should be discarded or the knotted area specifically excluded from the suture line (Table 4).

Table 4.
Effects of Surgical Manipulation on Suture Strength

	Control Segments	Kinked Segments	Knotted Segments
Number	18	18	18
Breaking Force (grams)	339.3 ± 12.3	323.9 ± 11.6	280.7 ± 10.2* ($p < .05$)

Describes the force necessary to break a 5-0 polypropylene suture extended between two holding clamps, and the modification of that required force by kinking the segment or by adding a stray knot within the segment. Stray knots significantly weaken the suture. (From Dobrin, P: Polypropylene suture stresses following closure of longitudinal arteriotomy. *J Vasc Surg* 7:423–28, 1988, with permission.)

Table 5.
Effects of Axial Twist on Suture Strengths

	Control Segments (0°)	1 Twist (360°)	2 Twists (720°)	3 Twists (1080°)	4 Twists (1440°)
Number	20	20	20	20	20
Breaking Force (grams)	333.1 ± 9.1	318.7 ± 12.4	312.6 ± 12.1	319.4 ± 14.0	315.4 ± 0.5

No breaking force was significantly different than control.

Describes the force necessary to break a 5-0 polypropylene suture extended between two holding clamps and the modification of that required force by axial twisting of the strand from 360° to 1,440°. There is no significant decrease in strength with up to four axial twists. (From Dobrin, P: Effects of surgical manipulation on the breaking strength of polypropylene sutures. *Arch Surg* 124:665–69, 1989, with permission.)

In further work, Dobrin has examined the relative strength of monofilament polypropylene suture before and after incorporation into a suture line. In studies of over 1,000 sutures, *no manufacturing or structural defects were ever noted,* indicating that it is the *surgeon* and what he/she *does* with the suture that is most responsible for suture line difficulties!

Infectivity of Suture

Tradition maintains that a monofilament suture is less likely to maintain infection than a braided one, based on the likelihood of bacterial sequestration in the interstices of the latter suture. However,

Scher has noted that the presence of surgical knots is probably more important than choice of suture, since the knot allows sequestration as does the braided suture. He noted that bacterial adherence of radioactively labeled *Staphylococcus aureus* to braided sutures was greater than to monofilament sutures, although the difference was not statistically significant. With the addition of surgical knots, the two sutures had nearly equivalent rates of bacterial adherance. His observation was that the purported anti-infective advantage of monofilament was perhaps not as real as some authors have suggested.

Reactivity of Sutures

Cavallaro and coworkers have presented data from a canine abdominal aortic grafting model to indicate that the tissue response to implanted sutures varies significantly. They looked at braided Dacron, polypropylene monofilament, and Teflon monofilament vascular sutures implanted as aortic anastomoses and harvested at 15 to 150 days. Although there was no gross difference in inflammatory response, braided Dacron showed an early intense inflammatory reaction that developed into a foreign body granulomatous reaction. A much lesser degree of acute inflammation leading to chronic connective tissue incorporation was seen with the monofilament sutures. The authors presented no conclusions relative to potential ill effects of the braided suture.[6] One can postulate problems with anastomotic collagen and elastin formation and perhaps a weaker anastomosis, but at this point all would be speculation.

Size of "Bite"

The actual construction of a vasclar anastomosis is highly variable between surgeons as to depth of bite, distance between suture bites, and whether or not adventitia should be excluded or included in the bite.

Pomposelli analyzed the theoretics of small (1 mm) versus large (2 mm) bites in augmenting or decreasing the induction of local wall stress at anastomoses as a function of conformational stress (see Chapter 5). Wall shear stress did not scale linearly with arterial size to which a constant size prosthesis was anastomosed, but rather reached a threshold point at which tension precipitously increased. Curves for tension vs. artery size were calculated for 1.0, 1.5, and 2.0 mm size suture bites, demonstrating a shift in the curves with decreasing size of suture bite (Fig. 12); the data would support the concept that smaller (1 mm) bites at the anastomotic apex are warranted, in order to decrease wall tension induced by conformational stresses.[7]

However, the absolute strength of an anastomosis in terms of its potential for disruption, is directly dependent on the size of each bite. We have performed strain gauge measurements of varying types of

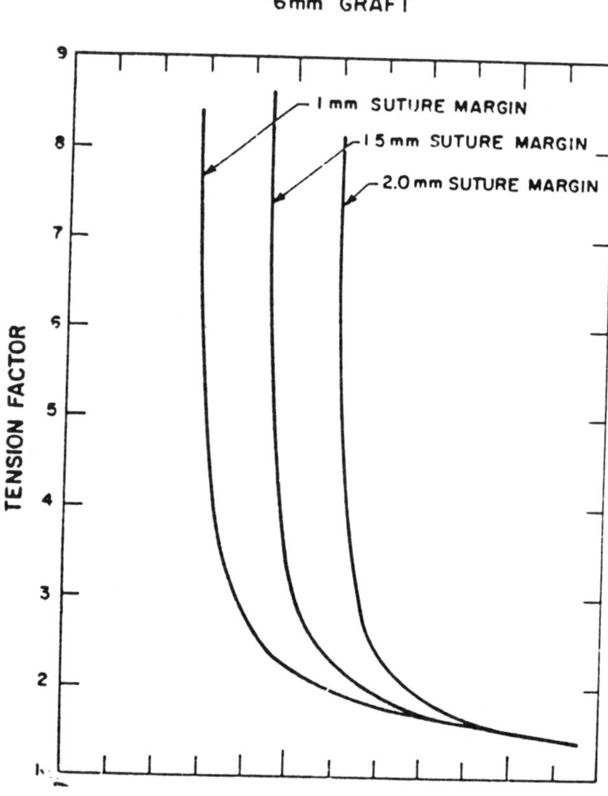

Figure 12. *Tension curves for arterial walls of vessels with diameters of 3 to 5 mm at an end-to-side anastomosis with a 6-mm synthetic graft, utilizing three different suture margins. Wall tension does not correlate linearly with the arterial outside diameter, but instead reaches a threshold at 4 to 4.5 mm. More tension is applied by a suture line of deeper (2 mm) bites than by one with smaller bites. (From Pomposelli, F, Schoen, F, Cohen, R, et al: Conformational stress and anastomotic hyperplasia. J Vasc Surg 1:525–34, 1984, with permission.)*

anastomotic techniques in both canine aortoiliac and atherosclerotic human femoropopliteal segments that shed further light on what is otherwise a matter of personal opinion and/or surgical tradition. One may utilize the data to support a variety of suture methods, although we feel that certain basic points are cardinal.[8]

Three types of bites were tested: 1 mm, representing a bite just at the intimal edge; 2 mm, being an average distance back from the intimal edge; and 3 mm, representing an excessive bite relative to the size of the vessels being studied. The grams of force illustrated in Figure 13 represent lateral tension to the point of disruption or suture pullout. It was evident to us that a 2-mm bite takes twice as much force as a 1-mm bite. However, there is a relative plateau above that, with 3-mm bites adding little additional strength. Table 6 shows the actual force exerted. It is of interest that in all situations, the force is less than the known tensile strengths of the commonly utilized sutures; in our experimental model, artery disruption always occurred prior to suture fracture.

We also studied the relationship of increasing numbers of suture bites, until the number approaches an anastomosis. It is of interest that there is essentially no synergistic effect of additional sutures; the anastomosis disrupts at roughly the same force as a single suture. This points to the necessity that every bite of an anastomosis must be equivalently strong, e.g., placed with equal care (Table 6).

Dissection of a vessel may proceed in an immediately periadvential plane or may utilize a thorough stripping/cleaning of the adventitia in the immediate area of the anastomosis. We further demonstrated that there is a remarkable increase in single suture pullout strength when the adventitia is included in the bite; arterial pullout still occurs at the same rough levels, but the adventitia holds to a greater total force. Our work demonstrates that this principle holds true for single, double, and triple sutures and for anastomoses. Furthermore, the contribution of the adventitia exceeds that of the vessel wall, such that a 1-mm suture with adventitia holds better than a 2-mm nonadventitial suture.

This would imply that arterial dissection either should *not* be performed in the adventitial plane or that the stripped layer of adventitia should be specifically included in the bite to add integral strength. Clinically we have seen this phenomenon when, unless adventitia is used, a suture tears through the wall of a relatively undiseased vessel during anastomotic construction. Whether or not long-term strength is

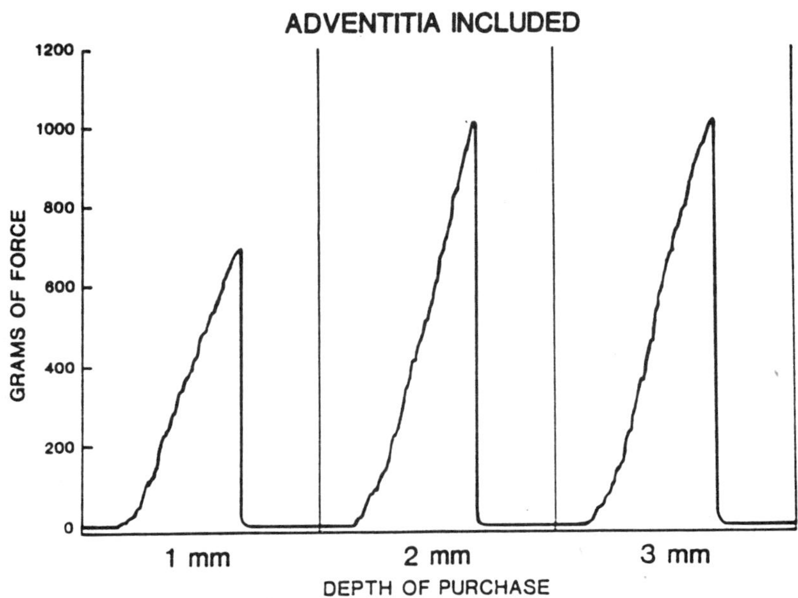

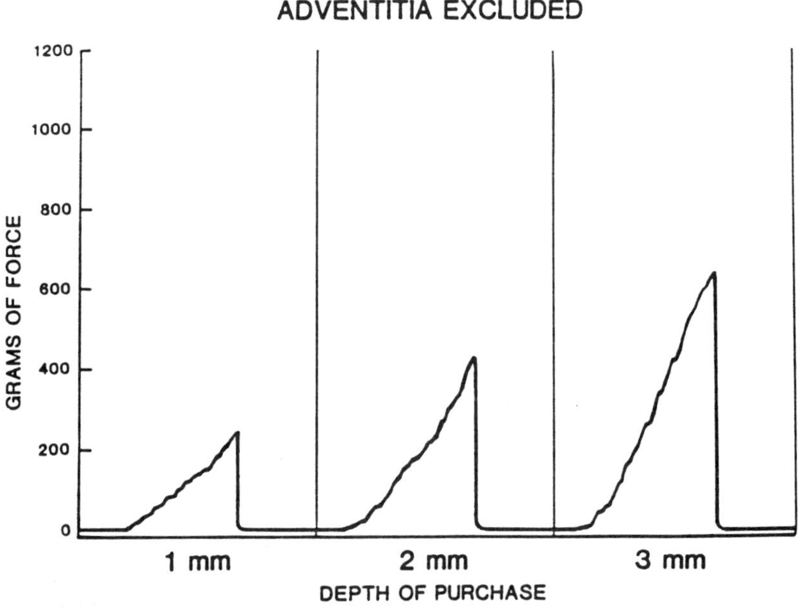

Figure 13A–B. *Strain gauge measurements of the lateral pullout strength of 5-0 polypropylene suture applied to canine iliac artery segments ex vivo at 1-mm, 2-mm, and 3-mm distances from the arteriotomy edge. (From Moore, WM, Bunt, TJ:* Vasc Surg, *in press.)*

180

Table 6.
Force Required for Arterial Anastomosis Disruption

	1 Bite	2 Bites	3 Bites	Anastomosis
1-mm $\bar{s}$ Adventitia	230	200	240	390
1-mm $\bar{c}$ Adventitia	700	675	750	1015
2-mm $\bar{s}$ Adventitia	415	400	400	505
2-mm $\bar{c}$ Adventitia	1010	1300	850	1250
3-mm $\bar{s}$ Adventitia	640	550	575	695
3-mm $\bar{c}$ Adventitia	1115	1100	1140	1100

All values represent mean grams of force.

also provided cannot be determined by those experiments, but it would seem clear that the long-term development of pseudoaneurysms due to suture pullout would be directly related to the type and sizing of the anastomotic bites.

Continuous Versus Interrupted Suture

As discussed in Chapter 5, performance of an end-to-end anastomosis of equivalent compliance index vessels at exact luminal match would theoretically result in an ideally matched mechanical transfer of energy: however, it has been demonstrated that the sutures themselves exert a measurable restraining influence and incite a local compliance mismatch. This may be minimized by the use of interrupted rather than continuous suture. (For details, see Chapter 5).

Recommendations

Optimal performance of an anastomosis begins with an appropriate selection of needle size (for strength and radius of curve) matched to suture size (for tensile strength vs. size vessel) matched to needle driver (to minimize needle injury). Technical performance of the anastomosis entails the details enumerated in Chapter 6, and a precise placement of successive sutures at appropriate depth and spacing related to the anticipated strength of the vessel or graft being anastomosed. One could say that indeed, it is not exactly "standard!"

We have found that in general, a BV needle handled in a Castrovieho or fine-nosed Ryder needle driver is suited admirably to small vessel anastomosis (tibial, radial/ulnar, internal carotid) where the small radius of curve of the needle allows precise instrumental adjustments. Ethicon (Somerville, NJ) currently is researching a BV sized needle in 6-0 and 7-0 polypropylene, with a 5- to 7-mm needle chord, which may prove to be ideal for anastomoses to tibial vessels. RB or CT needles on Ryder needle drivers are admirably suited to the majority of vascular anastomosis (carotid, femoral, popliteal, iliac) with needle driver length adjusted to the depth of the incision. SH or MH needles with their increased strength and broad radius of curvature are well suited to aortic and aneurysmal anastomoses, respectively.

The size of the bite should be at least 1.5 to 2.0 mm unless a 1-mm bite is critical (e.g., outflow at the anastomotic toe). If a smaller 1-mm bite is used, it should be driven obliquely from small intimal to larger adventitial inclusion. Conversely, the periadventitia should be specifically picked up and included in the bite for strength. This makes the 1-mm bite nearly as strong as the basic 2-mm bite.

In badly atherosclerotic vessels, a large bite may be taken, realizing that the media gives little additional strength and that this lays excessive graft over the exterior of the vessel rather than allowing its use within the flowing portion of the anastomosis. Conversely, a local endarectomy may be performed, followed by closure of the arteriotomy with what is essentially an adventitial suture. This is probably a better suture than one including a large bite of the plaque within the anastomosis.

Bites on a synthetic graft matrix should be no more than 1-2 mm since all except woven grafts have sufficient strength to hold at this depth, and the smaller bite allows more of the graft to be involved within the flow surface of the anastomosis.

References

1. Mason, RG, Mohammad, SF: A human model for study of blood vascular wall interactions. *Arch Surg* 115:952–8, 1980.
2. Guidoin, R, Dogon, B, Blais, P, et al: Effects of traumatic manipulations on grafts, sutures, and host arteries during vascular surgical procedures. *Res Exper Medic* 179:1–21, 1981.
3. Dobrin, PB: Some mechanical properties of polypropylene sutures. *J Surg Res* (In press).
4. Dobrin, PB: Effects of surgical manipulation on the breaking strength of polypropylene sutures. *Arch Surg* 124:665–69, 1989.

5. Dobrin, PB: Polypropylene suture stresses following closure of longitudinal arteriotomy. *J Vasc Surg* 7:423–8, 1988.
6. Cavallaro, A, Sciacca, V, Cisternino, S, et al: Experimental evaluations of tissue reactivity to vascular sutures: Dacron, polypropylene, PTFE. *Vasc Surg* 21:82–86, 1987.
7. Pomposelli, F, Schoen, F, Cohen, R, et al: Conformational stress and anastomotic hyperplasia. *J Vasc Surg* 1:525–34, 1984.
8. Moore, WM, Bunt, TJ: Evaluation of the strength of vascular anastomotic techniques. *J Vasc Surg* (In press).
9. Ethicon Suture Manual. Somerville, NJ, Ethicon Inc, 1984.

Chapter 7

Thoughts on Basic Peripheral Vascular Technique

T.J. Bunt

It is beyond the scope of this book to give the author's concepts of perfect vascular technique for each peripheral vascular operation; and all the more inappropriate when excellent texts concentrate their effort on precisely that. However, it is reasonable to give several pertinent examples of very commonly performed operations to underscore and illustrate the basic principles that are the concern of this book, namely, conscientiously performed, technically demanding vascular surgery. The concept of gentleness in technique and avoidance of the specific mechanisms of vascular injury that are otherwise elucidated is explicit; more implicit is the basic notion that the better a surgeon understands the complexities of the anatomy (and its variants) and the more thoroughly he/she comprehends not only the complications that may occur, but how to avoid them, then the more perfect the results. Vascular surgery to its devotees is a cut above general surgery because it is technically more demanding, the knowledge of relevant anatomy must be more precise, and it requires compulsive attention to detail in order to obtain excellent results.

Basic Instruments

There are a number of fine points to a well-conducted operation that either become second nature to a surgeon or (as is exemplified by

From *Iatrogenic Vascular Injury: A Discourse on Surgical Technique*, edited by T.J. Bunt, M.D. © 1990, Futura Publishing Inc., Mount Kisco, NY.

skilled cardiac teams) well-oiled cogs in a faithfully reproduced operative scheme. Beyond the psychological niceties of a quiet room, pleasant company, full stomach, and benevolent frame of mind, the apprentice surgeon needs to learn to have the patience to set up exactly and correctly before operating. Hurrying, trying to do without proper light or exposure, not waiting for the assistant, etc.—all are marks of an immature and impatient surgeon and lead inevitably to false starts or errors of technique. The rules are simple: do it right, do it carefully, and do it right the first time.

One must learn to position (and reposition) oneself for maximal effectiveness and be free to reposition constantly. It is important to be "square" to the table for a comfortable forehand technique, rather than forcing backhand dissection or suturing. Moving to and from opposite sides of the table is often useful (the "fempop shuffle"); one should be on the same side of the patient as the incision.

Instruments suited to each situation and of the appropriate length (defined as the ability to operate without one's hands bumping into the sides of the wound) should be used. A 5- or 6-inch needle driver might be suitable for an anterior tibial anastomosis, an 8-inch needle driver might feel more comfortable at the groin, and a 10-inch needle driver at the iliacs. Similarly, the less refined fascial/subcutaneous dissection can be done with Metzenbaum scissors, while the fine work of vessel dissection should be done with appropriately designed fine arterial (Shea, DeMartells) scissors (Fig. 1).

Careful inspection and palpation of a vessel can yield useful information as to anastomotic site; there are different qualities to a relatively undiseased segment (expansile, soft, yields with elastic recoil), a diseased thick walled segment (firm to palpation but still moderately elastic), a calcific stenosis (rock-hard, brittle appearing, rough/sharp edge, no elasticity), and a thrombosed segment (firm, unyielding, cordlike). Similarly, a visual inspection can broadly differentiate between translucent blue, minimally diseased vessels and the yellow discoloration of atherosclerotic plaques.

The angiogram should always be prominently displayed in the operating room, and reference made to it for a second check before deciding on levels of anastomosis. The angio should correlate with the noninvasive laboratory estimation of objective flow, which should correlate with the intraoperative assessment of the vessel at that level. All three parameters should be in agreement before decision is made for bypass, level of anastomosis, or length of endarterectomy.

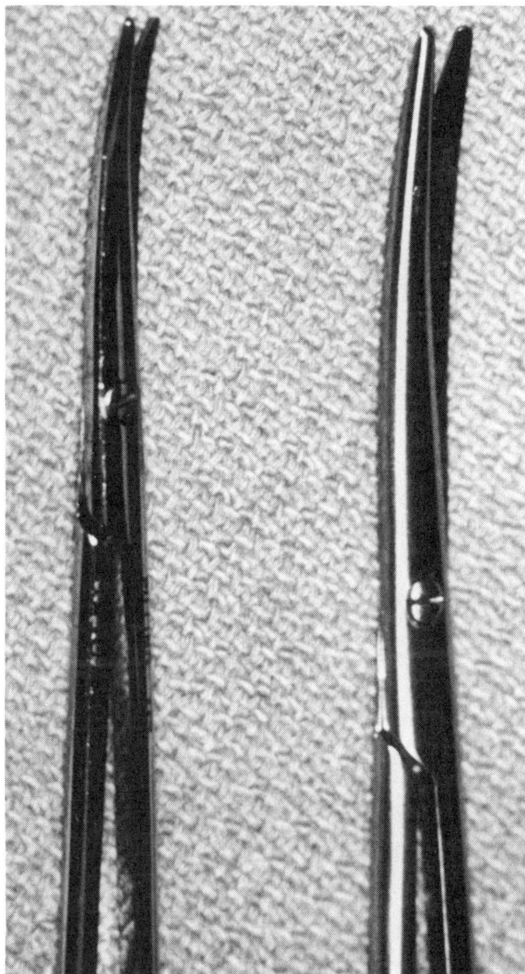

Figure 1A. *Two commonly utilized scissors for vascular dissection. The Metzenbaum scissors (right) have blunter, broader tips than Shea scissors (left), which are more suitable for small vessel dissection.*

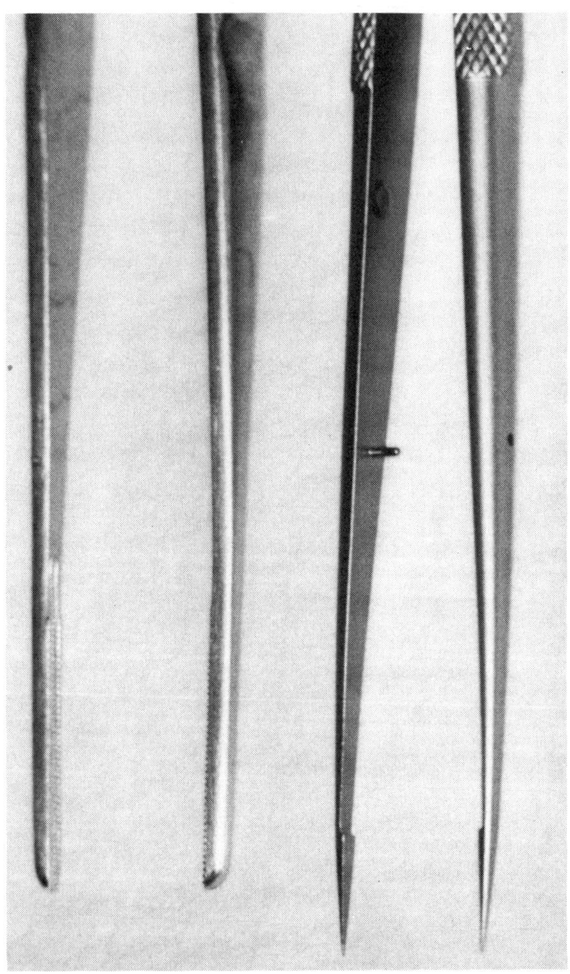

Figure 1B. *Two types of forceps: DeBakey (left) and needle points (right). The latter facilitate small vessel dissection.*

The operating surgeon should accept the inevitability (if not the inherent right) of "putting his/her nose" in the wound; the assistant by corollary should remain aloof from the field. By direct extension of this logic, the surgeon's light should be aimed from the head of the table, nearly directly above, while the assistant's light is angled from below onto a focus at the field, since he/she is less likely to interprose his/her head in its beam.

Saline or antibiotic solution soaked laparotomy pads laid around a wound after complete exposure and before beginning anastomosis aid immeasurably in preventing the suture catching on instruments/retractors and increase the visibility of the suture. All this is beyond the added benefit of keeping the tissue moist and protected from contamination.

Retractors should be carefully individualized to the depth of the wound and the necessity for wide or limited exposure. One should not work over the added depth of a retractor projecting out of the wound. Thus, we have found that Adson-Beckman laminectomy retractors work admirably for thigh level/popliteal exposure, since this jointed instrument allows exposure while keeping the "handle" of the retractor out of the field. Conversely, Meridines work better in the infrapopliteal position, with a blade depth selected dependent on the depth of the wound. Weitlander or Gelpe retractors work best in inguinal or related exposures, where subcutaneous (<2 inches) retraction is all that is required, and the incision plane is flat (Figs. 2A–2C). An Alm retractor is better than a mastoid for Cimino Brescia fistulae at the wrist, having very flat blades that do not project above the incision. Combined vessel-loop retraction and vascular control may also be utilized for side-to-side anastomoses (Fig. 3). In general, self-retaining retractors should be placed so that the handles are on the side opposite the dominant hand of the surgeon: e.g., from superior in groin dissections but inferior in popliteal dissections so that the surgeon does not have to work over them.

Use of Loupes

Magnification of small caliber vessels facilitates accurate placement of intimal sutures, but does so at a small price of encumbrance and loss of total visual field, even for individuals highly trained in their use. Simultaneous use of loupes with identical focal distances by both

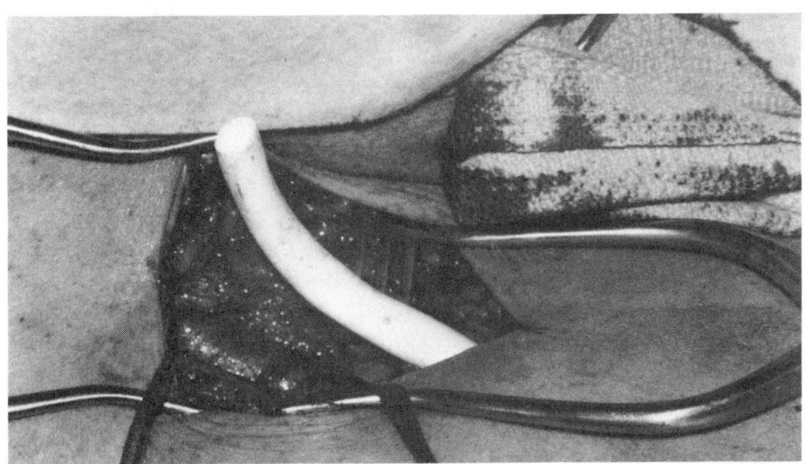

Figures 2A, B, C. *Depicts three types of retractors, and their selective use in three different incisions based on the principles of: (a) the arms should not project above the wound edge, and (b) the arms should not project into the wound. Either deficit impinges on the surgeon's view of and instrument handling within the incision. (A, above). Weitlander retractor in an inguinal incision.*

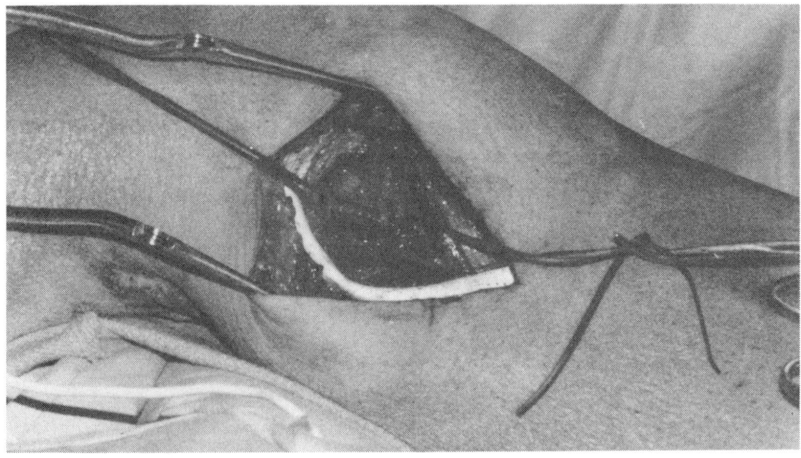

Figure 2B. *Adson-Beckman retractor in a popliteal incision.*

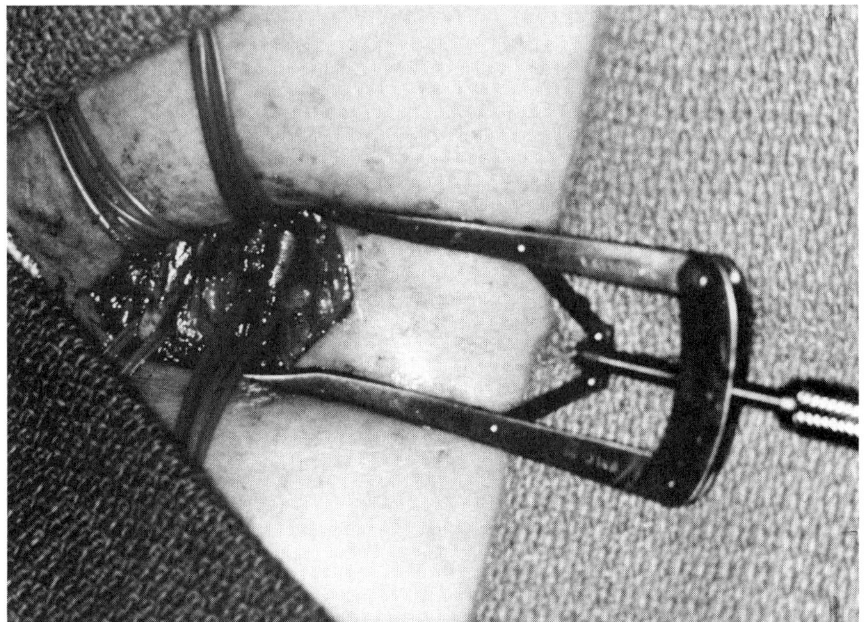

Figure 2C. *Alm retractor within a dialysis fistula incision.*

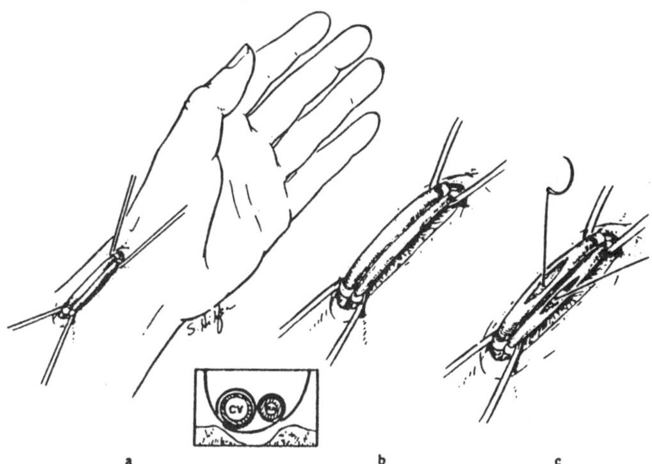

1. a, Silastic rubber vessel loop encircling both cephalic vein and radial artery. b, Close up monstrating simultaneous control, exposure and apposition vessels. c, Posterior row of anastomosis being initiated.

Figure 3. *Simultaneous small vessel occlusion and exposure may be obtained in preparation of a Cimino-Brescia fistula by looping both vessels with silastic vessel-loops. (From Bunt, T.J. et al: Vessel-loop combined exposure and control for Cimino-Brescia fistulae. Surg Gynecol Obstet 160:87:1985, with permission.)*

surgeon and assistant inevitably causes head-bumping; therefore perhaps the most logical solution is for the surgeon (who is suturing) to wear loupes and the assistant (who is controlling the operative field) to defer their use, or to use a set with a longer focal length.

Basic Dissection Techniques

Vascular Dissection

Since collateral circulation is so important in the long-term limb viability of patients with peripheral vascular disease, a general maxim is to preserve all branch vessels as potential collaterals. If ligation is performed, it should be just distal to a flush position with the adventitia to minimize intraluminal "crinkling" of the orifice, which causes intraluminal endothelial injury, and so as not to leave a blind pocket as a nidus for platelet deposition with secondary endothelial injury or thrombus formation. Gundry has noted a high incidence of luminal encroachment by ligatures applied flush to the vein wall during vein harvesting (see Chapter 3).[1]

Lymphatics accompany virtually all vessels currently accessible to the vascular surgeon, usually as discrete nodes and trunks closely approximating the vessel. Lymphocele formation in wounds may be the precedent for delayed wound healing and graft infection. In addition, Goldstone et al. have demonstrated that the lymph nodes at the inguinal site may harbor ascending infection from distal infected sites,[2] and Bunt has demonstrated that clinically benign lymph nodes harbor *Staphylococcus epidermidis* (a major cause of delayed graft infection) in 25% to 30% of cases. Hence, careful identification and ligation of lymphatics is important. If a lymph node is transected, it should either be resected with control of its afferent/efferent lymphangioles or its cut surface electrocoagulated thoroughly. We prefer the former technique.[3,4]

There are three major points to making an arteriotomy incision: the incision should be clean without crushing the vessel wall constituents; the incision should be made without creating a back wall injury; and it should be clear that the incision is actually within the arterial lumen. The incision may be made with a fine stilletto tip or hook blade scalpel, but should always be lengthened with Potts arterial scissors properly angled to maintain perpendicular relationships in all planes to the circumference and length of the artery. Visualization of the lumen may be facilitated by inserting/opening the tips of DeBakey forceps or by nerve hook distraction of the orifice (Fig. 4). If a back wall injury occurs, it should be repaired with double armed sutures placed from inside-out to prevent intimal flap formation or dissection.

An arteriotomy should be made only in the artery where careful preliminary palpation reveals a relatively soft wall and compressible (e.g., nonthrombosed) lumen. In areas where medial or lateral wall plaquing is characteristic, careful attention is necessary to ensure incision through normal wall with subsequent visualization of endothelium (e.g., lumen) before extending the incision—so that one does not incise deeply into a large plaque rather than into the lumen. Often the initial arteriotomy is thus made in a soft area and perhaps slightly lateral or off-center, and then extended with Potts scissors.

Integral to all of the discussion in this book regarding the ill effects of endothelial injury is the importance of gentle technique once the artery is open and the intima exposed. Efforts should always be made to prevent lengthy occlusive times with resultant ischemic injury. Similarly, the injurious efects of dehydration from prolonged intimal

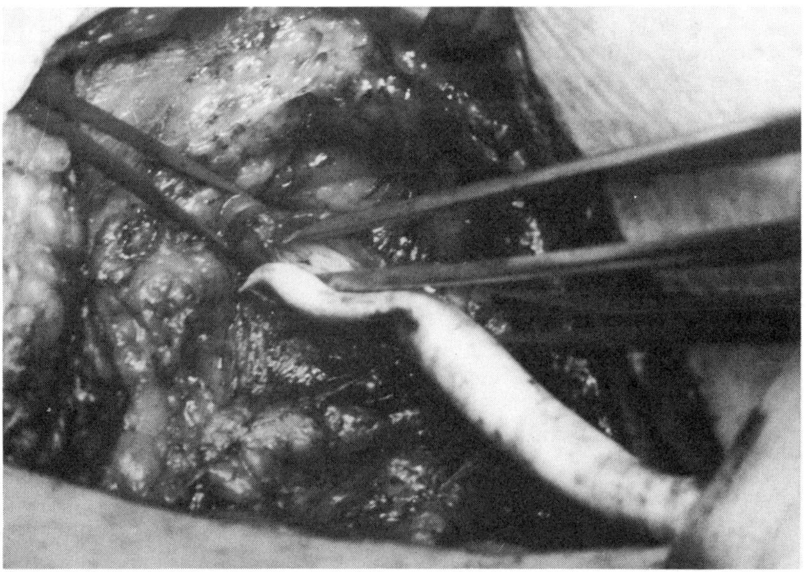

Figure 4. *An atraumatic method of luminal visualization. By insertion and spreading of vascular forceps, direct handling of the arteriotomy edge is avoided.*

exposure or toxic irrigants (e.g., povidone-iodine) should be avoided. It is an almost axiomatic, if often circumvented, rule of vascular surgery that one should never unnecessarily engage the intima with instruments; this should include direct forceps engagements of the arteriotomy or vein graft edge. It should *never* be necessary to actually "pick up" the intima! The arteriotomy may be exposed and the intimal edge visualized by a number of techniques illustrated on the accompanying pages; by displacement with a nerve hook or guy sutures placed in the arteriotomy, or by internal stenting with a DeBakey forceps. Once the suture line is placed, suture line displacement may be used to facilitate intimal visualization. Gentle upward traction on the running suture and countertraction laterally by holding the dome of the cobra head with pickups will show the intima. At the apex, "double-biting" with alternate lateral and medial displacement of the graft by the assistant will afford optimal visualization of each portion of the anastomosis.

The first assistant is directly responsible for the speed and efficiency of an operation. It is the assistant's ability to anticipate and facilitate each motion of the surgeon that makes an operation either easy or difficult. This individual's major duties are to provide and maintain exposure, facilitate the dissection by appropriate counter traction/suctioning/and hemostasis, and facilitate anastomosis by providing sequential and optimal exposure of the two structures being approximated, while keeping the suture free and clear of the surgeon's instruments and field.

In an anastomosis, the assistant should maintain gentle traction on the suture in a direction opposite to the axis of anastomosis and without pulling up tautly with one hand. With the other hand he/she alternately exposes either graft or artery edge by rolling its edge upward. The method used to do this varies with the size artery and where one is on the suture line.

A few pointers are to be considered. For suturing at the apex, insert the tips of a DeBakey forceps into the apex and open; thus spreading the arteriotomy (Fig. 4). Conversely, either at apex suturing or on the free edge, one may use a nerve hook to gently engage, elevate, and stabilize the edge for suturing (Fig. 5). On the graft side, heel sutures are facilitated by spreading an inserted forceps and angling the entire graft orifice upward. In addition, mid-length sutures on the graft side are facilitated by grasping the *hood* of the graft with forceps and laterally retracting while the assistant grasps the actual

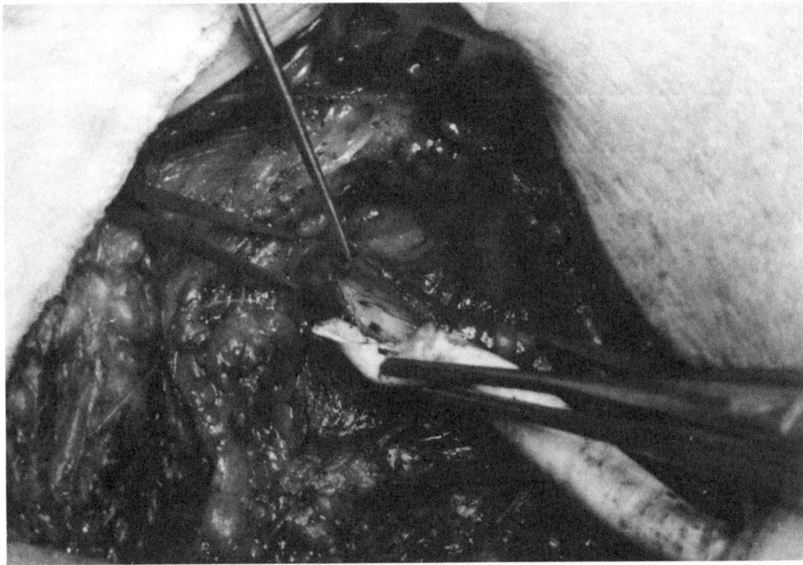

Figure 5. *An alternate method of atruamatic visualization of the lumen is demonstrated; gentle insertion/retraction with a nerve hook avoids direct handling of the arteriotomy edge.*

edge (Fig. 6C). After the heel and one side have been completed, apical sutures may be facilitated by the surgeon "double-biting" while the assistant rolls the graft medially for graft and laterally for open artery bites. Each of these techniques markedly increases intimal visualization (Figs. 6A–F).

As with any essentially judgmental decision, the extent of vascular dissection necessary and appropriate to any case is highly debatable. Certainly, exposure needs to involve a sufficient length of artery for occlusive control and subsequent arteriotomy/anastomosis. However, the routine wide exposure of vessels in the field probably is not optimal, particularly at popliteal and femoral locations. The incidence of "re-do" surgery is more than sufficiently high, and is made markedly more difficult by prior dissection. Therefore, a more limited dissection is preferable. In addition, such extensive dissection disrupts medial blood supply supplied by the adventitial vasa vasorum and thus leads to medial ischemia and an increased propensity for recurrent stenosis. Thus we favor a dissection limited to sufficient anterior exposure as is necessary for anastomosis and circumferential dissec-

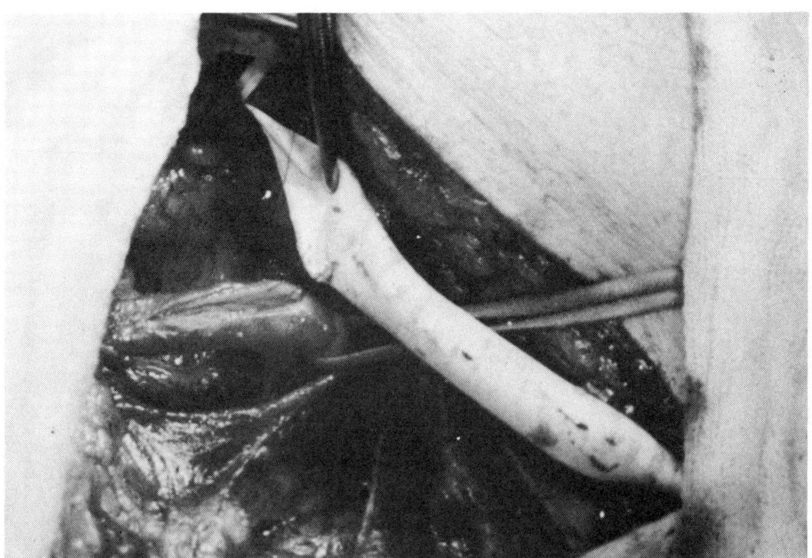

Figure 6A. *The heel is performed first, utilizing a parachute technique. The assistant holds the graft at its cobra head and rotates it away from the side being sutured and with gentle upward traction to keep the arterial lumen open. All sutures are placed with clear open visualization.*

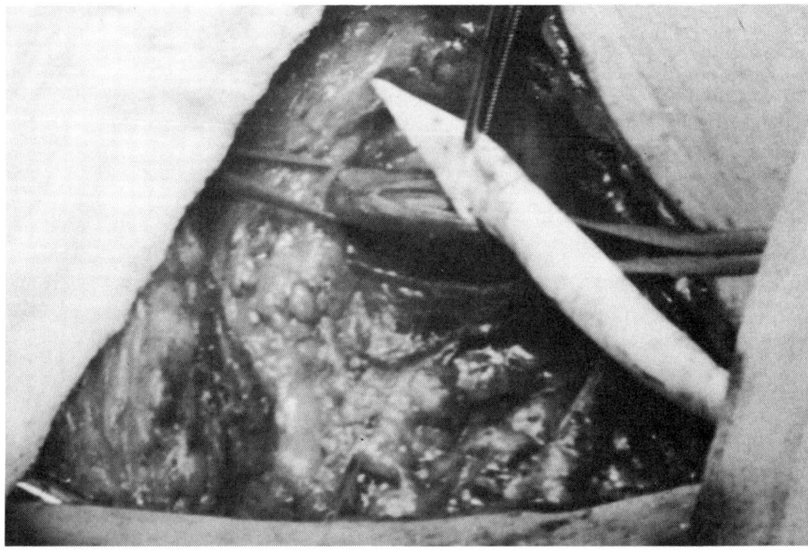

Figure 6B. *Once three or four sutures to either side of the heel have been placed, the graft is parachuted down. Now the first side of the anastomosis is facilitated by the assistant holding the dome of the cobra head and rotating the graft away and slightly upward: this holds the lumen open.*

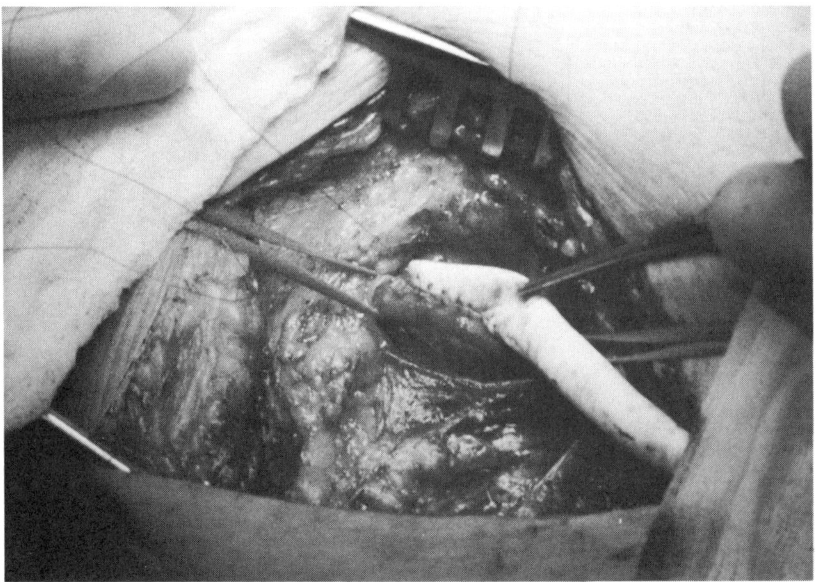

Figure 6C. *As the apex is approached, the assistant rotates the graft over the arteriotomy for graft "bites," and (see Fig. 6D)*

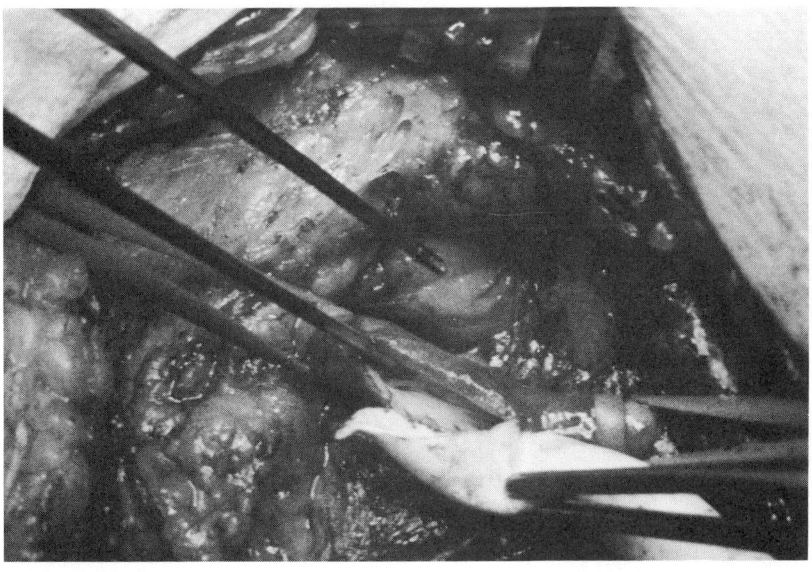

Figure 6D. *away from the artery to facilitate arterial "bites."*

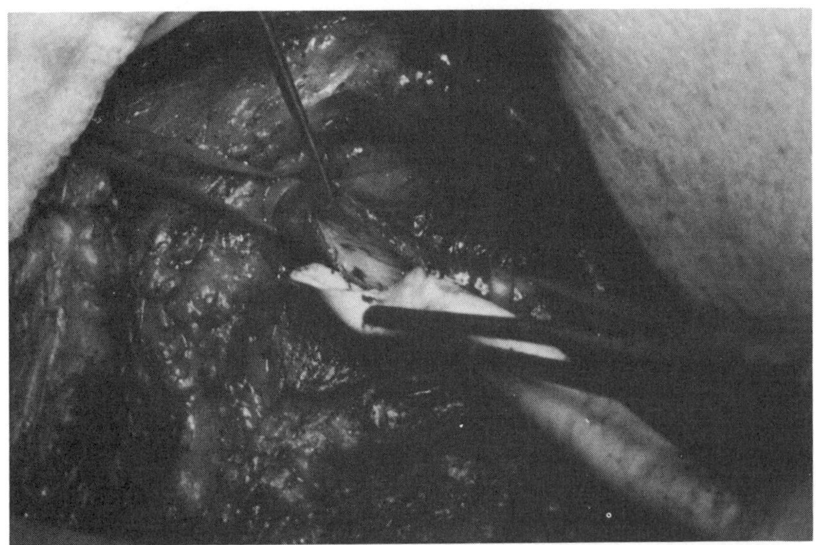

Figure 6E. *Complete visualization of the apex aterial lumen is afforded by rotating the graft away from the artery, parachuting the three apex sutures, and inserting a nerve hook into the arterial lumen.*

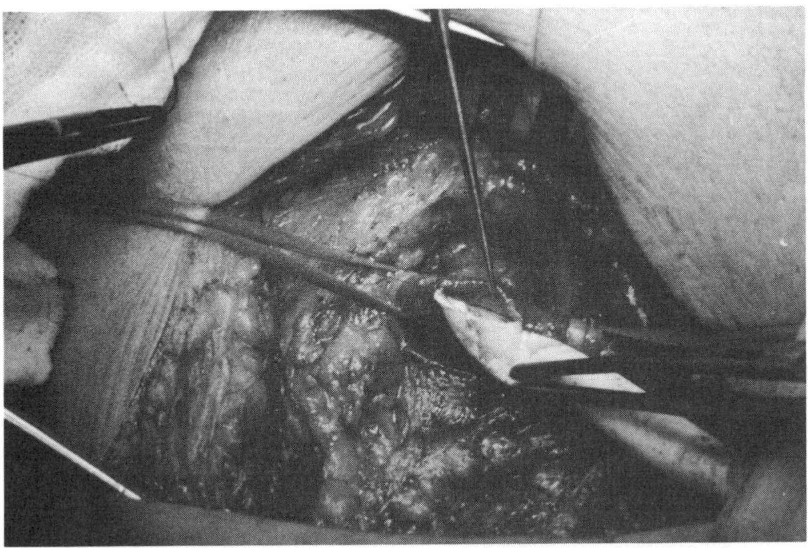

Figure 6F. *The second side is facilitated by 4-way distraction—upward/outward on both sutures, medially on the dome of the graft (by surgeon), and lateral on the arteriotomy with a nerve hook.*

tion limited to the proximal and distal points of occlusive control. In our opinion, extensive mobilization is detrimental.

Dessication of exposed tissues may lead to decreased infection resistance, particularly of exposed and relatively nonvascular subcutaneous fat. Measures to prevent dessication include frequent irrigation of the wound with physiological saline, packing an open but not currently utilized wound with a wet sponge, and temporarily closing the wound over a wet sponge with towel clips. This latter method is helpful in maintaining nondependent incisions such as the lateral or medial incisions in the leg used for femoropopliteal/femorodistal grafting.

Suturing

Basic teachings about suture techniques apply equally if not more convincingly to vascular surgery: the needle should be firmly advanced through tissue/graft in one smooth motion without rocking the needle and advancement should be made only in the curve of the needle. Failure to observe these simple precepts continuously and religiously results in a larger local endothelial injury at the artery and the potential for a leaky graft suture line (particularly with PTFE grafts).

Given the fact that suture strength is more than adequate at all sizes, the choice of needle is probably more important than suture size. The curve and size of the needle should lend themselves to manipulation within the narrow confines of the arteriotomy. Therefore, in general, the smaller the vessel, the smaller size and shorter radius of curve needle should be utilized (see Chapter 6).

Angling the needle in the needle driver is also a useful aid (Fig. 7). Placing it at right angles to the driver is ideal for suturing when the wrist can be placed parallel to the longitudinal axis of the artery. When rounding the apical corners, however, it is easier to change the angle of needle fixation than to change the angle of one's wrist supination. In these circumstances, 30°, 45°, and 60° forward angles facilitate suturing. In general, the optimal position for suturing is to place the needle in the driver jaws just forward of the halfway point and with a 30° forward angle (Fig. 7) since this duplicates the comfortable carrying angle of the supinated wrist.

Care should be taken when suturing calcific or dense fibrous plaques since they have a tendency to spontaneously dissect free of the

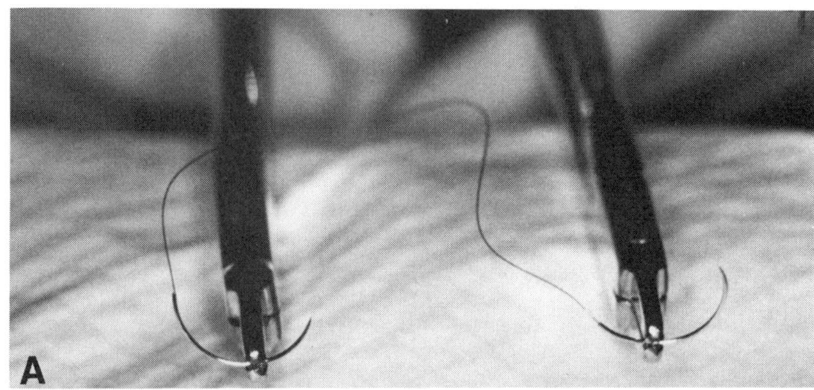

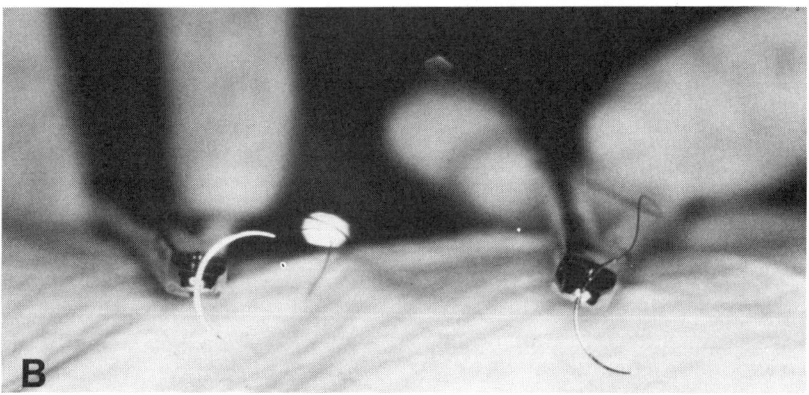

Figure 7A, B. *A needle driver should grasp the needle at the front third (left) rather than the back half (right) of the needle (A); with wrist supination (B), the needle tip is perpendicular without undue wrist supination.*

adventitia and cause local but poorly controlled endarterectomies. This may occur when the adventitia is grasped and retracted with forceps or when a suture is driven vigorously through the plaque. Two options are then available: (1) to perform a controlled limited endarterectomy and tack down the resultant intimal edges to prevent further dissection; (2) careful initial suturing to tether the plaque. The former technique weakens the anastomosis to some degree and has been variably

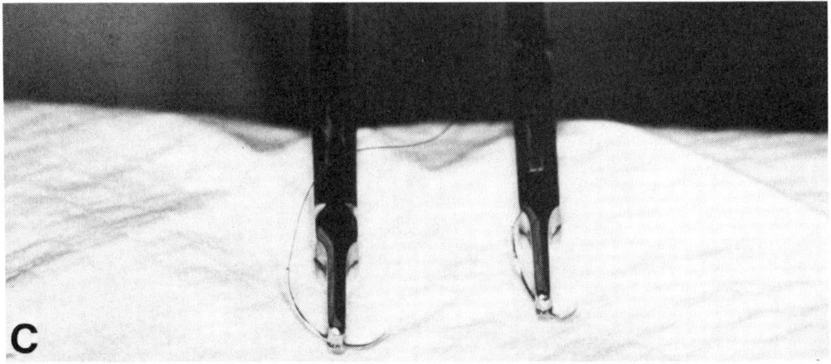

Figure 7C. *Rather than placing the needle at 90° angle to the driver (left), it should be angled 30° to 40° forward (right), so that the needle remains perpendicular to the arterial wall after wrist supination.*

associated with later pseudoaneurysm formations. In addition, it causes a discrete local conformational stress with deleterious local effects. It is useful to drive the needle against the external support of a Kuttner "peanut," rocking the needle gently rather than trying to forcibly drive it through. If such measures do not suffice, exlusion of the plaque via deeper placement of sutures is better than dislodgement/dissection of the nonyielding plaque.

When suturing, the needle driver jaws are not locked but simply closed ("palming"), which facilitates repetitive release. Careful work by Guidoin has demonstrated that needles and the suture/needle junction may be injured by locking the driver or by utilization of an excessively large driver. Such microinjuries on the needle increase the local endothelial and graft injury.[5] Similarly, the suture should never be directly grasped/engaged with the forceps or needle drivers since this may fray or weaken the suture. Dobrin has elegantly demonstrated that the strength of monofilament-extruded sutures is directly dependent upon the external circumstance and not the diameter of the suture. This relates to the extrusion process in which crystallization of the cooling fibers occurs in the lines of stress on the external surface, but is nonaligned throughout the central mass of the extruding suture. Consequently, microinjury to the external surface of the suture causes a disproportionate reduction in suture strength (see Chapter 7).[1,6]

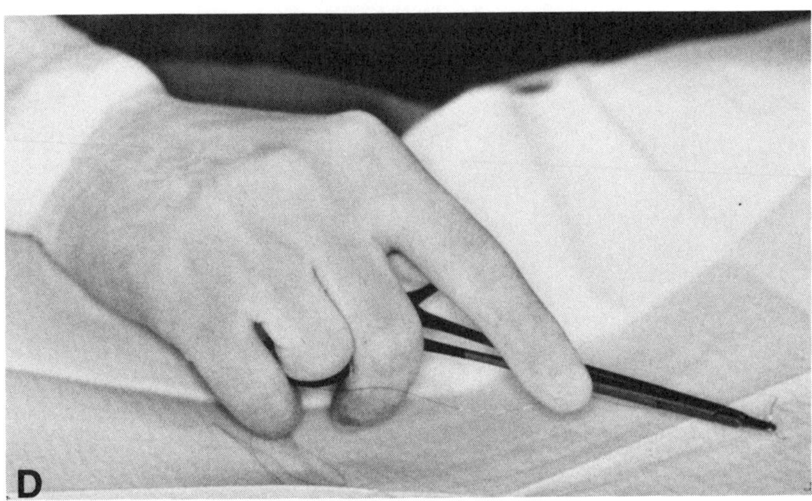

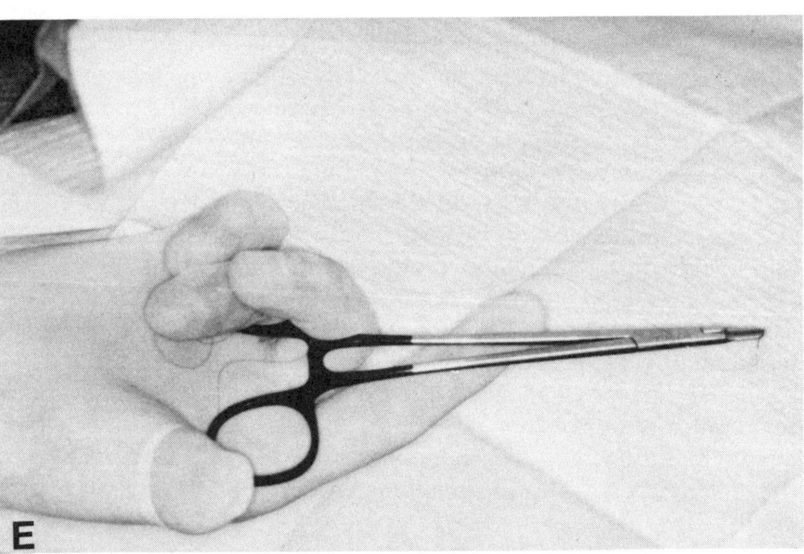

Figures 7D, E. *The wrist may be comfortably supinated only 80° to 90°. With the use of ½ or ⅔ circle needles, an uncomfortable oversupination of the wrist must occur if the needle is grasped at or behind its midsection.*

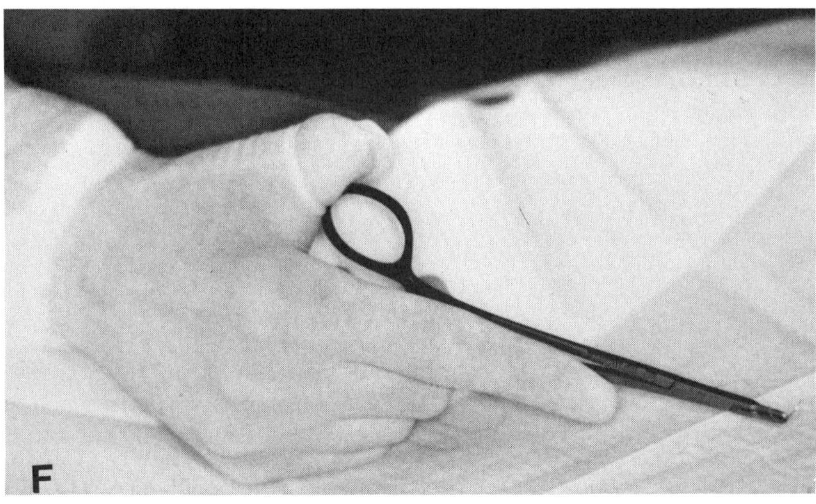

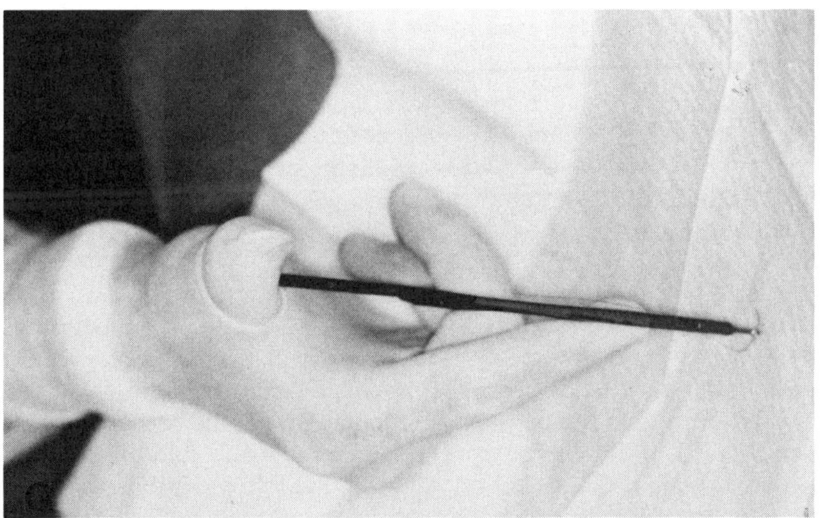

Figures 7F, G. *For comfortable perpendicular needle passage, the needle should be grasped forward of its midsection, usually at the junction of the first and middle thirds.*

The most accurate suturing at the heel and apex is obtained by open or semi-open techniques of "parachuting," that is, several throws of a continuous sutures are placed without pulling them taut with the assistant carefully gathering each and keeping the loops (Fig. 6).

The Groin Exploration

Indication

The groin exploration is implicit to a variety of operations; the proximal anastomosis of femoropopliteal or femorotibial bypasses; the distal anastomosis of axillofemoral, crossover femoral, ileofemoral, and aortofemoral grafts, femoral aneurysmectomy; repair of femoral pseudoaneurysm; femoral thromboembolectomy; and profundoplasty. As such, it is probably the most common dissection performed by peripheral vascular surgeons.

Preparation and Draping

Initial field preparation has great potential importance in determining complication rates. It is evident that exclusion of the obviously contaminated and potentially infectious perineum is particularly important. Indeed, the inguinal incision is well recognized as the major site of early synthetic vascular graft infections, particularly after "redo" cases.[3,7-9]

Exclusion of the perineum should follow thorough preparation of same. In addition an antiseptic soaked cloth can be placed over the perineum, which is then covered with a dry cloth. Exclusion is completed with an adhesive barrier drape. Conversely, the barrier towel may be sutured to the perineal skin to insure that the barrier stays in place. This is facilitated by towel clipping the inside fold of a doubly folded towel to pubis, then bringing the outer fold down over the clips to keep them out of the field. Simple draping of the perineum without these additional measures is not reliable. This is particularly true when the leg is abducted/flexed for popliteal dissection and the scrotum and perineal crease are frequently exposed, with wound contamination a real possibility. Similarly, an overlaid adhesive drape will not reliably exclude the perineum if the case is long (skin moistening), the patient obese, or recurrent leg abduction is performed.

Skin preparation may be performed with any of the antiseptic solutions. We prefer povidone-iodine but cannot argue against any particular agent. Small points to the prep include prepping the inguinal incision areas first, the leg second, and the foot and/or genitalia last with each sponge/brush. The leg should be held away laterally while prepping and draping to insure complete preparation of the perineal crease and posterior thigh. Careful preparation of the genitalia and proximal Foley catheter is also mandatory.

Incision

Although there is a "standard" incision for groin exploration, and it is probably utilized in more than 95% of the incisions made in actual practice, there is still room for discussion of the basic tenets of any surgical tradition, e.g., is it efficacious (does it provide the appropriate exposure in the minimum operative time)?; is it advantageous in terms of avoidance of problems or complications?; and is it appropriate in relation to known maxims of surgical therapy (healing well, cosmetically appealing, not prone to wound problems)? Surgeons should always ask these questions (heretical as they may sometimes appear) and make their own eclectic judgments as to the best incision. As is the philosophy of this book—there is less to be gained from dogma and/or tradition, than from independent analysis and judgment. Rather than make all patients fit to one incision, it is best to consider the advantages and disadvantages of each and choose for each patient and each operative situation.

The vertical incision has several advantages: it is parallel to or in direct line with the underlying vessels (give or take the 30° medial deviation of the artery as it passes under the inguinal ligament); therefore, it offers optimal exposure with minimum incision time and is in effect the "direct" approach much as the mid-line linea alba incision is to abdominal surgery. It may be extended downward to facilitate lengthy exposure of the profunda femoris artery or extended superiorly and laterally into a retroperitoneal exposure of the distal external iliac vessels. Disadvantages of the incision include the salient fact that the vertical incision violates Langer's lines of maximal skin stress. Therefore, it is theoretically more prone to disruption, poor healing, and wider scar formation than an oblique incision. It also courses a joint vertically in violation of basic plastic surgery principles. Thus, contracture formation is possible. We have seen several patients with painful thickened scars requiring Z-plasty revision. Furthermore, the vertical incision is poorly suited to the obese patient with a panniculus in which the superior aspect of the incision inevitably becomes macerated.

Oblique incisions are a second alternative. A formal transverse incision is rarely indicated, nor can it provide adequate exposure. However, an oblique incision may be made, coursing from lateral to the vessels at the inguinal ligament to a point medial to the saphenous vein. "Hockey stick" extensions may also be made to lengthen the basic incision. Such an incision more closely corresponds to Langer's lines with resultant decreased wound tension. It provides equivalent exposure to the vertical incision, particularly since only the skin and subcutaneous tissues are incised obliquely, and deeper dissection is performed vertically at all levels deep to and including the crural fascia. The plane of the incision also more closely corresponds to the axis of incisional extensions to the saphenous vein for harvesting or to a retroperitoneal iliac vessel approach. The incision does have disadvantages. Without careful planning, there is the potential for raising or undermining subcutaneous flaps. In addition, if there is not a palpable pulse present for early arterial location, an oblique incision is more difficult to orient directly over the vessels.

Dissection

Particularly in the absence of a readily palpable pulse, location of the vessels is facilitated by various maneuvers based on an appreciation of local anatomy. NAVEL is the well-known acronym from lateral to medial at the level of the inguinal ligament—nerve, artery, vein, "empty space," and lymph channels. Equally important gross anatomy is the fact that the artery courses under the inguinal ligament at the junction of the latter's middle and medial thirds, doing so at a 30° medially directed angle to the vertical plane of the leg (Fig. 8). A final anatomical method to localize the artery involves fairly constant anatomy: the saphenous vein (readily found in the subcutaneous tissue) penetrates the fascia at the level of the fossa ovalis and enters directly into the femoral vein, establishing both the position and depth of the femoral vessels (which is particularly helpful in re-do situations). Demonstration of the location of the fossa ovalis is facilitated by the constant branches of the saphenous vein at that level: the external superficial pudendal medially, the superficial epigastric superiorly, and the superficial lateral circumflex iliac laterally. The last named vein crosses in front of the common femoral artery at roughly the level of the bifurcation and may be used as a marker for same.

Dissection should be performed in as directly vertical a plane as possible. This provoides perpendicular tissue planes for later reapproximation without "dead space." Dissection should not be made bluntly or with wide spreading of the scissors since these measures only result in a much larger "dead space" than that produced by one clean vertical cut. If the surgeon knows where the vessel lays anatomically, he/she need not waste time plowing around in the subcutaneous tissues.

It is almost universally true in peripheral vascular surgery, that there are no (significant) branches of the artery coursing anteriorly at the levels of usual dissection (Fig. 9). (This the more irreverent may take as proof that God is either a surgeon or at least is benevolently inclined toward same.) An incision can thus be made vertically down to the periadventitial plane of the artery and, in general, can be extended in both directions with only slight scissor spreading to elevate the incisional plane from the underlying artery before incision. There are however known anatomical structures that lie in front of the vessels. These include the accessory obturator vein immediately subjacent to the inguinal ligament, the superficial lateral circumflex iliac vein just above the bifurcation, and the deep lateral circumflex femoral vein anterior to the profunda femoris artery 1 to 1.5 cm. distal to the bifurcation. In lengthy dissection under the sartorius muscle for exposure of the distal superficial femoral and profunda femoris arteries, motor branches of the femoral nerve to vastus medialis entwine about the profunda and cross anterolaterally. These branches must be kept in mind, avoided, and carefully retracted in such dissections (Fig. 10). Finally, the surgeon should look for and preserve two nerve branches. The medial branch of the anterior femoral cutaneous nerve, supplying the lower medial thigh, which may course from lateral to medial across the bifurcation at the level of the crural fascia and then perforates same between the sartorius and adductor magnus muscles to lie in the subcutaneous tissue. Division of this nerve may result in painful dysesthesia in the lower medial thigh. Similar injury may occur to the

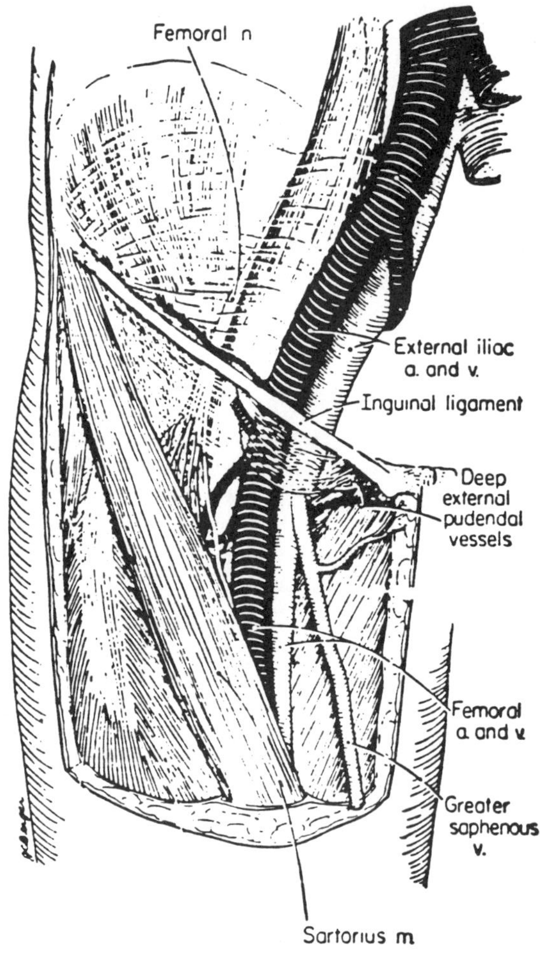

Figure 8. *Depicts the orientation of the femoral vessels to the inguinal ligament. After passing vertically through the thigh under the sartorius muscle, the femoral vessels turn medially at a 30° angle to pass under the inguinal ligament at or just lateral to the junction of its medial and middle thirds. The femoral nerve is single at this level, but quite lateral. As the femoral bifurcation is approached, the nerve becomes plexiform, and its medial branches pass increasingly closer to the profunda femoris. (Modified from Woodburne, R.T.:* Essentials of Human Anatomy, *ed 4. New York, Oxford Press, 1969, Fig. 406, p. 527).*

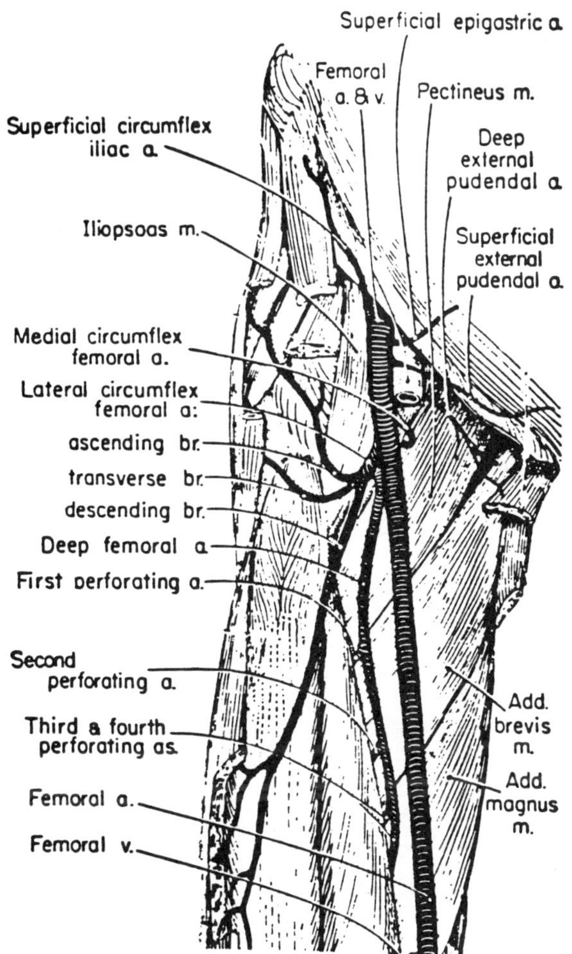

Figure 9. *Depicts the major branches and orientation of the femoral artery (with the sartorius muscle removed): a) branches of the common femoral are two small vessels, the superficial circumflex iliac and superficial external pudendal; b) the medial circumflex femoral usually exits from the posterior common at the bifurcation; c) the major branches of the profunda are the muscular and lateral circumflex trunks. (Modified from Wood-burne, R.T.:* Essentials of Human Anatomy, *ed 4. New York, Oxford Press, 1969, Fig. 418, p. 544.)*

femoral branch of the genitofemoral nerve in high subinguinal dissections. It enters the thigh under the inguinal ligament anterior to the femoral artery, pierces the femoral sheath, and descends with the saphenous vein through the fossa ovalis (Fig. 11).

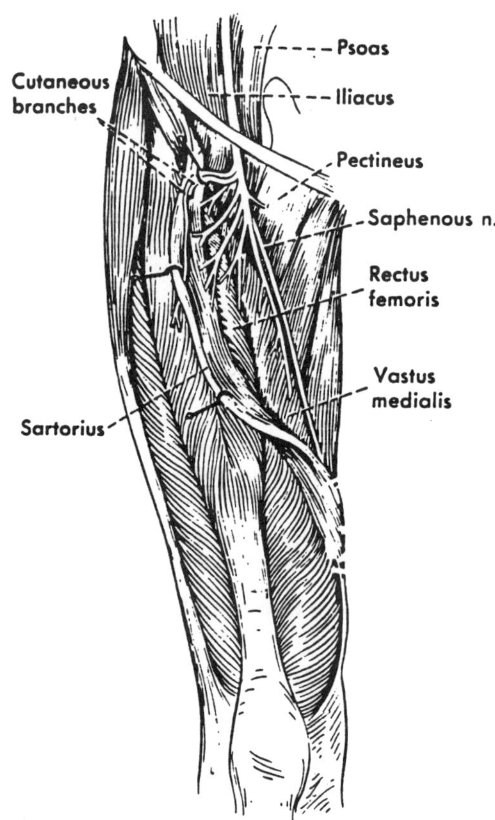

Figures 10A, B. *Depicts the orientation of the femoral nerve plexus to the profunda femoris artery (sartorius muscle and superficial femoral artery excised): The branches to the rectus femoris and vastus lateralis exit high and laterally, while branches to vastus medium and intermedius and the saphenous nerve are adjacent to or cross in front of the distal profunda femoris artery. (Modified from Hollingshead, W.H.:* Anatomy for Surgeons, *Volume 3. 1982, Fig. 8.57 and 8.70, pp. 692 and 708.)*

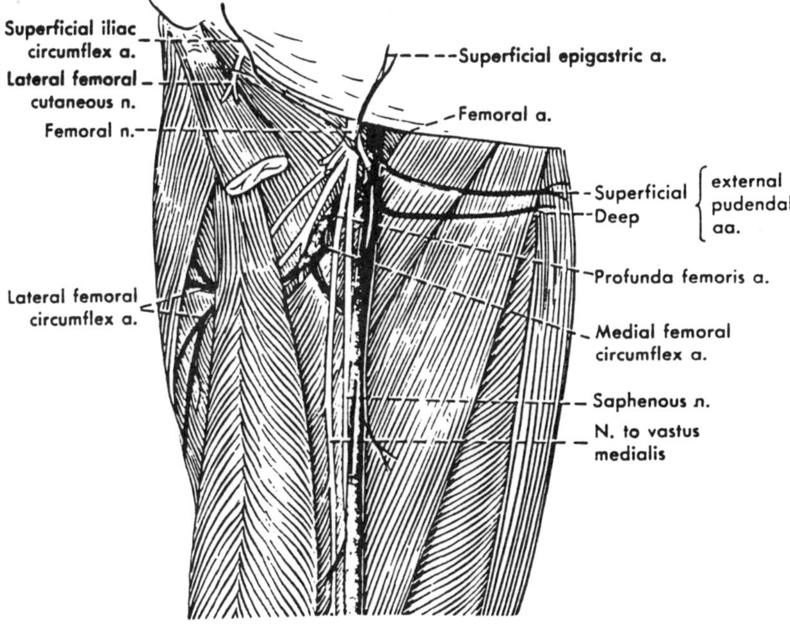

Figure 10B.

Arterial Dissection

Dissection of the artery should be done in the periadventitial plane to maintain the maximal tensile strength of the vessel and to preserve the vasa vasorum ramifications. The vasa vasorum themselves must of necessity be disrupted by separation of the artery from its investing areolar tissues. Extension of this logic would dictate that dissection not be universally (as is traditionally true) complete in that the artery is laid bare from inguinal ligament to beyond bifurcation with all branches looped. Such a needlessly extensive dissection does not aid in anastomosis, while it does cause maximal iatrogenic ischemia. Such ischemia increases the medial injury, with an increased tendency to fibrodysplasia (spell that ''late stenosis'') and is far more prone to scar in densely (spell that ''difficult re-do cases''). Dissection should be circumferential *only* where encirclement with loops is necessary. Dissection should include only sufficient length as is necessary for the arteriotomy and/or anastomosis and should *not* include the profunda unless profunda revascularization is to be performed or when encirclement is necessary for control of the distal common femoral artery. Re-do surgery is an unfortunate reality of any established vascular practice, and is markedly facilitated by preservation of "virgin" planes for secondary dissections.

Collateral arterial supply should be routinely preserved by gentle dissection and looping with small silastic tapes or singly (not doubly) looped zero silks held in place with *lightweight* (e.g., Heifetz) clamps. Dissection around a vessel should be done with a combination of gentle spreading (<2-cm excursions) parallel to the long axis of the artery to envision areolar planes of tissue that may then be sharply incised. Specific instruments for such dissection include the blunt-tipped but thin-bladed, small excursion scissors of Shea or Demartels. Metzenbaum scissors are heavier, blunter, larger, and with wider excursions, all of which tend to lend themselves to blunter, less precise dissection. One may dissect with a fine-tipped right angle or other clamp, but this does not allow simultaneous incision. The coincidental dual-action of dissection scissors is preferred.

Knowledge of the relevant anatomy and its variants is crucial if one is to avoid inadvertent injury (Fig. 8). The common femoral gives off a variable set of small superficial external pudendae collaterals. Usually, at least one pair is located at the mid-portion. The deep lateral may exit the common femoral slightly anteriorly, lending itself to injury during initial artery dissection. Sometimes three or four (2 pairs matched) vessels may be found. Under the inferior surface of the inguinal ligament and above the accessory obturator vein lie the superiorly directed superficial epigastric and superficial lateral circumflex arteries: these are usually not seen in standard dissections, but must be identified and preserved in dissections involving control at the external iliac level, e.g., femoral aneurysmorrhaphy. At the bifurcation, the superficial femoral artery (SFA) courses slightly mediad but otherwise in the same plane as the common femoral; the immediate size differential between the 2 vessels is an accurate clue to the level of the bifurcation and therefore to the more occult location of the profunda. There are no significant named branches of the SFA, but dilated unnamed collaterals should be looped and preserved.

Profunda femoris (PFA) anatomy may occur in one of three or four usual variants. The constant anatomy is a single-vessel trunk that bifurcates into a muscular profunda that continues into the thigh 1 cm posterior and 1 to 2 cm lateral to the SFA, joining medial branches of the femoral nerve after it gives off the first perforator, and a smaller lateral circumflex femoral exiting under the femoral nerve into the thigh and rapidly bifurcating into ascending and descending branches (Fig. 11). The main trunk of the PFA is only 1.5 to 2.0 cm long and is crossed by the deep circumflex femoral vein. The origin of the medial

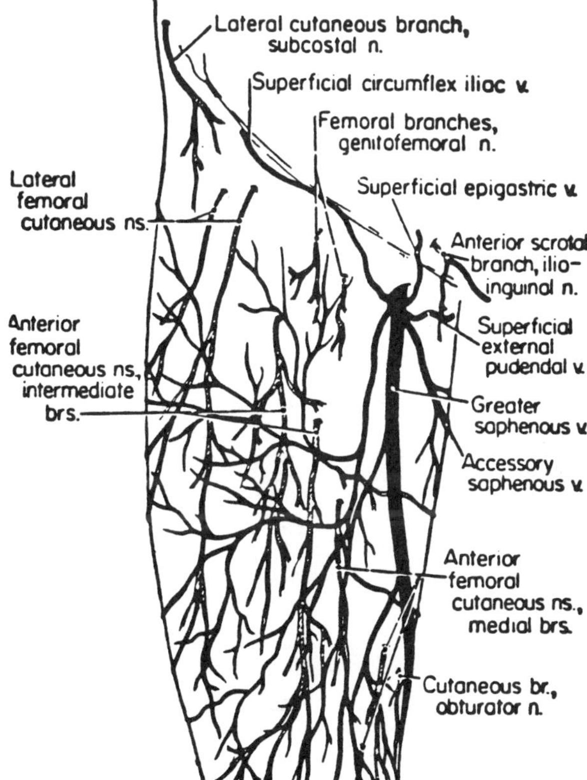

Figure 11. *Depicts the encountered superficial sensory nerves of the upper thigh and their relationship to the saphenous vein as a marker for the standard vertical inguinal incision. Branches of the anterior femoral cutaneous nerve are directly under the incision. When high exposure to the inguinal ligament is utilized, the femoral branches of the genitofemoral nerve may be encountered. (Modified from Woodburne, R.T.:* Essentials of Human Anatomy, *ed 4. New York, Oxford Press, 1969, Fig. 402, p. 521.)*

circumflex femoral artery is variable: it may exit from the muscular profunda above the first perforator and course medially, it may exit posteriorly from the proximal trunk of the PA, or most commonly, it may exit from the posterior CFA just above the bifurcation—a treacherous position where it is either overlooked or inadvertently injured during encirclement of the PFA (Fig. 8).

The danger areas in profunda control therefore are the inferoposterior aspect of the crotch between PFA and SFA and the posteriorly oriented medial circumflex vessel. Dissection of the PFA is thus most safely obtained by initial anterior dissection down to the lateral circumflex branch, with division of the deep circumflex iliac vein; dissection at the superior aspect of the crotch while gentle mediad traction is obtained by vessel loops on the SFA and CFA, looking at that juncture for the medial circumflex; and encirclement with a right angle aimed from lateral-superior toward inferior—the reverse facilitates inadvertent injury at the crotch.

Distal Dissection

The more distally the dissection is continued on the PFA or SFA, the more nerve branches are encountered (although the main femoral nerve plexus stays both lateral and more superficial) and the more anterior the superficial femoral vein becomes, crossing from medial to an almost anterior position relative to the SFA. It should be noted that at the level of standard inguinal dissection there is a femoral nerve *plexus* rather than a femoral nerve (Fig. 10).

Vascular Control

Silastic rubber vessel loops properly applied are the preferred occlusive device. Proximal femoral control on heavily diseased vessels, however, often requires clamp application, which should be done in accordance with the principles discussed in Chapter 2.

Wound Closure

Thorough cleansing of the wound should be performed and thorough hemostasis obtained. Careful inspection should be made for occult sites of oozing, lymphorrhea, devitalized tissue, and fragments of atheroma, etc. Wound irrigation with an antiseptic or antibiotic solution is optimal: studies by Lord and Pitt indicate that these are efficacious in reducing wound and graft infections.[5,10–12]

Closure of the wound seeks to reapproximate the anatomical layers (skin, subcutaneous tissue, deep fascia, and/or femoral sheath) incised at initial dissection, but must also take into account the graft traversing the area. Closure of the sheath is seldom possible if a graft was used. Closure of the deep and superficial subcutaneous tissue usually can be performed. The choice of suture size/needle type and suture class (running or interrupted) are probably of less importance than a careful reapproximation with equally spaced, equal depth bites.

Closure of the skin should afford the surest dermal reapproximation with the least potential for contamination. We prefer running buried subcuticular dermal closure reinforced with Steristrips®.

Closure of the wound is as important to the operative result as the anastomosis and should not be delegated to inexperienced assistants. Vein graft conduits require a closely coapted tissue for early and adequate reformation of vasa vasorum. Wound hematoma/seroma/lymphoceles impair that process and may lead to medial ischemia and later fibrointimal hyperplasia. Similarly, synthetic grafts require coapted tissues for early fibrous incorporations. Wound hematomas, etc., are associated with early graft infections.

Dressing

The purpose of the dressing is to keep the incision dry (by absorbing extruded serus or blood) and to minimize wound contamination by maintenance of a (relatively) sterile field until adequate inherent wound resistance is obtained in 48 to 72 hours. In the absence of absolute convincing evidence against various methods, we can only state a preference for closure with Steristrips® and wound exclusion with a minimal additional dressing, e.g., Telfa® or cotton gauze and tape.

Conduit choice and preparation are beyond the scope of this monograph. Readers are referred to Chapter 7 for the principles that should be followed in regard to anastomosis.

Carotid Endarterectomy

Isolation of the carotid vessels is particularly demanding in anatomical knowledge (mostly in terms of avoiding cranial nerve injury) and in observance of very careful vascular technique to avoid technical problems that might culminate in perioperative stroke.

Preparation and Draping

Position of the operating table in the room relative to lighting and anesthesia and positioning of exposure are critical starting points to this demanding operation. We have found that surgical assistance is optimal and most comfortably obtained by positioning the patient's head at the edge of the headrest with the long axis of the body shifted somewhat to the surgeon's side. We rotate the table to face crosswise in the room, with the assistant standing at the patient's head and anesthesia positioned on the contralateral side. This maximizes surgical access and minimizes back discomfort for the assistant. A "doughnut" cushion elevates and firmly holds the patient's head in place; gentle extension and contralateral rotation facilitate exposure. A shoulder roll is not necessary unless the patient is heavy set with a short neck and broad shoulders.

Skin preparation is limited to "painting." We avoid possible embolization of poorly adherent thrombosis from external manipulation associated wih scrubs, realizing of course that such is a rare occurrence and highly unlikely to be causally related to the prep. The converse truth is that wound infections are so rarely seen in clean neck incisions that even that potential risk is worth avoiding. Draping should include the anatomical landmarks of the operation: the lobe of the ear (for styloid process), the angle of the jaw (for marginal mandibular nerve), the thyroid cartilage (for level of the omohyoid), and the sternal notch (sternocleidomastoid insertions). Whether the field is excluded with sutures, clips, or an adhesive drape is a matter of preference.

Incision

Two basic incisions are used for carotid exposure, each with its strengths and weaknesses. The oblique incision seems to be the standard incision for carotid endarterectomy (CEA), running along the anterior border of the sternocleidomastoid muscle from just below the angle of the jaw and to the level of the thyroid cartilage. If necessary, it can be extended to the sternal notch or into a median sternotomy for extensive innominate or aortico-carotid reconstructions. Extension superiorly for high internal carotid lesions should involve a posteriorly oriented hockey stick incision aimed behind the ear lobe, which keeps the deeper aspect of the incision out of the parotid gland and minimizes chances for injury to the great occipital nerve.

Advantages of the oblique incision are its direct approach to the carotid sheath and its correspondence with the course of same, making extensions for additional access very easy. The oblique incision also has several disadvantages. Although placed in an obviously cosmetic area, it is *not* cosmetic and indeed violates plastic surgical principles by crossing Langer's lines. At worst, it can heal with a fibrous contraction that requires Z-plasty release to allow free extension of the neck (we have seen two cases of this). Additionally, it results in a relatively large anesthetic area of skin at the neck and along the jaw due to sacrifice of two or three branches from the cervical plexus, a fact that should be pointed out in preoperative patient discussions.

The transverse incision is the other incision of choice for CEA. The primary advantage of the transverse incision is that it is more cosmetic since the incision is placed more closely within Langer's lines. However, there is less optimal exposure for superior or inferior extensions of the disease process, but this can be alleviated by more vertical extension of the incision as needed.

Since a significant proportion of the bleeding incurred by cervical incisions occurs at the subdermal plexus and since we prefer to perform such technically demanding surgery in a bloodless field, it has been our policy to "score" the skin down to the visible subdermal vessels and then complete the skin incision with electrocautery. This obviates persistent skin bleeding and has not proven cosmetically disadvantageous.

Dissection

The exposure of the carotid vessels requires a detailed understanding of the anatomical variants and the exact courses of the related structures (seen and unseen) in order to minimize inadvertent cranial nerve injury. In addition, the handling of the artery requires knowledge of all the principles outlined in this book to maximize postoperative patency and minimize intraoperative embolization, both of which may result in clinical stroke.

The usual exposure extends from the omohyoid muscle inferiorly to the posterior belly of the digastric muscle superiorly. Dissection should always be performed sharply, vertically, and only after clear definition that what is being incised is "areolar" and does not contain any other structures. The surgeon should not be stopping to find and control bleeders at every turn. The composition and depth of the investing areolar tissues vary widely, with filmy tissue in some patients and gristle in others. The more carefully the dissection is done, the less chance there is for surgically embarrassing injury. Retractor placement is equally important, since the majority of hypoglossal and mandibular nerve injuries are felt to be secondary to retractor pressure rather than actual nerve division. The importance of accurate retractor positioning is underscored by our remarkably low (0.5%) incidence of clinically apparent cranial nerve injuries in 250 of our cases. For inferior wound retraction, we utilize a Weitlander carefully placed on the inferior wound so as to engage the free edge of the incised carotid sheath laterally (thus retracting the jugular vein without injury) and carefully placed medially in the sternocleidomastoid fascia above the ansa and therefore away from the superior laryngeal nerve as it enters the larynx (Fig. 12).

Superiorly oriented retraction varies depending on the depth of the neck and the necessity for distal internal carotid dissection. In standard cases we utilize a second Weitlander carefully placed to again engage the carotid sheath edge laterally (with retraction of the jugular vein) and *very* careful positioning in the digastric belly *above* the plane of the hypoglossal nerve. A Mayo Collins triblade retractor may be utilized, but has a disadvantage in that all three blades are deep and the superior third blade in particular tends to slip into positions of direct pressure on the hypoglossal and/or vagus nerves. Similarly, although we use a vein retractor to medially and superiorly retract the hypoglossal as the distal internal carotid is dissected, we never leave this retractor (particularly with a medical student affixed) in place, since the prolonged vigorous upward traction on the hypoglossal seems to be associated with a high incidence of temporary paresis.

We limit the initial skin incision and dissection to the middle and inferior thirds, dissecting first to find the carotid low in the neck where cranial nerve injury is unlikely. Once the plane of the artery (and therefore the hypoglossal, superior laryngeal, and vagus nerves) (Fig. 13) is established, we carefully extend the incision through all layers in a plane paralleling the medial border of the internal jugular vein.

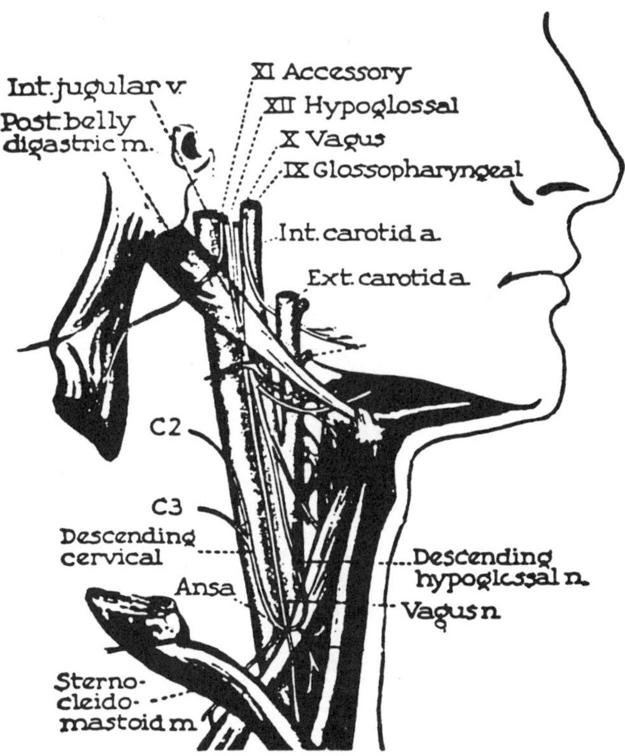

Figure 12. *Depicts the commonly encountered cranial nerves and their relationship to the carotid vessels. All are deep, lying at the level of the vessels. All descend vertically and then bend medially/anteriorly to cross diagonally downward from lateral to medial. (Modified from Thorek, P.:* Anatomy in Surgery, *ed 2. Philadelphia, J.P. Lippincott Company, Fig. 127, p. 170.)*

Several superficial nerves are encountered. The great occipital, which crosses diagonally upward from lateral to medial on the sternocleidomastoid at the superior aspect of the incision, should be preserved, since severance gives anesthesia behind and at the base of the ear. There are two or three cervical plexus sensory nerves that also cross diagonally and more horizontally from lateral to medial from over or through the sternocleidomastoid. Two of these will require division for adequate carotid exposure, but additional branches above and below should be preserved if possible (Fig. 13). The marginal mandibular nerve is the lowest branch of the facial nerve and innervates the

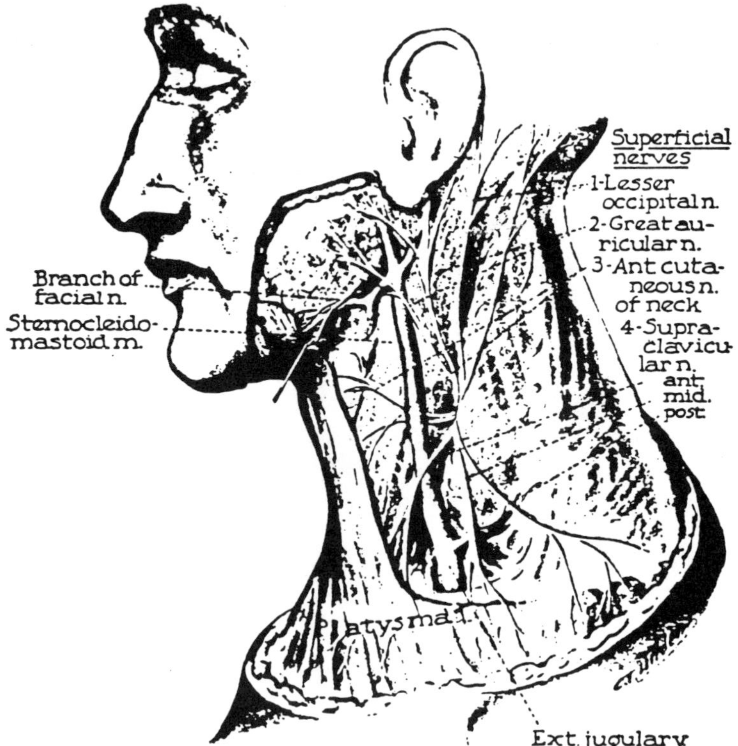

Figure 13. *Depicts the superficial sensory nerves of the face and neck encountered in a standard carotid exploration; all are deep to platysma. In contrast to cranial nerves (descending diagonally from lateral to medial), encountered nerves of the superficial cervical plexus ascend diagonally or transversely from behind/through the sternocleido-mastoid muscle from lateral to medial. Two or three of these are commonly divided. Also note that the lesser occipital and great auricular nerves of this plexus ascend more vertically at the mid to posterior aspect of the sternocleidomastoid belly. (Modified from Thorek, P.:* Anatomy in Surgery, *ed 2. Philadelphia, J.P. Lippincott Company, Fig. 126, p. 169.)*

musculature of the corner of the mouth. It runs in the tissues deep to the platsyma, but superior to the level of the common facial vein and courses along the inferior border of the posterior mandible from the parotid. However, in 19% it may course through the submental triangle to the facial artery and vein. It is uncommonly visualized. Avoidance of injury is dependent on three maneuvers: posterior angulation of the superior incision following the parotid fascia; division of the common facial vein flush with the jugular without dissection along its bifurcation into anterior and posterior facial communicators; and careful medial placement of retractors at a deeper level that engages the digastric belly superiorly and the larynx inferiorly.

The dissection should begin in the lower portion of the incision, dividing the plastysma with electrocautery over a small clamp. It should continue through the fascia at the anterior border of the sternocleidomastoid and then *behind* the anterior third of that muscle toward the palpable carotid pulse. It is useful to leave a film of fascia on the muscle to facilitate its retraction with a Weitlander. The omohyoid belly is identified coursing upward diagonally from medial to lateral; inferior extension of the dissection can be performed in the areolar plane between the sternocleidomastoid and omohyoid. There are inevitably branches of the anterior accessory jugular vein crossing at the inferior apex of this plane that require careful division.

As the carotid sheath is approached, the ansa cervicalis should be found just mediad and dropping vertically through the incision. Entry into the carotid sheath should be made *lateral* to the ansa, preserving it and utilizing it as an absolute guide to the depth and anatomical location of the hypoglossal. The ansa drops inferiorly and laterally from the hypoglossal trunk, so that dissection tracing it back along its lateral side will prevent hypoglossal injury. Single trunks, double trunks in a loop, or two trunks with cross connectors are all variations that can be seen in the ansa anatomy. We always preserve the ansa and divide branches to the sternocleidomatoid that obscure the field. Routine division of the ansa should not be necessary. Although it can theoretically result in impaired swallowing (particularly after bilateral division) since the ansa innervates the strap muscles that elevate the larynx during deglutition, this is not usually a problem.

As the carotid sheath is approached at the common carotid level, the common facial vein will be found crossing diagonally upward from lateral to medial from the internal jugular vein—it is a fairly constant marker for the level of the carotid bifurcation. The vein is dissected and ligated flush with the jugular.

Visualization of the carotid sheath should be carefully performed prior to entry to determine if there is an anterior vagus nerve just under the sheath: this occurs in 4% to 5% of cases. If the anterior vagus nerve is present, entry is made *medial* to it, and the vagus dissected and retracted laterally and posteriorly to its normal position. If the vagus is in its normal position posterolaterally in the sheath, it should be carefully identified and avoided during circumferential dissection and encirclement of the common carotid. Gross encirclement including posterior tissue may cause inadvertent clamp injury to the vagus, which can result in unilateral cord paresis.

Having identified and encircled the common carotid (CCA), we carefully dissect up to the bifurcation and encircle the superior thyroidal and external carotid (ECA). Dissection of the carotid is performed with sufficient anterior vessel to allow clear visualization for arteriotomy but avoiding circumferential dissection (with its medial injury and long-term fibrodysplasia) and distractions and manipulation of the artery that might result in embolization. The artery is simply left in its normal plane and never lifted out of that plane. One should encircle the ECA from medial to crotch, rather than from lateral to medial, since the heel of the right angle clamp inadvertently compresses the internal carotid artery (ICA) at the bulb in the latter maneuver and may cause an embolus.

Encirclement of the superior thyroid artery (STA) and ECA should be preceded by careful sharp dissection of what is usually a more fibrous investing tissue. Gross encirclement may result in superior laryngeal nerve injury as this nerve courses behind the STA/ECA crotch and joins the STA to course inferiorly to the thyroid gland. The nerve is small and not usually seen. Preservation is a matter of careful dissection close to the vessels and restricted to their origins.

With the CCA and ECA encircled, dissection is made into the critical area of the distal ICA. This area is critical for nerve injury and iatrogenic vascular injury. The hypoglossal nerve drops from superior to inferior and superior to medial from below the digastric muscle and in juxtaposition to the vagus superiorly, crossing the external carotid at a plane within 1 cm or less of its adventitia. The absolute depth is indicated by the previously visualized ansa cervicalis. Preservation requires recognition of all of these factors and avoidance of sustained superiorly oriented retraction (Fig. 12).

The vagus nerve descends vertically in the angle between jugular vein and the posterolateral edge of the distal ICA and is essentially "out of harm's way," invested in a portion of the sheath. Engagement of the lateral leaf of the incised carotid sheath with the retractor visualizes and retracts it. The superior laryngeal nerve descends from the vagus in the sheath posterior or posteromedial to the distal internal carotid. It is seldom visualized because of its small size, and prevention of injury simply requires that dissection of the ICA be done in an immediately periadventitial plane (Fig. 12).

Dissection of the ICA is performed to a level that corresponds on three clinical grounds to a *normal* distal artery, by visualization of a translucent blue rather than yellow tinge, by gentle palpation of a soft elastic compressible artery distal to firmer plaque, and by confirmation by reference to the angiogram, which should be available in the operating room. All dissection on and manipulation of the ICA and bifurcation are done without disturbing the artery from its anatomical plane. Perineural xylocaine block of the nerve of Hering is seldom necessary. If bradycardia occurs, it may be aborted with IV atropine/scopolamine. Division of the nerve should only be required in very high dissections in which the nerve actually tethers the bifurcation superiorly: otherwise, our dictum is to preserve all structures. When intraluminal debris or thrombus is suspected, distal ICA control is obtained and/or a shunt placed before formal dissection of the diseased ICA segment is carried out. This will reduce the chances for inadvertent embolization during further dissection.

Endarterectomy

We use silastic vessel loops rather than clamps for vascular control, based on the findings in Chapter 2. If distal control requires a clamp, we use a 75-cm pressure baby bulldog if a shunt is not used or a small Javid clamp if a shunt is used. Although we usually utilize an intraluminal shunt, discussion of that method versus EEG, awake anesthesia, or stump pressures is beyond the scope of this monograph.

Endarterectomy is initiated distally, with careful Potts scissor division of the distal edge unless "feathering" occurs in a readily visible plane well within the arteriotomy site. We prefer to control this distal intima edge first so that more proximal endarterectomy manipulations do not cause inadvertent undermining and extension of the endarterectomy plane to a level beyond the arteriotomy site. That is, we clearly incise the distal intima circumferentially first, then complete the more proximal aspects of the endarterectomy. We routinely use intimal tacking sutures (unless "feathering" has occurred) placing three mattress sutures at the quadrants of the vessel in the longitudinal plane of the artery so that no additional constriction of the vessel lumen occurs.

Closure of the arteriotomy is facilitated by using a 6-0 BV-1 (small short curve) needle superiorly. However, a 5-0 RB-7 (larger, stouter) needle should be used on the CCA where the denser plaque makes suturing with a BV-1 needle more difficult.

Since we use a shunt, initiation of the suture line at the ICA apex is facilitated by first placing an adventitial bite right on the apex and using this as a "guy" to lift up the apex, thus allowing direct visualization of the apex intima to facilitate the formal first suture through all layers. The alternative method is to use both needles of a double-armed suture, placed from inside-out on each side of the arteriotomy. We have found the former to be easier, particularly in small distal ICAs essentially filled by the intraluminal shunt.

Flushing techniques, use of intraoperative Doppler, and details of eversion endarterectomy of the ECA are standard and need no further elaboration here.

Closure

After checking patency with intraoperative Doppler, duplex scan, or angiogram and thorough hemostasis is obtained, closure of the wound may be obtained in three layers: loose reapproximation of the sternocleidomastoid fascia with several interrupted sutures, platysma closure, and skin, which we perform with a subcuticular absorbable suture.

Dressing

We prefer simple Steristrips® to allow inspection of the neck for hematoma postoperatively.

Summary

A thorough review of the surgical approach to the femoral and carotid vessels has been utilized to illustrate the principles of this book—avoiding iatrogenic injuries by observance of careful technique.

References

1. Dobrin, PB, Jorgenson, RA: Balloon embolectomy catheters in small arteries III: Surgical significance of eccentric balloons. *Surgery* 93:402–8, 1983.
2. Rubin, JR, Malone, JM, Goldstone, J: The role of the lymphatic system in acute arterial prosthetic graft infections. *J Vasc Surg* 2:92–98, 1985.

3. Bunt, TJ, Wooldridge, ND, Doerhoff, CA: Vessel-loop combined exposure and control for cimino-brescia fistulae. *Surg Gyne Obstet* 160:87, 1985.
4. Dobrin, PB: Balloon embolectomy catheters in small arteries II: Comparison of fluid-filled and gas-filled balloons. *Surgery* 91:671–79, 1982.
5. Guidoin, R, Dogon, B, Blais, P, et al: Effects of traumatic manipulations on grafts, sutures, and host arteries during vascular surgical procedures. *Res Exper Med* 179:1–21, 1981.
6. Dobrin, PB: Balloon embolectomy catheters in small arteries I: Lateral wall pressure and shear forces. *Surgery* 90:177–85, 1981.
7. Bunt, TJ: Sources of Staphylococcus Epidermidis at the Inguinal Incision During Peripheral Revascularization. *Am Surg* 52:9:472–74, 1986.
8. Bunt, TJ, Mohr, JD: Incidence of Positive Lymph Node Cultures at Time of Peripheral Revascularization. *Am Surg* 50:10:522, 1984.
9. Bunt, TJ: Synthetic Vascular Graft Infections: Part I. *Surgery* 93:733–46, 1983.
10. Lord, JW, Ross G, Daliana M: Intraoperative antibiotic wound lavage: An attempt to eliminate postoperative infection in arterial and clean surgical procedures. *Ann Surg* 185:634–38, 1977.
11. Pitt, HA, Postier R, MacGowan, N, et al: Prophylactic antibiotics in vascular surgery. *Ann Surg* 192:356–61, 1980.
12. Gundry, SR, Jones, M, Ishihara, T, et al: Optimal preparation technique for human saphenous vein grafts. *Surgery* 88:785–94, 1980.

Chapter 8

Microvascular Surgical Technique

Harold I. Friedman, Peter C. Haines, Glen Strickland, Jason B. MaGee, and William M. Moore

The advent and refinement of microvascular surgical techniques during the past twenty years has markedly expanded the reconstructive options available to surgeons who are well versed in these operative modalities. Replantation of severed digits, hands, and arms has become almost routine procedure in many centers. Transfer of tissues, such as muscle, bone, subcutaneous tissue, and skin from one area of the body to another with immediate revascularization has greatly improved the functional consequences and cosmetic appearance of traumatic injuries or previously performed ablative surgery. The use of microvascular techniques has also greatly reduced the number of operative stages required for a given reconstruction, as well as the cost of hospitalization and loss of work income. Reconstructive surgeons trained prior to the advent of microvascular surgery are all too familiar with the loss of a tubed pedicle flap upon final division of its pedicle after multiple staged procedures to move it from one body area to another. Instead, the microvascular surgeon has substituted this concern with one of re-establishing blood inflow and venous drainage across a suture anastomosis of only 1- to 2-mm diameter—a procedure that entails perhaps 6 to 8 hours. Thus, the development of microvascular technique has been paralleled by a recognition of the technical problems encountered in satisfactorily manipulating small vessels to prevent the iatrogenic complications observed in larger vessel surgery.

From *Iatrogenic Vascular Injury: A Discourse on Surgical Technique*, edited by T.J. Bunt, M.D. © 1990, Futura Publishing Inc., Mount Kisco, NY.

Furthermore, additional problems unique to microvascular surgery have been identified and methods found to minimize trauma to the vessels and maintain patency and flow through them.

Training in Microvascular Surgery

The development of the field of microvascular surgery has been dependent on the parallel advances made in operating microscopes, suture materials, and instrumentation. Jacobson was the first to demonstrate that small vessel anastomosis could be reliably accomplished under the microscope. Subsequently, several investigators demonstrated the feasibility of free flap transfers in experimental animals.[1-6] In 1965, the first report of successful reanastomosis of severed digital vessels in an ischemic thumb was presented by Klienert and Kasdan.[7] Restoration of a totally amputated thumb at the metacarpal phalangeal joint level was successfully achieved 3 years later by Komatsu and Tomai.[8] However, even these pioneers admitted to a number of failures prior to their first success. At that time, the surgeons used a Zeiss operating microscope and a relatively large suture material (8-0 monofilament nylon, and 7-0 braided silk). In 1972, McLean and Buncke performed the first free tissue transfer in a human by successfully revascularizing an omentum flap for coverage of a large scalp defect.[9] The following year, Daniel and Taylor, and O'Brien independently transferred vascularized island flaps from the groin for reconstruction of traumatized lower extremities.[10,11] During the past decade microvascular surgery has advanced from being a new field with occasional spectacular triumphs, to one in which replantation of digits and free tissue transfers are fairly commonplace in most major medical centers. These procedures are performed by orthopedic and plastic/reconstructive surgeons with a very high percentage of success.

The rapid dissemination of technical expertise amongst surgeons in the United States is perhaps related to two factors. The first was the standardization of techniques and equipment for operating on 1-0- to 0.5-mm diameter vessels. The second was the establishment of numerous courses in microvascular surgery throughout the country. These courses provided the opportunity for surgeons with little experience in microvascular techniques (over a 7- to 14-day period) to initiate a process of proficiency development that would enable them to return to their parent institutions, where, with additional practice in laboratory animals, they might gain sufficient skills to achieve a fairly high and consistent rate of success in replantation and free tissue transfer surgery. However, most surgeons trained in microvascular surgery do not see an adequate volume of cases to limit their practice entirely to this operative field. Furthermore, the fine hand and eye coordination required to perform microvascular surgery dictates frequent practice to maintain proficiency. Therefore, many surgeons have opted to establish some form of laboratory environment in which microvascular surgery can be performed on rodents to maintain skills between actual clinical cases.

The decision to begin training in microvascular surgery also necessitates a commitment to the establishment of a team approach.[12] The specialized equipment (instruments, sutures, operating microscopes, etc.) mandate a nursing staff intimately familiar with the use, care, and maintenance of the equipment and a familiarity with the specialized requirements for the pre- and postoperative patient care and monitoring of the vascular anastomoses. Finally, it is important to consider the fact that microvascular surgery requires not only a surgeon capable of technically performing the operation, but an *assistant* who is *equally* well versed in the techniques. The requirements for replantation of multiple amputated digits are even greater. Given the fact that replantation of a single digit takes 4 to 6 hours to accomplish, if one multiples these hours by the number of amputated fingers, it becomes readily apparent that fatigue alone will mitigate against a successful outcome. Ideally, a team of trained microvascular surgeons should be employed for multiple digital replantations.[12] In the latter instance, the teams can rotate every several hours, thereby reducing failure secondary to operative fatigue. This type of team approach is difficult to establish in local community hospitals. Therefore, replantation centers are often relegated to university hospitals where staff surgeons, residents, and fellows-in-training can provide sufficient manpower for the effort required. As in other areas of surgical endeavor, there is a direct correlation between successful outcome and the experience of the team performing the procedure. This fact also argues for a "center" approach to replantation surgery.[13]

Equipment

As in any highly specialized surgical field, it is pointless to begin a procedure without immediate access to the critical instrumentation that makes the operation feasible. Uninitiated residents ask if the operating microscope is necessary or if procedure could be done using loupes? The allowable margin of error in the anastomosis of vessels diminishes in proportion to the luminal diameter. Whereas, 1 or 2 mm of narrowing in a proximal leg vessel may go unnoticed, half a millimeter of narrowing in a vessel of 1.0-mm diameter is a catastrophy. Similarly, a small adventitial tag in contact with the lumen of a large artery may result in a clinically unnoticed small thrombus; a similar-sized thrombus in a digital artery will occlude the entire lumen. The likelihood of a successful outcome is therefore predicated on magnification. Although anastomosis of a 2.0-mm vessel may be possible using loupe magnification, an operating microscope is essential when working on vessels 1 mm or less.

Microvascular techniques demand adequate surgical exposure because of the small room for error. The operating microscope must be satisfactorily positioned over the operative field. The light emanating from the scope has to be bright at high magnification. The operating surgeons must be totally familiar with the particular microscope used including all positioning controls. The interpupillary distance on the binocular eyepieces must be appropriately adjusted. The focus of the eyepiece must be exact. If any of the abovementioned factors are not perfect, they will plague the surgeon throughout the procedure and interfere with the prospect of a superb result. Other preoperative aspects are also critical to a good outcome. The operative field must be completely dry of blood. If the surgeon or his assistant have to constantly interrupt their concentration on the anastomosis to clear blood from the field, it will be extremely difficult to suture a proper anastomosis. Both surgeon and assistant must be comfortable. There can be no back or neck strain secondary to improper positioning of the eyepieces or seat level. The seats must be comfortable to reduce both buttock and leg pain fatigue. The normal smooth passage of a needle through the vessel wall imparts a significant amount of trauma to the vessel wall. If the surgeon's forearms are not supported and resting comfortably, tremor in the fingers will increase, leading to further vessel wall damage, thrombus formation, and possible occlusion of the vessel.

These factors all relate to taking an extra few minutes prior to beginning the procedure to maximize the opportunity for perfectly performed vascular anastomoses.

A number of fine operating microscopes are available commercially that have certain features in common. They incorporate a beam splitter allowing both surgeons to see precisely the same field. Most microscopes have motorized controls for focusing and change of magnification that are activated by either foot pedals or hand controls. This feature allows change from high magnification (approximately 30 to 40×), which is required for suture placement, to a lower magnification (10 to 5×) with a wider field, which facilitates suture tying. Such microscopes maintain their focus throughout the range of magnifications.

Instruments required for microsurgical repairs are few in number and vary somewhat with the preference of the operator. Since these tools will come into contact with the vessel wall, they must be perfectly maintained, particularly the vascular clamps (see below). Rust or clotted blood on the instruments will make them incapable of holding a 10-0 suture, thereby frustrating the surgeon when he/she is attempting to tie knots and endangering the vascular repair. After each use, the instruments are washed with water to remove any saline solution and are polished, oiled, and demagnetized. The instruments are placed in an instrument case that is wrapped for gas sterilization. The instruments include sets of jewelers forceps (#3 and #5), needle holders of the nonlocking Castroviejo type (curved and straight), vessel dilators and irrigating needles (blunt type), spring-loaded scissors of various sizes, and microvascular clamps of varying design, including those that are attached to a bracket to allow vessel approximation. (These clamps will be discussed in greater detail later in this chapter as they have been found to produce varying degrees of intimal damage.) A bipolar coagulator using fine microforceps is also essential. A demagnetizer is needed as magnetized instruments make control of the fine needles very frustrating.

Suture and Suture Technique

Monofilament nylon is the suture of choice for microvascular procedures. The most frequently used sizes are 8-0 through 11-0, with 10-0 commonly used for most routine microvascular anastomosis. Buncke and Schulz developed a technique for electroplating the end of a 10-micron nylon suture to eliminate the diameter change between the suture material and the drilled end of a conventional needle.[4] Unfortunately, this technique did not provide strong enough needles. Today, however, several companies make smoothly swaged on needles without a "step" between needle and suture, which has eliminated the need for electroplating. The commonly used needle for microvascular anastomosis is 70 microns in diameter or 50 or 30 microns, useful for smaller veins. A three-eighths circle to the needle is frequently used.

Passage of a needle through a 1-to-1 mm vessel causes local damage to the vessel wall (Figs. 1 and 2). Pagnanelli et al.[14] identified four types of lesions with the scanning electron microscope. The lesions included: (1) a large internal hole in the intimal surface where the needle penetrated the vessel wall; (2) an intimal tear surrounding and continuous with the needle hole; (3) a variable number of satellite

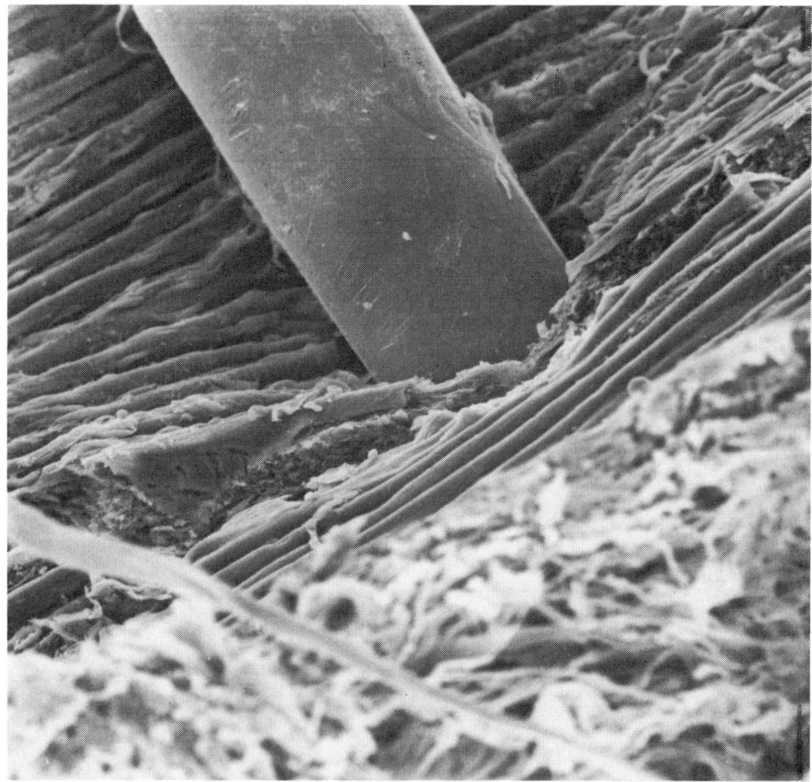

Figure 1. *Scanning electron micrograph of a microvascular needle passing through the rat femoral artery. Endothelial ridges have both been separated and pierced by the needle. 300×*

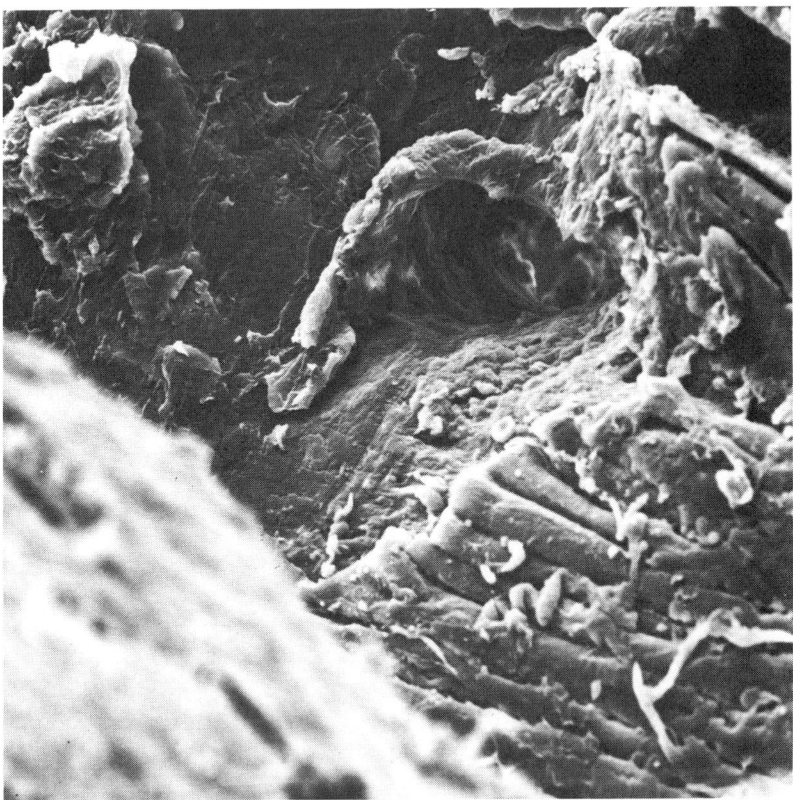

Figure 2. *Hole made by complete passage of a needle through the arterial wall. Note the exposure of all layers of the vessel wall, the disruption of the endothelial ridges, and desquamation of the endothelium. 440×*

patches of denuded subendothelium surrounding the hole and extending from it; and (4) a variable degree of platelet aggregation and white blood cell adhesions extending from the needle hole over a wide area of the vessel. These lesions occurred regardless of the needle diameter (50, 75, 100, or 130 microns). Needle diameter did influence the *size* of the hole. The other three classified lesions, however, were independent of needle diameter dimension and were produced equally by blunt and tapered pointed needles. Of interest was the fact that the point where the needle penetrated the vessel intima on the way out of the vessel clearly suffered less damage than the intima at the point of entrance into the lumen from the outside. In a later study, Apkarian et al. analyzed the scanning electron microscopic features of vessels pentrated by a variety of needles produced by several manufacturers.[15] The majority of tapered needles appeared to spread apart internal folds as they passed through the vessel walls. Newer specially designed cutting needles tended to cut through the endothelium and tear off endothelial cells surrounding the wound, thereby exposing the internal elastic membrane.[15] The clinical significance of these findings was not delineated.

Clearly, if this much damage is done to the vessel wall by a needle and suture just passing through it in the experimental condition, actual performance of an anastomosis under difficult or pressured circumstances will increase the potential for injury. For this reason, the surgeon's hands must be comfortably positioned. Most microvascular surgeons refrain from drinking coffee prior to operating since hand tremor while passing the needle through the vessel wall will cause severe vascular injury intolerable in the microvascular situation, which will presumably lead to early postoperative thrombosis of the repair. Perhaps the key to atraumatic technique in microvascular suturing is not to attempt suture placement until the exposure is perfect and the surgeon is satisfied that the needle can be passed through the vessel wall at the appropriate distance from the cut end of the vessel on the first attempt. As seen in Figure 2, repeated attempts at suturing will leave holes in the vessel wall that will create nuclei for thrombus formation.

Vascular Clamps

Just as inappropriate passage of a microvascular needle through the vessel wall can damage the vessel and result in vascular compromise, microvascular clips can also harm the vessel if not carefully applied and removed within a reasonable period of time. Vessel wall damage is directly proportional to the pressure of the clamp, duration of clamp application, and the surface area over which it is applied.

One of the first studies of the effects of microclamps on small vessel integrity was performed by Thurston et al. more than a decade ago. These investigators studied the parameters of clamp pressure and width over a constant 1-hour period of application. The vessels were examined at varying periods of time after removal of the clamp. Clamps tested demonstrated jaw pressure of up to 200 g and produced an aneurysmal-like dilatation of the vessel wall within 20 minutes of clamp removal. In the case of clamps exerting greater than 30 g of pressure, this area of dilatation progressed to endothelial sloughing with platelet and white cell adherence to the damaged wall. In those vessels clamped with less than 30 g of pressure the vessel dilatation resolved within 4 hours of clamp removal while the endothelial surface remained normal. The vessel dilatation was postulated to produce local turbulent flow and boundary separations that could be responsible for subsequent thrombus formation and vessel occlusion. Vessels exhibiting endothelial sloughing (clamp pressure greater than 30 g) had complete resolution of the damage by 7 days.[16]

Slayback et al. demonstrated the same vessel endothelial and internal injury with vascular clamps exerting high pressures (100 to 190 g).[17] Blaschke et al.[18] in a study of the effects of microvascular clamps suggested that the edges of the clamps produced the greatest amount of vessel injury and therefore recommended dispersing the pressure over a wider area with a broader clamp surface. Finally, Richling et al. demonstrated the importance of the length of time of vessel occlusion by microvascular clamps for a given amount of pressure.[19] With clamps exerting up to 35 g of pressure, the length of time the clamp was applied (up to 3 hours) correlated directly with the amount of intimal damage. Clamps with pressure 45 g or greater produced significantly more damage correlating with the greater the amount of pressure, even with short periods of clamping (10 min).

The type of clamp injury can be seen in Figures 3 through 6, which demonstrate the normal vessel wall and vessel wall after clamping for periods of 8 and 12 hours, respectively. The clamp pressure applied was approximately 25 g.

Our recommendations are to use clamps exerting pressures of approximately 20 to 25 g and to avoid, if possible, vessel occlusion by these clamps for more than 90 minutes. If a greater period of time is required, then the position of the clamp on the vessel wall should be moved to a nontraumatized portion of the vessel in an effort to diminish the possibility of a more permanent injury, and therefore an increased risk of subsequent thrombosis.

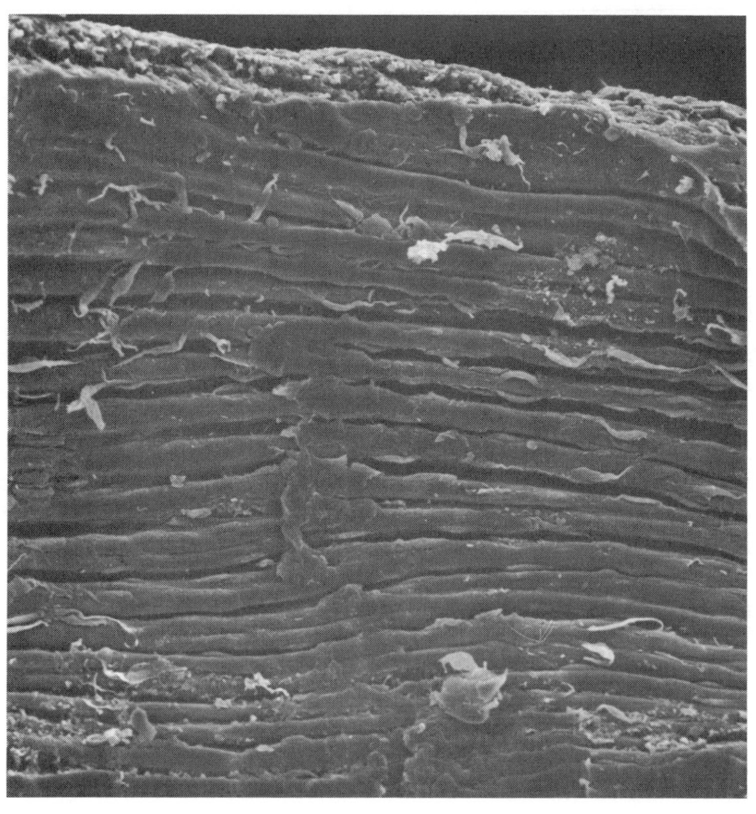

Figure 3. *Normal arterial endothelial ridges and endothelium.* 260×

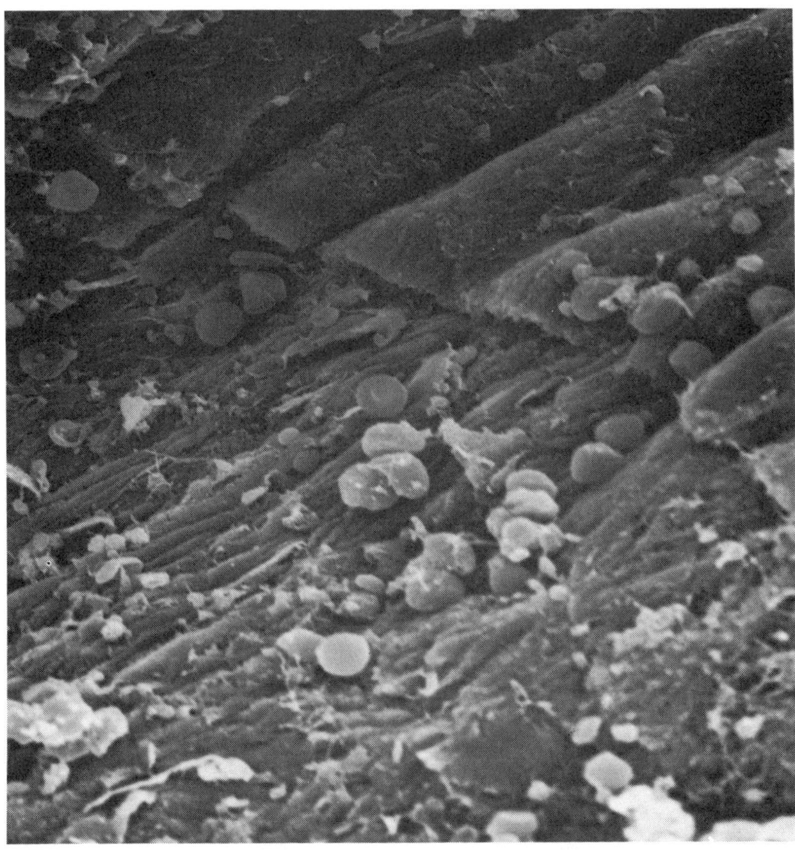

Figure 4. *Appearance of vessel wall after 8 hours of continuous cross clamping with a microvascular clamp. Note the junction of normal endothelium with the denuded cross-clamped areas. 1200×*

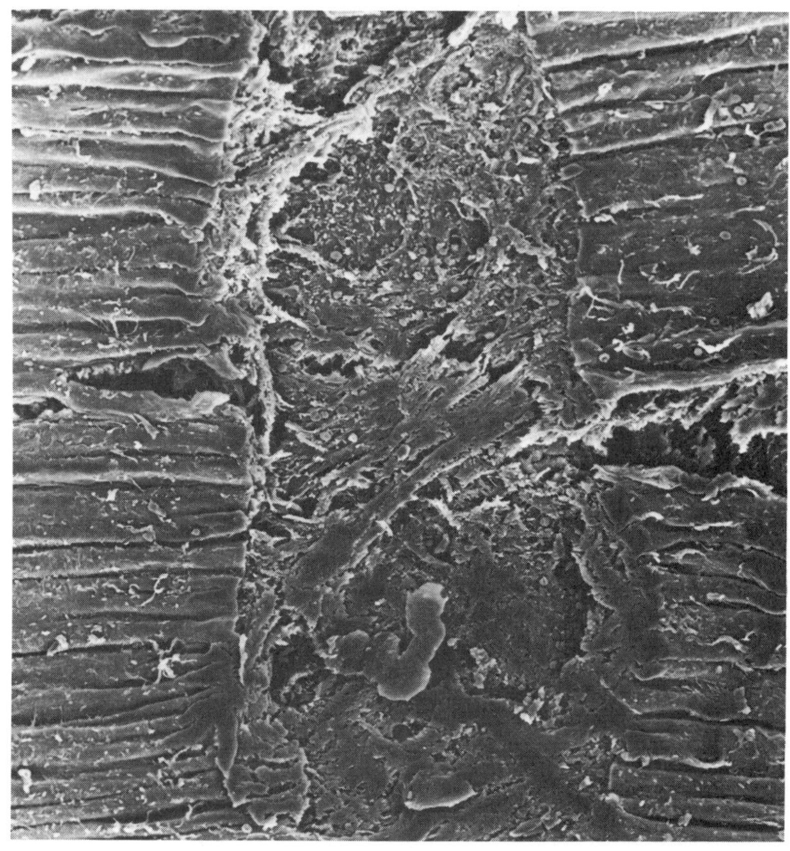

Figure 5. *Vessel wall 12 hours after cross clamping. The defect observed at 8 hours has progressed, exposing a deeper trough in the vessel wall. 200×*

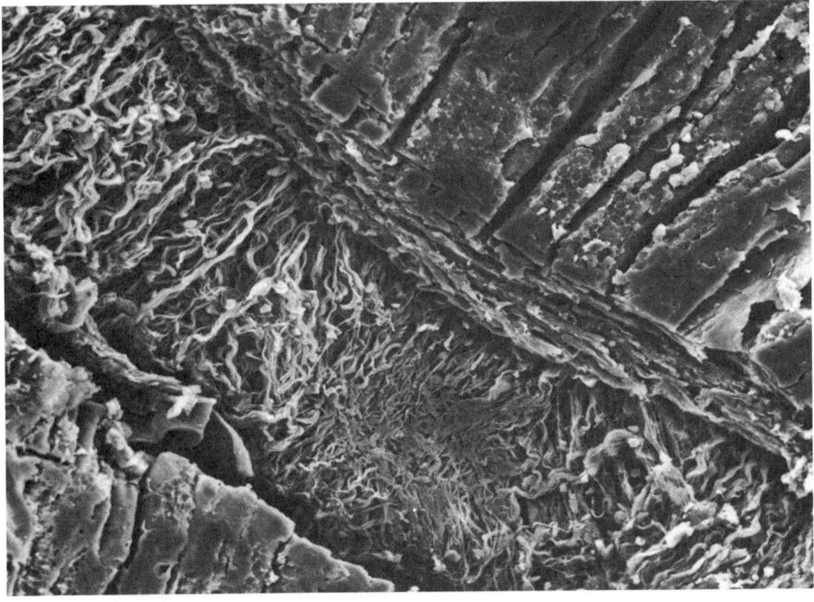

Figure 6. *Vessel wall 12 hours after cross clamping. Although this period of time does not represent what one might see clinically, the pressure effect of the clamp is obviously progressive, exposing the underlying collagen matrix. 200×*

Microvascular Anastomosis

One of the prime caveats in microvascular surgery is not to attempt suture repair of irrevocably damaged vessels. Thus, the microvascular surgeon beginning an anastomosis must first determine if the vessels are so badly damaged as to preclude a successful outcome. The nature of the injury often predicts the amount of vessel damage. For example, simple, clean lacerations due to a knife would have relatively minimal trauma at the separated vessel ends. However, crush or avulsion injuries produce extensive damage to the vessel walls at considerable distances from the point of actual vessel separation.[20] If either vessel end is occluded by adventitia, there is no flow from the proximal artery or vein, there is separation of the intima from the media, or there are intimal flaps, the vessel should be resected back to a more normal anatomical appearance and/or flow. Van Beck et al. described a "ribbon sign" or tortuosity of the artery found 0.5 to 1.0 cm from the site of transection associated with an avulsive injury. This sign was associated with intimal disruption and the recommendation was made to resect the vessel back to normal contour and interpose a vein graft if necessary. Similarly, a "red line" sign indicates intraluminal thrombosis and also requires resection of the vessel.[21]

The need for resection of damaged vessel ends raises the question of suture line tension. Simply stated, the two vessel ends must be copated under minimal tension. If an excessive amount of force is used to bring the vessel ends together, the anastomosis will almost uniformly fail. Thus, the surgeon must be prepared to harvest vein grafts from the wrist or foot to bridge the gap created by resection of the damaged vessel. Alternatively, in replantation surgery, resection of a small amount of bone from the phalanx may shorten the distance sufficiently to allow a direct anastomosis without a vein graft. If doubt exists, it is usually wiser to interpose a vein graft and perform two anastomoses without tension than a single one with a high likelihood of failure.[22,23] Attempting to suture the vessel ends under tension results in: tearing of the suture through the vessel wall, intimal disruption, and spaces between the sutures where the vessels are not approximated. These spaces form clots that serve as a nidus for further thrombus propagation and possible complete occlusion. The probability of occlusion is directly proportional to the vessel size and flow, such that smaller vessels with low flow states are the most affected. Furthermore, in an effort to approximate vessels under tension, crushing forces will be applied by forceps and other instruments that also damage the vessel walls. Bremer has documented the gross and histopathological changes of small vein grafts used in the microarterial circulation in experimental animals.[24-26]

Prior to placement of the first suture, it is usually necessary to remove a small amount of adventitia from the ends of each vessel. Failure to do so will result in the inadvertant incorporation of pieces of highly thrombogenic adventitia into the lumen. The recommended clearance of adventitia is usually 1 to 1.5 mm from the vessel ends. Resection of greater than 3.0 mm may compromise the blood supply to the media.[27] During this maneuver and the subsequent suturing of the vessel wall, the vessel should never be grasped with forceps. The latter injure the media and induce fractures of the intima allowing for initiation of platelet thrombi.[25]

The number and placement of sutures required to provide a leak-free anastomosis is important. As mentioned previously, each passage of the needle may significantly damage the vessel wall. Fortunately, the endothelium has a rapid rate of repair.[16] The repair mechanism may be significantly stressed, however, when multiple passes are made for a single suture or because of malplacement of the suture with respect to the edge of the vessel. The latter results in large amounts of intraluminal suture that acts as a foreign body interrupting laminar blood flow and initiating platelet thrombi. Ideally, the number of sutures to close an anastomosis should be the smallest number required to provide vessel approximation and limit leaking. Lower flow vessels usually require fewer sutures. However, all sutures should be placed accurately at a uniform distance from the cut end of the vessel to limit the amount of exposed suture or subendothelium and the amount of lumen constriction. Both of these factors contribute to decreased vessel patency. The anastomosis usually is accomplished with approximately 6 to 12 sutures in a 1-mm artery and approximately 4 to 8 in a 1-mm vein. The most common technique employed is one of triangulation at 0°, 120°, and 240° with one to two sutures being placed between each of the triangulation sutures. This method provides tension-free, nonconstricting apposition of the vessels' cut ends. As luminal size increases, suture number tends to increase as a function of the increase in wall circumference. Thus, there is a higher predisposition to gapping between sutures.

Since recipient and donor vessels do not always coincide in diameter, multiple techniques have been developed to adjust for size discrepancy. These include spatulation, sleeve invagination, differential vein graft, and plication of vessel wall. Probably the most common, however, is placing the smaller vessel in an end-to-side configuration to the larger vessel. This method dictates a technically more difficult anastomosis than the classic end-to-end anastomosis. It also results in a more turbulent blood flow and thus a higher thrombosis rate even if the quality of anastomosis is ideal. However, studies attempting to document the best angle of anastomosis have been inconclusive.[32] There is documentation that turbulent eddy currents are present at all angles that deviate from 180° and that the ideal angle of anastomosis varies depending on vessel size and flow.

There is some difference of opinion regarding the continuous suture technique versus the use of interrupted suturing. Clearly, continuous suturing reduces operative time[28] and may provide patency rates equivalent to the interrupted technique.[29] Some investigators have reported better results with interrupted techniques,[30] and others feel interrupted techniques have fewer technical problems relative to the actual performance of the anastomosis.[31] More than likely excellent patency rates can be provided by either method if gentle tissue handling and precise suture placement techniques are followed.

During the microsurgical repair, all vessels should be irrigated (with heparinized saline) with a blunt tip angled 30-gauge needle to insure removal of any luminal clot and establish evidence of adequate inflow. A small amount of this saline solution should remain in the lumen to prevent intraluminal thrombosis during the repair. The repair should be as expedient as possible to limit the above phenomenon, which is an ongoing process. Intraluminal irrigation and cannulation is not without complication. Hydraulic injury from too forceful an irrigation or dissection of the vessel layers may occur due to inadvertent canula placement. Either of these complicate what should be an exacting process and increase the risk of failure.

Trauma to vessels has long been noted to cause spasm, and microvessels are not an exception. Multiple vasoactive medications have been utilized to limit and reverse this phenomenon.[32,34,35] A 1-mm arterial vessel can easily constrict to less than 0.2 mm with trauma and manipulation. With such a decrease in vessel size, accurate anastomosis is impossible. Thus, vasodilation and relaxation of vessel smooth muscle are essential for vessel repair. The most commonly used drug for this purpose is lidocaine. Recent studies have indicated that a dose response curve exists for lidocaine with respect to degree and resolution of vascular spasm such that low doses of the drug induce vasospasm, while high doses cause vasodilation.[33,34]

After completion of the anastomosis and removal of the vascular clamps, there remains the question of determining actual vessel patency. Determination of vessel patency is perhaps most difficult for the venous side of the anastomosis. With a replanted digit, the presence of capillary refilling in the distal portion of the digit or nail bed is perhaps the best indication of an open anastomosis. The same finding would pertain to a free flap with a cutaneous skin paddle. With a transferred muscle, the presence of bleeding from the edges of the cut muscle is also an indication of an open arterial anastomosis. For further confirmation, intraoperative Doppler examination may be helpful. Venous obstruction is indicated by bluish discoloration, rapid capillary refill, and a slowing of arterial inflow.

For many years microvascular surgeons would strip the vessel to determine patency across the anastomosis. This procedure involved grasping the vessel between forceps, stripping the vessel with a second pair of forceps in a proximal direction, and watching for vessel re-distention across the anastomotic site. This patency test has been shown to be too traumatic for clinical microsurgery as it causes massive endothelial sloughing and may adversely affect the result.[36] It is mentioned for historical note only and is strongly condemned.

Anticoagulation in Microvascular Surgery

Postoperative anticoagulation is an important consideration in the overall management of vascular anastomosis. The repair or anastomosis of smaller vessels carries an increased risk of postoperative thrombosis primarily through damage to the intima, some of which is perhaps unrecognized by the surgeon at the time of repair. Again, a small thrombus in a large vessel may be tolerated, while the same thrombus in a vessel 1–2 mm in diameter may result in the loss of a finger or the loss of a free flap transfer.

Several drugs have been recommended and used in the postoperative period to prevent thrombosis of microvascular anastomoses. At the current time there is no uniformity of opinion amongst microvascular surgeons as to the necessity or efficacy of any given drug. Various protocols are used with anecdotal success at different centers. However, it is clear that thrombus formation is initiated by contact between platelets and exposed collagen in a damaged intima. Therefore, the majority of drugs used clinically are those that inhibit platelet function. The three most commonly used drugs are heparin, aspirin, and dextran.

Heparin accelerates the action of antithrombin. Although this drug is used extensively in the treatment of venous thrombosis and pulmonary embolism and in the past has been used liberally in microvascular surgery, it has several disadvantages that currently limit its routine use. The profuse bleeding that follows its use in replanted digits can result in significant blood loss requiring several transfusions. Furthermore, the exsanguinated blood tends to then soak into and eventually cake on the dressings, resulting in a constricting ring that can embarrass venous return. Ketchum et al. have demonstrated that the patency rate of vessels repaired using heparin adjunctively is no better than that of untreated controls.[37] However, mini dose heparin (5,000 units subcutaneously b.i.d.) has fewer side effects in terms of postoperative bleeding and may prove valuable in combination with other drugs. Unfortunately, prospective randomized studies of subcutaneously injected heparin have not been done.

Aspirin inhibits subendothelial collagen-induced platelet aggregation by inhibition of the release of platelet ADP. Inhibition is detectable after ingestion of 3 mg/kg and persists for 4 to 7 days. Aspirin also decreases thromboxane synthesis, and at higher doses, inhibits prostacyclin synthesis by endothelial cells. Prostacyclin itself has a powerful antiplatelet aggregation effect. Therefore, doses of 3 to 5 mg/kg are recommended. Many centers use aspirin for the postoperative treatment of patients undergoing microvascular procedures.

Dextran markedly decreases ADP-induced platelet adhesiveness. Dextran-70 has the greatest effect, peaking 2 to 5 hours after infusion. It also increases local tissue blood flow by decreasing viscosity and alters the fibrin structure of a clot making it more susceptible to fibrinolysis.[38] However, it antagonized PG12 inhibition of platelet aggregation.[39] Again, many centers use dextran as part of the postoperative regimen, but its efficacy in randomized studies has not been determined.

In a worldwide survey of microvascular surgeons in 73 centers in 22 countries, equal success rates of 89% were reported for free flaps performed with or without the aid of anticoagulation.[40] The probable reason for the high success rate without the help of anticoagulation relates to two factors: (1) the relative large size of the vessels used for free flap transfer (2.0 mm or greater); and (2) the fact that these vessels had not been previously traumatized. In contrast to the variance of usage for free flaps, all but three of the centers used anticoagulation for limb replantation. Those centers that did not use anticoagulation for replantation had lower success rates (76%) than centers that did use anticoagulants (89%). However, the sample size was too small for the centers that did not, and the severity of trauma was not categorized, making meaningful comparisons of the data difficult. The reasons for anticoagulation being used in replantation operations are again threefold: (1) the relatively smaller size of digital vessels (1.0 and less); (2) antecedent trauma to the vessels during the amputation, which can be extensive along the length of the vessel and may be underestimated by the surgeon if only the intima is involved; and (3) the prolonged length of ischemia, which often cannot be controlled.

With the available information we now have, it would seem reasonable to recommend the use of some form of anticoagulation following digital replantation and in free tissue transfer if there has been any mechanical or iatrogenic factors recognized at the time of operation that might lead to an enhanced probability of vessel thrombosis. Anticoagulation would involve some combination of dextran-10 and aspirin; however, it must be remembered that until well-designed prospective randomized trials are performed the use of anticoagulation is purely empiric.

Postoperative Monitoring

Technical excellence is essential for optimal postoperative results and high patency rates; however, monitoring of the postoperative course is equally essential to insure the continued patency of the anastomosis. Multiple methods have been tried; each of which, unfortunately, has shortcomings.

The classic parameters of warmth, color, and capillary refill have been utilized as indications of adequate blood supply to revascularized tissue. These parameters, however, are qualitative, not quantitative, and are highly subjective. Accuracy depends to a large degree on the experience of the observer. Therefore, different mechanical devices including temperature probes, dermatofluorometry, Doppler and magnetic flow meters, radioactive washout, labeled microspheres, tissue O_2 saturation, percutaneous PO_2 monitors, and laser Doppler capillary flow meters have been used to provide a more uniform and quantitative measurement.[41-44] The deficiencies of presently available monitoring systems can be highlighted by considering what would be an ideal system. This system would be reproducible, have the capability to be attached to and stabilized on the tissue in an easy and secure fashion for repeat measurements, a high sensitivity (e.g., filter extraneous input to limit false-negatives), a direct correlation to tissue survival and vascular flow, and be simple to read and interpret. To date there is no system that accomplishes all these criteria. Some of the more promising systems include tissue O_2 saturation monitors[41] and laser Doppler flow meters.[45] Both of these measure the capillary system. Presently, however, each is cumbersome and lacks a simplified engineering design so as to be widely used clinically.

Tissue failure can result from either lack of adequate inflow (arterial) or obstruction to outflow (venous). It is important to determine which is the major factor to decide upon the course of action. Decreased arterial inflow is characterized by decreased temperature, increased capillary refill time, pallor, decreased O_2 saturation, and decreased capillary blood flow. This phenomenon may be secondary to a decrease in the pressure available to perfuse the tissue (decreased systolic blood pressure, decreased cardiac output, or vascular compression) or an increase in resistance to flow in the tissue (increase in endothelial swelling, increased tissue ischemia, membrane and protein degradation) or external pressure on the tissue itself (constrictive dressing or direct pressure from positioning). Venous obstruction, however, is characterized by little or no skin temperature change, increased tissue swelling and cyanosis, rapid capillary refill (less than 3 sec), decreased O_2 saturation, and decreased capillary blood flow. The etiology can usually be related to obstruction of outflow via intraluminal sources (venous hypertension, intraluminal clot, or endothelial swelling) or extraluminal sources (external compression of the venous system). It is important to determine the cause since many of the etiologies are reversible without reoperation and should be attempted as initial treatment. However, if a nonoperative course is instituted, a watchful eye should be maintained on the result of such intervention as *rapid* benefit should follow from corrective manipulation. Unless there is measurable evidence of improvement, expedient operative exploration is mandatory to limit ischemic tissue injury.

Despite the drawbacks of presently available monitoring systems, some type of monitoring of all vascularized tissues is essential as thrombosis of either the arterial or venous anastomosis can be corrected if documented early (to limit warm ischemia of the tissue supplied). However, if the thrombus has become adherent to the vessel wall or there is significant warm ischemia causing increased membrane damage, endothelial swelling, and cellular death, the revascularized tissue will fail despite a patent anastomosis.

Summary

Technical performance of microvascular surgery is directly and causally related to results. There are numerous ways in which the microvascular surgeon can modify his/her technique to allow as minimal an iatrogenic injury as possible.

References

1. Jacobson, JH, Suarez, EL: Microsurgery in anastomosis of small vessels. *Surg Forum* 9:243, 1960.
2. Jacobson, JH, Miller, DB, Suarez, E: Microvascular surgery: A new horizon in coronary artery surgery. *Circulation* 22:767, 1960.
3. Krizck, TJ, Tani, T, Desprez, JD, et al: Experimental transplantation of composite grafts by microsurgical vascular anastomosis. *Plast Reconstr Surg* 36:538, 1965.
4. Buncke, HJ, Schulz, WP: Total ear reimplantation in the rabbit utilizing microminiature vascular anastomoses. *Br J Plast Surg* 19:15, 1966.
5. Goldwyn, RM, Lamb, DC, White, WL: Experimental study of large island flaps in dogs. *Plast Reconstr Surg* 31:428, 1963.
6. Strauch, B, Murry, DE: Transfer of composite graft with immediate suture anastomosis of its vascular pedicle measuring less than 1 mm in external diameter using microvascular techniques. *Plast Reconstr Surg* 40:325, 1967.
7. Kleinert, HE, Kadsan, ML: Anastomosis of digital vessels. *J Kentucky Medical Association*, 1965.
8. Komatsu, S, Tamai, S: Successful replantation of a completely cut-off thumb. *Plast Reconstr Surg* 42:347, 1968.
9. McLean, DH, Buncke, HJ: Autotransplant of omentum to a large scalp defect with microsurgical revascularization. *Plast Reconstr Surg* 49:268, 1972.
10. Daniel, R K, Taylor, G I: Distant transfer of an island flap by microvascular anastomosis. A clinical technique. *Plast Reconstr Surg* 52:111, 1973.
11. O'Brien, B M, MacLeod, A M, Hayhurst, J W, et al: Successful transfer of a large island flap from the groin to the foot by microvascular anastomosis. *Plast Reconstr Surg* 52:271, 1973.
12. Biemer, EW, Daspiva, E, Herndl, W, et al: Early experience in organizing and running a replantation service. *Br J Plast Surg* 31:9, 1978.
13. Furman, DW, Silabian, AH, Achauer, BM: Genesis of replantation program. *Am J Surg* 136:21–25, 1978.
14. Pagnanelli, DM, Pait, TG, Rizzoli, HV, et al: Scanning electron micrographic study of vascular lesions caused by microvascular needles and suture. *J Neurosurgery* 53:32, 1980.
15. Apkarian, RP, Burns, JT, Acland, RD: Scanning electron microscopic study of disturbances in arterial walls following microsurgical needle perforations. *Scan Electron Microsc* 2, 781, 1982.
16. Thurston, BJ, Bunke, HJ, Chater, NL, et al: A scanning electron microsurgery study of micro-arterial damage and repair. *Plast Reconstr Surg* 57:197, 1976.
17. Slayback, JB, Bowen, WW, Henshaw, DB: Internal injury from arterial clamps. *Amer J Surg* 132:183, 1976.
18. Blaschke, MJC, Osgood, CP, Huston, JS: Laboratory study of commonly used microvascular clips. *J Maine Med Assoc* 69:339, 1978.

19. Richling, R, Griesmayr, G, Lametschwandtwer, A, et al: Endothelial lesions after temporary clipping. *J Neurosurg* 51:654, 1979.
20. Morrison, MG, Papadopoulos, A, O'Brien, B McC: Experimental avulsion study on rabbits. *Br J Plast Surg* 38, 278.
21. Van Beck, AL, Kutz, JE, Zook, EG: Importance of the ribbon sign, indicating unsuitability of the vessel, in replanting a finger. *Plast Reconstr Surg* 61:32, 1973.
22. Alperti, BS, Bunchke, HJ, Brownstein, M: Replacement of damaged arteries and veins with vein grafts when replanting crushed, amputated fingers. *Plast Reconstr Surg* 61:17, 1978.
23. Fujikawa, S, O'Brien, B: An experimental evaluation of microvascular grafts. *Br J Plast Surg* 28:244, 1975.
24. Chater, N: Microsurgical vascular bypass for occlusive cerebrovascular disease. In Rand R W (ed): *Microsurgery*. St. Louis, CV Mosby pp 363–378, 1978.
25. Osgood, CP, Dujouny, M, Faille, R, et al: Early scanning microscopic evaluation of microvascular maneuvers. *Angiology* 27:96, 1976.
26. Bremer, E: Vein grafts in microvascular surgery. *Surgery Ann Acad Med* 19:382, 1979.
27. Corbet, JR: Microvascular surgery. *Surg Clin North Am* 47:521, 1967.
28. Acland, M D, Acland, R D: Continuous-suture technique in microvascular end to end anastomosis. *J Microsurg* 2:238, 1981.
29. Firsching, R, Terhaag, PD, Müller, W, et al: Continuous and interrupted suture technique in microsurgical end to end anastomosis. *Microsurgery* 5:80, 1984.
30. Chase, MD, Schwartz, SL: Consistent patency of 1.5 millimeter arterial anastomoses. *Surg Forum* 13:220, 1962.
31. Hamilton, RG, O'Brien, BM: An experimental study of microvascular patency using a continuous suture technique. *Br J Plast Surg* 32:153, 1979.
32. Szilagi, DE, Whitcome, JG, Scherkivene, W, et al: The laws of fluid flow and arterial grafting. *Surgery* 46:55, 1960.
33. Puckett, CL, Winters, RRW, Geter, RK, et al: Studies of pathologic vasoconstriction (vasospasm) in microvascular surgery. *J Hand Surg* 10A:343, 1985.
34. Johns, RA, DiFazio, CA, Longnecker, DE: Lidocaine constricts or dilates rat arterides in dose-dependent manner. *Anesthesiology* 62:141, 1985.
35. Geter, RK, Winters, RRW, Puckett, CL: Resolution of experimental microvascular spasm and improvement in anastomotic patency by direct topical agent application. *Plast Reconstr Surg* 77:105, 1986.
36. Petry, JJ, French, AB, Wortham, BA: The effect of "patency test" on arterial endothelial surface. *Plast Reconstr Surg* 77:960–963, 1986.
37. Ketchum, LD, Wenner, WW, Masters, FW, et al: Experimental use of pluronic F68 in microvascular surgery. *Plast Reconst Surg* 53:288, 1974.
38. Ketchum, LD: Pharmacological alterations in the clotting mechanism: Use in microvascular surgery. *J Hand Surg* 3:407, 1978.
39. Eldor, A, Weksler, B: Heparin and dextran sulfate antagonized PG12 inhibition of platelet aggregation. *Thromb Res* 16:617, 1979.

40. Davies, DM: A world survey of anticoagulation practice in clinical microvascular surgery. *Br J Plast Surg* 35:96, 1982.
41. Serafin, D, Lesesne, CB, Mullen, RY, et al: Transcutaneous PO_2 monitoring for assessing viability and predicting survival of skin flaps: Experimental and clinical correlations. *J Microsurg* 2:165, 1981.
42. Jones, BM, Sanders, R, Greenhalgh, RM: Monitoring skin flaps by color measurement. *Br J Plast Surg* 36:88, 1983.
43. Jones, BM, Greenhalgh, RM: The use of the ultrasound Doppler flowmeter in reconstructive surgery. *Br J Plast Surg* 36:245, 1983.
44. Jones, BM: Monitors for the cutaneous microcirculation. *Plast Reconstr Surg* 73:843, 1984.
45. Morrison, WA, O'Brien, BM, MacLeod, AM: Evaluation of digital replantation—A review of 100 cases. *Orthop Clin North Am* 8:2, 1977.

Index